Resources for Teaching Mindfulness

"A deep, supportive, and challenging dive into the art of teaching mindfulness, including the science of it, in the form of MBSR and other mindfulness-based interventions. Highly experienced contributors offer a cornucopia of inspiring, instrumental, and non-instrumental perspectives on the multi-dimensional topology of the classroom in vastly different contexts and cultures. Of particular note is the intimacy of one's own embodied sharing and exploring of the practice with others as the instructor — with the welcome mat for what arrives within us and between us firmly rolled out in not-knowing, coupled with deep listening, creativity, imagination, daring, and caring."

Jon Kabat-Zinn
Founder of MBSR
Author of *Full Catastrophe Living and Coming to Our Senses*

"This book is a wonderful and vital contribution to the field of mindfulness training. The editors have brought together a hugely impressive team of experienced trainers from across the world. Together the authors explore both the general demands that such training requires and the specific needs of particular groups and cultures. This book will find itself at the heart of required reading for students, teachers and trainers of mindfulness-based approaches.

MarkWilliams
Emeritus Professor of Clinical Psychology
University of Oxford

Donald McCown • Diane Reibel
Marc S. Micozzi

Resources for Teaching Mindfulness

An International Handbook

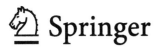 Springer

Donald McCown
Center for Contemplative Studies
West Chester University of Pennsylvania
West Chester, PA, USA

Marc S. Micozzi
Department of Physiology and Biophysics
Georgetown University School of Medicine
Washington, DC, USA

Department of Medicine
University of Pennsylvania School
  of Medicine
Philadelphia, PA, USA

Diane Reibel
Mindfulness Institute
Jefferson-Myrna Brind Center
  of Integrative Medicine
Thomas Jefferson University Hospitals
Philadelphia, PA, USA

Emergency Medicine
Sidney Kimmel Medical College
Thomas Jefferson University
Philadelphia, PA, USA

ISBN 978-3-319-30098-6   ISBN 978-3-319-30100-6   (eBook)
DOI 10.1007/978-3-319-30100-6

Library of Congress Control Number: 2016943054

Printed on acid-free paper

This Springer imprint is published by Springer Nature
The registered company is Springer International Publishing AG Switzerland

Introduction: Meeting Mindfulness Teachers "Where They Are"

It is the time of the teacher, at last. After decades of growth of the mindfulness-based interventions (MBIs), the importance of the person and skills of the teacher has come to the fore. The demand for well-practiced and well-trained teachers has accelerated, as the MBIs have become more established through the elaboration of a scientific evidence base and are now recommended and even preferred for many clinical applications.[1]

This demand has brought the more senior teachers and trainers of teachers within the MBIs together in order to seek agreements on MBI integrity, standards for good practice, and assessment of training and teaching competency. This effort is worldwide, involving organizations in more than a dozen countries in Europe, as well as North America, the Australasia region, and Africa, so far. Such efforts and agreements are, of course, of great importance in establishing a community of scholars and practitioners with common concerns and aspirations. Finding common ground and making descriptions and definitions of the basic skill sets and core characteristics is essential to ensuring the competence of MBI teachers and maintaining the established pedagogy.

Yet, there are differences in the context of any MBI class that must also be recognized and allowed. Teachers must be encouraged to "grow into" the skills and characteristics within their very specific relationships to persons, places, and cultures. This requires an exacting balance. On the one hand, the teacher's own ongoing practice of mindfulness must be encouraged. Practice deepens the teacher's understanding of what we call the "key move" of the pedagogy, which is to help participants *turn toward and be with and in their experiences of the moment in a friendly way.* Every pedagogical move can be weighed, measured, and reflected on in its relation to this move. On the other hand, the teacher's deepening understanding needs to be enlivened by encounters and experiments with different pedagogical

---

[1] Note that our interest here is in the clinical applications of mindfulness, as the broader applications in organizations, businesses, education, and other social environments are too varied and too freighted with their own theoretical and practical issues to be effectively addressed. We believe it is best for MBI teachers to continually keep in mind that the clinical applications of mindfulness may differ significantly from other contexts, in background, theory, motivation, and intention.

theories, styles, and techniques. This is how teachers and the pedagogy itself will continue to mature and evolve.

With such growth and change inevitable in a global undertaking, another requirement is to capture the ongoing unfolding of pedagogical possibilities. As teachers co-create mindfulness with their class participants, meeting them where they are, the teachers are continually learning from class to class how to negotiate the key move in their emerging context. Such moments of discernment, of knowing something very particular, are transformative for the teachers; yet, only when they can share them with other teachers do they have the power to help the pedagogy of the MBIs evolve.

The intention of this book is to support the ongoing development of established MBI teachers and the evolution of the pedagogy through a simple strategy of sharing teachers' insights and ideas from a rich variety of sources and contexts. Our work as teachers is to tend and extend relationships in the classroom. As editors, through our curious, careful, contemplative relationships with the chapters presented here, we have been touched, moved, and changed in our approaches to our classrooms, practices, and lives. We invite you to join in and experience your own relationships to this work that our colleagues have so generously shared. Explore what is here. Live with it. Allow it to influence you, as you influence others. With one hand on the key move of the pedagogy, the other forever reaching out, reaching toward, and ultimately grasping what is needed in the moment.

Vitality and Variety

This book is meant as a contribution to the ongoing co-creation of the pedagogy of the MBIs. The authors of these chapters represent a living, thriving range of geographical, cultural, philosophical, theoretical, and practical positions on the pedagogy. To read any chapter is to enter the community of teachers through a particular door and to see the pedagogy from a unique perspective. The variety of perspectives offers us vitality. You may be comforted to encounter perspectives aligned with your current ideas. You may be challenged when you meet other positions and postures that have evolved in different contexts. And you may be inspired and encouraged as you come upon the stories of teachers who find their own way, even when the way seems difficult or lost.

This book is not designed to deliver basic knowledge about teaching in the MBIs. Rather, it offers possibilities for growth in the practice of the pedagogy. Chapters are arranged to expand on four domains of teaching.

Part I: Honing the Skills of MBI Teachers

Here you'll find what might be thought of as "master classes" in the skills of the teacher, as they are originally defined in the book *Teaching Mindfulness: A Practical Guide for Clinicians and Educators* (McCown et al., 2010). Don McCown starts with stewardship, the most basic yet least definable skill, which is focused on the space and relationships in the classroom. He offers ways of conceptualizing the MBI class and the activities of the co-creation of the pedagogy of mindfulness, making connections to the ethics of the practice, as well as to the all important atmosphere of the gathering in the room.

Next, Aleeze Moss, Diane Reibel, and Don McCown present the skill of guiding practices as a way of catalyzing the co-creation of the pedagogy, through four dimensions of skill in guidance that culminate in the key move of being with and in the experience of the moment in a friendly way. With precision, they provide and analyze a script for seated yoga—which becomes a resource as a practice and as a training.

Saki Santorelli, a pivotal thinker at the UMASS Center for Mindfulness, particularly in the development of inquiry, delivers a truly masterful class on that skill. Inquiry may be described as a dialogue of teacher and participant, leading to what Santorelli calls "remembrance"—participants' inner realizations that they have the capacity to transcend their inherited and self-imposed limiting views, ideas, and opinions about who and what they are and to gain a vastly larger perspective on their own capabilities. The verbatim dialogues and the penetrating discussion of the types of questions that may open participants to such realizations must be returned to again and again.

Florence Meleo-Myer, also contributes from the UMASS CFM, adding a new, emerging skill of leading interpersonal practices. These practices turn participants toward one another to explore mindfulness in a closely focused spoken encounter.

Willoughby Britton covers the skill of homiletics—speaking to the group—with meticulous regard for how to keep up with, review, and bring into easily understood language the vast range of scientific evidence supporting the MBIs. Offering valuable insights and examples for presenting this material, the chapter can expand not only your skills in developing and delivering talks, but also can deepen your understanding of the effects and applications of the practice.

Rebecca Crane and Barbara Reid round up the skills section with a unique form of reflection for users of this book, from their position in the academic/clinical mindfulness community in the UK, where government health policies have driven increasing demand for MBI teachers, and qualifications are critical. Whether you wish to consider your own development, or that of teachers you are training, the comprehensive assessment they outline creates a useful opportunity for considering competence—and it is commensurate with the values and ethos of the MBIs.

Part II: Teaching MBI Curricula Everywhere—International Contexts

In this section, the contributors help to probe the big question: What is it like to be an MBI teacher? They offer perspectives from a range of geographical sites, giving us thick descriptions of how it is to bring mindfulness to groups of participants with very different national or cultural positions—who are often together in one classroom. These chapters are not meant to exclude readers—"I'll never live there; I don't need to know about that"—but rather to include us all in thinking about the differences any teacher may overlook and avoid encountering in her own classroom. Each chapter illuminates another facet of how the key move of the pedagogy becomes possible for participants and how it touches and moves them.

Heyoung Ahn, teaching in Seoul, South Korea, has thought and experimented intensely to create ways of bringing a curriculum that was built in the extreme individualism and anti-authoritarianism of the USA to a culture that is more collectivistic and accepting of hierarchy. An MBSR class looks the same, but different as he leads it—one hand on the key move, one hand reaching outwards.

Among other powerful appraisals, Fabio Giommi and Antonella Commellato reflect on differences between participant and teacher attitudes and affect in Italy and the "normative" ones of more often described US and UK participants and teachers. Explanations of how and why American teachers, say, can seem inauthentic in a European MBI context may generate considerable soul-searching questions.

Dina Wyschograd's elegant personal essay on teaching MBSR in Israel opens with the question, "If missiles are fired at Jerusalem and the air-raid sirens go off during class today, is there enough space in the shelter for my MBSR group?" There is conflict, cultural contrasts, and challenges, and at the center, the key move of being with and in the present moment in a friendly way—she has learned so much and shares it transparently.

In an anglophone country close to the cultural and religious diversity of Southeast Asia, the MBIs can be positioned with less concern for the exoticism of their Buddhist references. Timothea Goddard and Maura Kenny describe a growth and reception of the MBIs and the differences from the US/UK norms that continue to affect teaching and to generate new approaches.

Simon Whitesman and Linda Kantor reflect from South Africa on the demands that an enormously heterogeneous population, dynamic economic situation, and dramatic social challenges place on the teaching of the MBIs. They offer vignettes of the developing practices of teachers in different niches in the culture—describing the kinds of reaching out to experiment with great richness.

The challenges of diversity insist on the two-hand approach to evolution of the pedagogy. The need to hold fast to the key move while reaching out with an open hand to build a friendly atmosphere in the classroom is sensitively addressed in Rhonda Magee's personal and potent essay, "Teaching Mindfulness with Mindfulness of Diversity." Written from the USA, the spirit nonetheless may pervade the pedagogy everywhere.

Part III: Teaching MBI Curricula to Everyone—Special Populations

In this section, contributors share their expertise, developed through long and deep commitments in working with particular audiences, from inner-city populations to clergy and religious and from frail elders to participants with trauma in their personal histories. These chapters are not presented to encourage or support teachers to become specialists, but rather to help them become better generalists. Through the detailed sharing of these experts, teachers can develop their own abilities to understand and work in their diverse classes with participants who may benefit from the pedagogical ideas and approaches generated and refined within these focused categories. What's more, the ideas and approaches may generate further new ways of thinking about and practicing the pedagogy.

Beth Roth, through decades of teaching inner-city populations on the US East Coast, has discovered pedagogical turns that make the MBIs more accessible. This is a highly creative undertaking. As Roth remarks, "I consider myself an artist engaged in a vital art form: meeting others' full and imperfect humanity with my own, for the explicit purpose of growth and healing."

Lucia McBee's long engagement with elderly populations has resulted in more comprehensive recasting of the MBSR curriculum than required in many other instances. The challenges are large and the demands are layered. Teaching frail elders actually requires teaching frail elders and their caregivers, and each audience experiences the world differently and needs the teacher to meet them where they are and draw everyone together. The work has been done.

The potential of mindfulness pedagogy to bring about reduction in anxiety and accompanying shifts in behavior in folks diagnosed with developmental and intellectual disabilities is profound. Nirbhay Singh and Monica Jackman have been in the vanguard of this work that is so specific and yet so applicable in any class because it is simple, memorable, and effective. The "soles of the feet" practice belongs in every teacher's repertoire.

Some issues are highly prevalent in MBI participants in MBI groups, such as chronic pain, anxiety/depression, and trauma history. The more a teacher can learn and practice, the richer each class will be. Lone Overby Fjorback and Else-Marie Elmholdt Jegindø specialize in chronic pain. Their chapter offers a balance of thorough, scientific analysis of the biopsychosocial experience of such conditions with the "not knowing" inherent in the practice of the pedagogy. Susan Woods brings practiced discernment to working with anxious and depressed participants. Among many insights her chapter offers a grounding in the benefits of the teacher's own mindfulness practice for her participants and inquiry dialogues that capture nuances of the work. Trish Magyari describes how, for participants with trauma in their personal history, the teacher can make the key move of the pedagogy possible through subtle shifts in timing and language, as well as use of self. Examples of "anticipatory guidance" for participants to stay out of distress, and demonstrations of skillful ways of addressing such distress in class or home practice, will influence teachers' classroom practices.

Jean Kristeller and Andrea Lieberstein speak to a further issue of prominence in the makeup of MBI classes, participants' relationships to food and eating. In describing the curriculum of a specialized MBI for this issue, they show how practices involving food and eating are powerful explorations of the interaction of mindfulness and personal choices.

We learn much more at the extremes than through engagement with the center. Susan Bauer-Wu works with participants with life-limiting illness and at the end of life. The adaptations and additions she has made are sensitive, beautiful, and—perhaps surprisingly—widely applicable for any MBI class.

This section ends with two chapters dealing with participants who have vocations: health-care professionals and clergy. These choices, perhaps, have interest to the MBI teacher, as this work is a calling, as well. Mick Krasner describes a specific curriculum that investigates resilience as a dynamic force and incorporates mindfulness practices, with a focus on the self-care of the health professional. There is much for teachers to use in the classroom and to explore on their own. Don Marks and Chris Moriconi consider the same ground, from a perspective that includes both the religious and the spiritual. Here, again, teachers may be doubly touched, exploring new possibilities for participants and themselves.

Part IV: Practices and Scripts for the Classroom and the Teacher

One way to get started in thinking through and exploring new directions in the pedagogy for your specific context as an MBI teacher is to start with someone else's idea. The editors invited any contributor who was so moved to offer a practice, and we were rewarded with variety and vitality. As a result, the final section of the book is a trove of practices written for adoption in the classroom to explore a new direction or adoption by the teacher for work on self-development. Yet each practice is more than that, more than simply a template to apply. Each is also offered to be analyzed, rewritten, reconfigured, tested, retested, and ultimately transformed to meet participants—and teachers—right where they are, wherever that is in the world or in life, and to lead them on.

Unshakable and Evolving

Resources for Teaching Mindfulness has been created to deliver just what it says for teachers with sufficient grounding in their own mindfulness practice to grow in the two-handed way that helps the pedagogy of the MBIs to continue to evolve. Whether the teacher connects with the master classes in the broad skill sets of teaching in the MBIs or the detailed personal reflections on how it is and what it means to be an MBI teacher across a wide range of geographic and cultural positions or the finer points of teaching specific populations, one hand must remain unshakably on the key move of the pedagogy—turning toward and being with and in the experience of the moment in a friendly way—while the other hand reaches out to try, to adapt, to touch, and to evolve.

West Chester, PA, USA   Donald McCown
Philadelphia, PA, USA   Diane Reibel
Washington, DC, USA   Marc S. Micozzi
Philadelphia, PA, USA

Contents

Editors and Contributors

Editors

Donald McCown, Ph.D., M.A.M.S., M.S.S., L.S.W. Associate Professor, Health; Co-Director, Center for Contemplative Studies; Program Director, Minor in Contemplative Studies, West Chester University of Pennsylvania, Sturzebecker Health Sciences Center, #312, West Chester, PA 19383, USA, dmccown@wcupa.edu

Marc S. Micozzi, M.D., Ph.D. Adjunct Professor, Department of Physiology and Biophysics, Georgetown University School of Medicine, Washington, DC, USA

Department of Medicine, University of Pennsylvania School of Medicine, Philadelphia, PA, USA, marcsmicozzi@gmail.com

Diane Reibel, Ph.D. Director, Mindfulness Institute, Jefferson-Myrna Brind Center of Integrative Medicine, Thomas Jefferson University Hospitals, 1015 Chestnut Street, Suite 1212, Philadelphia, PA 19107, USA

Clinical Associate Professor, Emergency Medicine, Sidney Kimmel Medical College, Thomas Jefferson University, Philadelphia, PA 19107, USA, diane.reibel@jefferson.edu

Contributors

Heyoung Ahn, Ph.D. Ed.D. Director, Korea Center for MBSR; Professor, MindBody Healing; Vice-President, Seoul University of Buddhism, 1038-2, Doksan-Dong, Geumcheon-Gu, Seoul 153-831, South Korea, mbsr1@hanmail.net

Susan Bauer-Wu, Ph.D., R.N., F.A.A.N. President, Mind & Life Institute, 210 Ridge McIntyre Road, Suite 325, Charlottesville, VA 22903, USA, susan@mindandlife.org

Willoughby B. Britton, Ph.D. Assistant Professor, Department of Psychiatry and Human Behavior, Brown University Medical School, Providence, RI 02906, USA

Assistant Professor, Department of Behavioral and Social Sciences, Brown University School of Public Health, 185 Brown Street, Providence, RI 02906, USA, willoughby_britton@brown.edu

Antonella Commellato, M.A. Associazione Italiana per la Mindfulness, Via Piranesi 14, Milano 20137, Italy, antonella.commellato@gmail.com

Rebecca S. Crane, Ph.D. Director, Centre for Mindfulness Research and Practice, School of Psychology, Bangor University, Brigantia Building, Bangor, Gwynedd LL57 2AS, UK, r.crane@bangor.ac.uk

Else-Marie D. Elmholdt Jegindø, Ph.D. Development consultant, Research Clinic for Functional Disorders and Psychosomatics, Aarhus University Hospital, Barthsgade 5, 3rd floor, Aarhus DK-8200, Denmark, else-marie@cfin.au.dk

Lone Overby Fjorback, M.D., Ph.D. Psychiatrist, Director, Danish Center for Mindfulness, Aarhus University Hospital, Aarhus University, Barthsgarde 5, Aarhus 8200, Denmark, lonefjor@rm.dk

Fabio Giommi, Ph.D. Associazione Italiana per la Mindfulness, Via Piranesi 14, Milano 20137, Italy, fabiomario.giommi@gmail.com

Timothea Goddard, B.A., Dip. Psychotherapy (A.N.Z.A.P.) Clin Mem P.A.C.F.A. Mindfulness Training Institute of Australasia, Suite 807/251 Oxford St, Bondi Junction, NSW 2022, Australia, tim@openground.com.au

Monica Moore Jackman, O.T.D., M.H.S., O.T.R./L. Little Lotus Therapy, 3242 SW Fillmore Street, Port Saint Lucie, FL 34953, USA, mjackman2317@gmail.com

Linda Sara Kantor, B.A. (HONS.), M.A. Psychology Director, Institute for Mindfulness South Africa; Lecturer, Mindful Leadership, University of Cape Town Graduate School of Business, Cape Town, South Africa

Lecturer, Post graduate Certification in Mindfulness-Based Interventions, Faculty of Medicine and Health Sciences, University of Stellenbosch, 503 Rapallo, 292 Beach Road, Sea Point 8005, South Africa, lindakantor@icloud.com

Maura A. Kenny, M.B.Ch.B., M.R.C.Psych., F.R.A.N.Z.C.P. Mindfulness Training Institute Australasia, maura@mtia.org.au; Centre for the Treatment of Anxiety and Depression, SA Health, 30 Anderson Street, Thebarton, SA 5031, Australia, maura.kenny@sa.gov.au

Michael S. Krasner, M.D. Professor of Clinical Medicine, University of Rochester School of Medicine and Dentistry, 42 Lilac Drive, #8, Rochester, NY 14620, USA, michael_krasner@urmc.rochester.edu

Jean L. Kristeller, Ph.D. Professor Emeritus of Psychology, Department of Psychology, Indiana State University, Terre Haute, IN 47809, USA, jkristeller@indstate.edu

Andrea E. Lieberstein, M.P.H., R.D.N., R.Y.T. Mindfulness-Based Registered Dietitian Nutritionist, Mindfulness Meditation Teacher, Founder of Mindful Eating Training, Novato, CA, USA, andrea@mindfuleatingtraining.com

Rhonda V. Magee, M.A., J.D. Professor of Law, University of San Francisco, School of Law, 2130 Fulton Street, San Francisco, CA 94117, USA, rvmagee@usfca.edu

Trish Magyari, M.S., L.C.P.C., N.C.C., R.Y.T.-200 Institute Trainer and MBSR Mentor, Mindfulness-based Professional Training Institute, UC San Diego Center for Mindfulness, 5060 Shoreham Place, Suite 330, San Diego, CA 92122-0980, USA, trish@trishmagyari.com

Donald R. Marks, Psy.D. Assistant Professor, Department of Advanced Studies in Psychology, Kean University, 1000 Morris Avenue, Union, NJ 07083, USA, domarks@kean.edu

Lucia McBee, L.C.S.W., M.P.H., C.Y.I. 207 West 106th Street, Apartment 12C, New York, NY 10025, USA, lucia@luciamcbee.com

Donald McCown, Ph.D., M.A.M.S., M.S.S., L.S.W. Associate Professor, Health; Co-Director, Center for Contemplative Studies; Program Director, Minor in Contemplative Studies, West Chester University of Pennsylvania, Sturzebecker Health Sciences Center, #312, West Chester, PA 19383, USA, dmccown@wcupa.edu

Florence Meleo-Meyer, M.S., M.A. Director, Train-the-Trainer Program, Oasis Institute for Mindfulness-based Professional Education and Training, Center for Mindfulness, University of Massachusetts Medical School, 38 Dragon Hill Road, Shelburne Falls, MA 01370, USA, florence.meyer@umassmed.edu

Christine D. Moriconi, Psy.D., L.M.F.T., P.M.H.C.N.S-B.C., R.N. Associate Professor, Nursing; Co-Director, Center for Contemplative Studies, West Chester University of Pennsylvania, 930 E. Lincoln Highway, Suite 100, Exton, PA 19341, USA, cmoriconi@wcupa.edu

Aleezé S. Moss, Ph.D. Associate Director, Mindfulness Institute, Jefferson-Myrna Brind Center of Integrative Medicine, Thomas Jefferson University Hospitals, 1015 Chestnut Street, Suite 1212, Philadelphia, PA 19107, USA, aleeze.moss@jefferson.edu

Diane Reibel, Ph.D. Director, Mindfulness Institute, Jefferson-Myrna Brind Center of Integrative Medicine, Thomas Jefferson University Hospitals, 1015 Chestnut Street, Suite 1212, Philadelphia, PA 19107, USA

Clinical Associate Professor, Emergency Medicine, Sidney Kimmel Medical College, Thomas Jefferson University, Philadelphia, PA 19107, USA, diane.reibel@jefferson.edu

Barbara Reid, Ph.D. Teacher and Trainer, Centre for Mindfulness Research and Practice, School of Psychology, Bangor University, Brigantia Building, Bangor, Gwynedd LL57 2AS, UK, beereid@googlemail.com

Beth Robins Roth, A.P.R.N., S.E.P. Hummingbird Trauma Resolution, L.L.C., bethroth@snet.net

Saki F. Santorelli, Ed.D., M.A. Professor of Medicine; Director, Mindfulness-Based Stress Reduction Clinic (MBSR); Executive Director, Center for Mindfulness in Medicine, Health Care, and Society, University of Massachusetts Medical School, 222 Maple Avenue, Shrewsbury, MA 01545, USA, saki.santorelli@umassmed.edu

Nirbhay N. Singh, Ph.D. Clinical Professor of Psychiatry and Health Behavior, Medical College of Georgia, Augusta University, Augusta, GA 30912, USA, nisingh@augusta.edu

Simon Whitesman, M.B.Ch.B. Programme Director: Certificate Training in Mindfulness-Based Interventions, Stellenbosch University; Chairperson, Institute for Mindfulness South Africa, Christiaan Barnard Memorial Hospital, Longmarket Street, Cape Town, South Africa, simonw@lantic.net

Susan L. Woods, M.S.W., L.I.C.S.W. Advisor, Trainer, Supervisor, Mindfulness-Based Stress Reduction and Mindfulness-Based Cognitive Therapy, P.O. Box 3565, Stowe, VT 05672, USA

Diane (Dina) Wyshogrod, Ph.D. Founder and Director, MBSR-ISRAEL, the Israeli Center for Mindfulness Based Stress Reduction, Licensed Clinical Psychologist, Private Practice, Dan 12, Jerusalem 9350912, Israel, dr.dina@breathedeep.net

Part I
Honing the Skills of MBI Teachers

Chapter 1
Stewardship: Deeper Structures of the Co-created Group

Donald McCown

The Primary Skill of the Teacher

What is it like in the room right now? This question is the key, the core, and the constant one for teachers in the mindfulness-based interventions (MBI). It is a question of *atmosphere*, which in everyday speech refers to vague, indeterminate, intangible characters of persons, objects, and environments (Böhme, 1993, 2011). Yet somehow, despite this vagueness, we can still answer the question quickly and easily. We all walk into the room and know, through body sensation and affect, that the atmosphere is tense, or friendly, or calm, or maybe a little sad. And furthering the mystery, we find that we have a very rich vocabulary at hand to describe it. Atmosphere is not something objective, entirely "out there," although the experience comes to us in that way. Nor is it something entirely subjective, available to oneself alone. Rather, it is available to us from both without *and* within, through an undivided relationship between self and other (Böhme, 1993, 2011; Bollnow, 2011; Ingold, 2015). Thus, a group can agree on, and even engage in dialogue about, what it is like in the room at a particular moment. Atmosphere, then, is what we attend to as MBI teachers, while tracking the unfolding of a class session moment by moment. The character of atmosphere is evident not only to teachers but also to participants, making it a valuable and valid measure for the relational state of the group, which the teacher tends through stewardship activities.

This chapter uses the concept of atmosphere to explore the skill set that comprises stewardship, the first of the four skill sets of the teacher, together with homiletics, guidance, and inquiry, as defined in the book *Teaching Mindfulness* (McCown,

D. McCown, Ph.D., M.A.M.S., M.S.S., L.S.W. (✉)
Center for Contemplative Studies, West Chester University of Pennsylvania,
Sturzebecker Health Sciences Center, #312, West Chester, PA 19383, USA
e-mail: dmccown@wcupa.edu

© Springer International Publishing Switzerland 2016
D. McCown et al., *Resources for Teaching Mindfulness*,
DOI 10.1007/978-3-319-30100-6_1

Reibel, & Micozzi, 2017). The concept of atmosphere allows us to venture more deeply into the ways that the stewardship skills contribute to the co-creation of an MBI class, and provides us entrée into emerging areas of concern. We examine seven stewardship skills that interlock, overlap, and allow the shared and unspoken experiences of participants and teacher to be revealed in the atmosphere—how it is in the room in the moment. These skills and their actions range from massively concrete to subtly intuitive. They are less conceptual and less language dependent than the other three skill sets of teaching, making them the first in the list, yet perhaps the last to be fully mastered.

The seven stewardship skills or actions are:

1. *Caring for place*: The most concrete skill, involving rooms, tables and chairs, lighting and HVAC systems, and the greater environment as it impinges on class participants.
2. *Attending to bodies*: Curricula in the MBIs are directed in a variety of ways to helping participants become more aware of and engaged with their corporeal experiences; indeed, through corporeal experience they often come to understand the benefits of mindfulness.
3. *Maintaining relationships*: The practice of mindfulness is a relational undertaking; therefore, an important skill is helping participants to find ways to "be" along with others, to have a sense of co-created experience in silence and in speech.
4. *Learning from and in the atmosphere*: Participants develop the potentials of mindful presence through dwelling in the place that mindful presence happens and among the ones with whom it happens. Teachers are shaped by the atmosphere of mindful presence, as well; the actions of the other skills of homiletics, guidance, and inquiry are responses to the atmosphere. Atmosphere not only teaches participants, it teaches the teacher.
5. *Tending the ethical space*: The practice of teaching and learning mindfulness in clinical applications is inherently ethical. The space that participants and teachers co-create becomes a first-order morality. When that space is threatened or collapses, the teacher has the necessary resources to repair it or shift to a different but sufficient professional ethic.
6. *Sensing sublime moments*: The atmosphere of the class is, in a way, a gauge for its value to participants. When it supports mindfulness—the turning towards and being with the experience of the moment—it has a particular character. We might use an aesthetic term to name it: the sublime. The presence of sublime moments in a class, then, suggests that it is possible for participants to find the potential to be with and in their experiences, even when aversive, and to live differently.
7. *Positioning the self for teaching*: As much as possible, teachers in the MBIs need to live in the atmosphere and ethical space of the class, to "steep" in it in a corporeal and affective way. This process of steeping, a key to teacher training, engenders new potentials for being, or perhaps new versions of the self to be accessed in the classroom. How these potentials become available to the teacher in any particular moment is a question worth addressing under the heading of stewardship.

As we move through each of these skills and actions, the concepts of atmosphere, relationality, and the meaning of the word stewardship will become clearer. It may even become a synonym for teaching.

> **Box 1.1: The Word "Stewardship"**
> Derived from Old English words *stig* and *weard*, or more familiarly *sty* and *ward*, the word stewardship clearly points to one who is a servant with significant responsibilities. The ward of the sty, or hall, must guard it to keep it safe from what is outside, and to serve those who are inside. This implies watchfulness and care.
>
> The steward is one who is in charge while the true ruler is away, and who is expected to keep all of it safe—and to make it prosper—until the ruler's return. The MBI teacher takes on the democratic version of this task, stewarding the co-created mindfulness of the group until the group can teach and maintain itself. Teachers do well to remember the admonition to the wise steward of the Gospels: *"Every one to whom much is given, of him will much be required..." (Luke 12:48, RSV).*

1. Caring for Place

No skill is more humble. The MBI teacher, in a tradition stretching back to Jon Kabat-Zinn's first MBSR classes in the basement of UMASS Medical Center, is often the one who repurposes some general use space, taking down tables and setting up chairs in a circle to create a possibility of togetherness and comfort. That circle is emblematic of the stewardship skill set. It defines the group. It has an outside, which defines the group, and an inside, which belongs to the group. The circle also suggests a meeting of equals, in the way of King Arthur's Round Table. Stewardship skills are applied on both sides of the circle.

In caring for place, we focus on "outside" skills that define the space and the circle itself. Such skills are concrete—finding a meeting space, recruiting and organizing participants, and tending the space before and after the session.

Worldliness, compromise, and even business acumen come into play in these outside skills. Depending on the teacher's situation, the possibility of running a class may hinge upon entrepreneurial skills, from gaining institutional support for a program, to securing time and space on the calendar. Certainly, resources for marketing, public relations, and advertising are required; lacking institutional support, teachers often take on much of this responsibility. (For a structure to consider, see sidebar, "Marketing Mindfulness.") And, of course, as participants join the program, all the administrative tasks of enrollment, payment, orientation, and continuing contact must be accomplished. Again, often by the teacher.

How can the teacher make all this happen—often as only a small part of ongoing professional commitments—while maintaining a mindful balance? This facet of stewardship may be more challenging than it appears. The idea that teachers must live what they teach—mindfulness in the midst of life's tumult—is a constant truth. Not so much a choice as a necessity!

Screening Participants

After recruiting, screening participants is perhaps the most important stewardship skill outside the circle. Screening may be done in short conversations before or after a group orientation session, or through intake questionnaires, followed up by phone or face-to-face conversation, if needed. What must be decided is not so much who is appropriate for the group as who may be *inappropriate*. Success at screening out those very few potential participants who have a potential to be disruptive is unseen by the class, yet it is essential for their safety, comfort, and possibilities for transformation.

Well-honed clinical skills are an advantage in screening. A teacher's honest appraisal of her own skill in maintaining the central move of the pedagogy is paramount—helping participants to turn towards and be with and in the experience of the moment, no matter how difficult. Only the teacher can decide what she can handle. Hayes and Feldman (2004) suggest that what must be judged is the participant's ability to face his own

> **MARKETING MINDFULNESS**
>
> However large or small your local market, it may be valuable to do the analysis that will let you speak clearly about why people should choose your programs. Here are four points to consider, and some telling questions to get you started (McCown, 2005).
>
> 1. **Identity**: Defining who is offering what. Are you marketing yourself, as a teacher? Or your organization? Are you offering a defined, recognizable program (say, MBSR or MBCT)? Or do you have a new proposal?
> 2. **Audience**: Defining specific target groups. With whom would you like to work? Consider demographics, psychographics, psychometrics, and potential alliances with organizations.
> 3. **Position**: Differentiating your offering. What other programs and practitioners are in your area? Is what you do in a new category? Is it a fresh approach? Does it emphasize different features and benefits than what is in the market now?
> 4. **Communication**: Defining the language and imagery most appropriate for a specific target audience. How do they prefer to get information? (e.g., adolescents and social media; folks with chronic illness and referrals from organizations and online news groups.) What propositions are most persuasive? Scientific evidence? Participant testimonials? Professional endorsements?

negative material while suspending use of his current coping strategies to try on new possibilities. This requirement is a tall order for anyone. The teacher must feel confident that, with her help as required, the participant will be able to do this. As such, a teacher's exclusion parameters will no doubt change over time, and with more experience become more and more inclusive.

For beginning teachers, some rules of thumb may be useful. The exclusion criteria used by the UMASS Center for Mindfulness (Santorelli, 2014) are clear, and offer confidence for teachers with differing levels of clinical training. They specifically exclude folks in active addiction or in recovery less than a year; patients with suicidality, psychosis (refractory to medication), post-traumatic stress disorder, major depression, other psychiatric disorders if they interfere with group participation, and social anxiety unworkable in a group environment. Exceptions are individualized and enrollment may be considered if the participant is highly motivated, engaged in supportive professional treatment, agrees to the teacher communicating with the professionals, and the professionals agree to act as primary caregivers and first contacts in emergencies. Meditation practice may be contraindicated in some cases, as adverse effects are possible and recorded in the literature (for an overview, see Britton, Chap. 5). More prosaic exclusion criteria include language comprehension, logistical barriers to attendance (not related to physical impairment), and scheduling issues that could result in missing three or more classes. Ultimately, the teacher's intuitive feel for the participant and confidence in her own skills are the most important factors.

Returning to the concrete skills, caring for place means working with the room and its furnishings. A teacher works to make the room as comfortable and attractive as possible. However, there are logical and pedagogical limits. Being overly "fussy" about room décor, or attempting to control all temperature fluctuations and outside noise may undermine the central teaching point—to be with and in the experience of the moment, whether pleasant or aversive. More pedagogically valuable than exercising excessive overcontrol would be to use the less-than-satisfactory characteristics of the meeting space as an opportunity to talk about mindfulness. A teacher can call participants' attention to the balky heating or air conditioning system, or to the traffic noise outside the room, not to make excuses, but to highlight how the practice helps us in real-life situations, which are seldom perfect or even the way we would prefer. The message that most supports the pedagogy is that "we do what we can, and accept what we must."

2.   *Attending to Bodies*

Stewardship is about tending to living, breathing, moving people, whose bodies are responsive in profound ways to the others and "othernesses" in their inner and outer environments. It is about creating conditions under which participants may come to greater awareness of, and possibly control over, their responsiveness. Right from the start, MBI curricula are designed to sensitize participants to their corporeal experiences (McCown et al., 2010). The first formal practice is the body scan, in which participants are asked to bring attention to all the areas of the body in turn, without the editing and ignoring of regions as often determined by social, cultural, and personal history. Further, sitting meditation is introduced with emphasis on physical sensations of the breath, while mindful movement practices bring focus to the body in motion in space, developing interoception (feeling the body from inside) and proprioception (feeling the body in space) in tandem. In any curricular situation, the body is the gateway to the present moment.

As participants begin to better connect to corporeal experience, they often notice differences in their engagement with the world. One participant wrote,

> This class's focus on getting in touch with our bodies helped me start to bridge the gap and repair the damage of being disconnected from my body. I started to notice things that I never had before (feelings, emotions, reactions, etc.). Now, I am more in tune with my body and notice physical changes more quickly than I had before. Now, I can recognize feelings for what they are instead of reacting without knowing what the motivating force behind the reaction was. This class helped catapult my understanding of my head and heart connection to a higher degree (McCown, 2015).

Stewardship skills facilitate this in concrete ways, by making the place in which the class meets amenable to corporeal learning.

Beginning from the definition of mindfulness that participants hear in the first session—paying attention, on purpose, from moment to moment, and nonjudgmentally,—the teacher establishes ground rules for the classroom. Such rules are specifically shaped by institutional considerations and cultural expectations. Yet, they might be expressed (to borrow from *Star Trek*) as a prime directive: "Take care of yourself." This directive is very much applicable when it comes to bodily needs—drinking water, going to the lavatory, moving the body, shifting postures. It applies as well to participating, or not, in activities that may be physically or emotionally challenging. Such emphasis on discernment and self-care may contribute to an atmosphere in which self-compassion becomes a possibility for participants. Research has suggested self-compassion may be strongly transformative (Feldman & Kuyken, 2011; Kuyken et al., 2010; Van Dam, Sheppard, Forsyth, & Earleywine, 2011).

The Buddhist and Taoist literatures identify four postures to illustrate the whole range of possible postures of the human body—traditionally said to number 80,000. These iconic postures of *walking*, *standing*, *sitting*, and *lying down* are often referred to as the *four dignities*, and are used for meditation practice. Stewardship makes the classroom accessible for all four dignities and the thousands in between. In fact, it is an example of stewardship for the teacher to be open to participants using any of the postures for meditation at any time. Suggesting, for example, that sitting meditation, or the body scan requires a certain bodily form militates against the prime directive, not to mention the broader teaching point that mindfulness is bringing attention to however it is in the moment.

Walking and standing must be also accommodated. There must be open floor space for participants to travel to the circle where the class gathers in the event members are using canes, walkers, wheelchairs, and other supportive devices. Ideally, there will be space that can be cleared for walking meditation for all participants, or another space nearby with the proper characteristics that may be used. When outdoor spaces are available, a choice to remain inside should be offered and supported by teaching staff, mitigating issues with weather, terrain, and any added physical effort.

Sitting is perhaps the most varied, and contested, of the four graces in the MBIs. Certainly, how we sit, the furnishings we use, and our expectations of "sitting meditation" are culturally derived. In western cultures, we spend far more time sitting in chairs than on the floor. We emphasize particular postures, and know that certain postures are expected in certain kinds of chairs. We even offer children smaller versions of chairs, so they can learn to sit up "correctly." In Eastern cultures (from which, for the West, popular "orientalist" images of meditation have been derived), it is common to sit on the floor, and there are furnishings and accepted postures for particular situations, including meditation.

Teachers should simply furnish their classes for the culturally preferred ways of sitting. This point is based on two strong ideas. First, ways of sitting are deeply ingrained and not easily, quickly, or comfortably changed. As the early twentieth century sociologist Mauss (1934/1973) noted, sitting is a technique of the body that is deeply learned and highly variable by culture. The contemporary anthropologist Tim Ingold expands upon Mauss's view and suggests that humans grow into such techniques as a body-mind-environment complex. That position makes the preferred technique(s) not something learned, but a noncognitive potential of being (e.g., Ingold, 2008; see section "Learning from and in the Atmosphere" of this chapter for detailed discussion). Second, we are teaching mindfulness practice for use in the everyday world. It is therefore sensible to teach sitting meditation in the participants' preferred posture(s), so that practice is as "close" to the everyday moment as possible. In this way, formal and informal practices have a powerful continuity. What is achieved in formal practice becomes available even when literally just "sitting around."

Lying down, the fourth grace, requires floor space and comfort, and can be encouraged by making yoga mats and/or blankets available. This posture is suggested (although not required!) for the body scan, the first formal practice of most MBI curricula, and also for the floor yoga that is practiced as part of the mindful movement in the curricula. Rarely do clinical or educational programs, biased towards the cognitive, include lying quietly on the floor as a regular activity. Such an unusual action can be seen to help catalyze the idea for participants that the MBI class holds the potential for discovering new possibilities of experience (McCown et al., 2010). The literal change of perspective that accompanies lying down is simple yet dramatic. It can transform the atmosphere in the room, bringing curiosity and anticipation into the foreground.

3. Maintaining Relationships

We can begin right at the top of the head with defining relationships—in the mirror neurons in our brains. These neurons allow us to feel the movements and even the intentions of those who are with us (Gallese, Fadiga, Fogassi, & Rizzolatti, 1996; Gallese & Goldman, 1998). A "resonance circuit" through the brain makes the connection (Siegel, 2007). We notice an action or expression in another person, and our mirror neuron system duplicates it. Then, our superior temporal cortex predicts how it will feel. That information is processed by the insula and limbic system, in turn, to define its emotional tone. This tone is returned through the insula to the prefrontal cortex, which interprets it—and voilà, we come to know the situation and to feel what others are feeling. In fact, we can read their intentions and attune to them. Through this circuit, infants bond to caregivers, family and lovers bond, and social connections are made (Carr, Iacoboni, Dubeau, Mazziotta, & Lenzi, 2003). From an evolutionary perspective, this neural process is what allows us to cooperate and compete, to make love, and to fight (Cozolino, 2006).

This circuit is active in the pedagogical situation of the MBIs. When we add mindfulness practice into the mix, the space and place change further. Meditators attune to their own intentions and resonate with themselves. The resultant activity in the prefrontal cortex calms the limbic system, particularly the "fearful" right amygdala (Creswell, Way, Eisenberger, & Lieberman, 2007; Lieberman et al., 2007). A physiological shift may be potentiated that results in what participants report as peace or relaxation—with attendant changes in body posture, vocal tone, gesture, and expression.

Now consider that during a formal group practice, participants may come to experience this kind of physiological shift. When the practice ends, participants begin to look around the group. Even if they are not peaceful themselves, their mirror neurons react to the attitudes of all those who are. Everyone has a chance to "try on" each other's feelings—to experience the atmosphere.

We can explain this characteristic situation of the MBIs in some detail, through Stephen Porges's "polyvagal theory" (2011). His theory posits that we have not only the two subcortical reflex reactions to awareness of threats in the environment—"fight/ flight," or "freeze"—but we also reflexively react to awareness of safety. This third reaction is mediated by the evolutionarily newer branch of the vagus nerve, which enervates the internal viscera, including the heart and the muscles of the head and neck. When our subcortical threat detection system perceives a safe environment, such as with a group of peaceful meditators, the "fight or flight" reflex is suppressed, the heart rate slows, and we become ready for social engagement. That is, our eyes open further to exchange glances, our hearing tunes to the frequency of human voices, our face and neck muscles are prepared to make finely distinctive facial expressions and gestures, and we are ready for articulate speech. Also important in this context is release of the "love hormone" oxytocin which encourages approaching and even embracing.

The characteristic atmosphere of the MBI class is "clearer" now in terms of physiology. Again and again, through formal and informal mindfulness practice, the group together creates an environment that feels safe. Changes in expressions, postures, voices, and gestures may help even those who are struggling move towards social engagement. That response may flow around and throughout the group, creating an atmosphere in which approach and embrace of the moment is possible. In such an atmosphere, participants become more free to explore their aversive, painful experiences of the moment, and to meet them with friendliness.

Stewardship Inside the Circle

Let's consider now the circle of participants, this time looking at the "inside" skills of stewardship. As the capacity develops for the group to stay with the central move of the pedagogy, it is often tested by the environment, dramatic distractions, emotions, or conflicts, within the gathering. The teacher's skills here provide ways of bringing the pedagogy of mindfulness to bear, by helping participants to turn towards difficult experiences as they arise, or to let go of attractive experiences as they pass.

A simple example of an aversive distraction that cannot be avoided is a series of fire engines passing with sirens blaring in the street. In a loud enough voice, the teacher can ask the group to "drop in" to meditation and notice to what they are aware from moment to moment. With the distraction over, the group can then speak together in small subgroups or the full group about the experience. An extraordinary experience can thereby be turned to an ordinary example of mindfulness practice.

If the group is tested in its dialogues by conflict, cross talk, or dominating participants, the teacher may invoke stewardship skills of a formal approach to conversation that may equalize the situation. One approach is to remind participants that listening is the mindfulness skill in dialogue, and then introducing a formal dialogue practice.

A simplified version of the subgrouping technique from Systems Centered Therapy (Agazarian, 1997) may be valuable. Three instructions can be given: First, come to awareness of the body, and maintain that awareness throughout the process of listening and speaking. This practice helps ensure that the group is present focused. Second, when one person speaks, all others listen in a specific way. Listeners attempt to make a connection between what is said and their own present-moment experience. Third, if they find a connection, they may choose to voice it to the group. However, if they do not find a connection, they may hold their own truth, in silence, listening while those who have connected explore their topic. As dialogue continues, it may be that they do find a connection and may speak. If not, the teacher may make time for those who have been silent to speak. Slowly and supportively, all sides of a topic may find a voice.

Council Circle (Zimmerman & Coyle, 1996) may also be used in such situations. It too makes listening a mindfulness practice—so participants may become more aware of their own reactions and "inner" dialogues (also known as thinking). The process involves a talking piece that progresses around the circle. Whoever holds the talking piece speaks or offers silence; the others listen. There are four instructions: (1) speak the truth from the present moment; (2) really listen—be wholly present to what the speaker offers; (3) be concise—omit stories or analyses; (4) be spontaneous—just listen, you'll know what to say when it is your turn.

Both these practices offer the option for the participant to choose to be silent—perhaps the most important option offered as part of stewardship. It is not easy to define or discern who is participating in the group, and when. One may be silent during spoken dialogues and yet be deeply engaged. Participants may be transformed by what looks like simply sitting in the circle.

A Hidden Dimension

The fact that we learn mindfulness *together*, that mindfulness is a relational achievement, has been obscured for decades in the scientific literature. We might trace this obscurity to the kind of scientific research that has grown over the past three decades, and is being further elaborated year after year. Research modeled on (or aspiring to) the so-called gold standard of the randomized controlled trial (RCT) is still widely perceived to endow scientific legitimacy. However, its approach to outcomes is positivist, reductionist, and individualist (Micozzi & Cassidy, 2015). It attempts to set up some property of mindfulness in analogy to a pharmaceutical compound, making it an external object to be placed "inside" to change the individual patient.

While this kind of research approach has elaborated a powerfully persuasive evidence base that has encouraged adoption of mindfulness for a wide range of clinical applications, much potential understanding has been lost. As professionals attempting to describe the pedagogy have suggested (Crane et al., 2014; Crane, Kuyken, Hastings, Rothwell, & Williams, 2010; McCown, 2013; McCown et al., 2017; McCown & Wiley, 2008, 2009), the discourse of this kind of MBI research does not match the concerns of pedagogical study and teacher training. In fact, the research discourse all but ignores the relational dimensions of mindfulness. Even the little bit of data that might be considered from a relational perspective nevertheless focuses on individual outcomes: Imel, Baldwin, Bonus, and MacCoon (2008) looked at data from 60 groups. Through multi-level statistical modeling they calculated the effect on symptom change of the others in the group, factoring out teacher effects, and adjusting for pre-intervention symptom severity. The reported effect accounts for 7 % of variability in outcomes. To put that in perspective, consider that the most significant predictor of outcomes in psychotherapy, the client-therapist alliance, accounts for only about 5 % of variability in outcomes (Horvath & Bedi, 2002).

To better connect with the relational dimension, my colleagues and I have been working with a social constructionist view (e.g., Gergen, 2009, 2015), pioneered in *Teaching Mindfulness* (McCown et al., 2017), to describe the pedagogy of the MBIs. The power of being together has always been obvious to teachers, who hear first hand how participants find it so much easier to practice with others, and how "close" they feel to people with whom they've actually spent precious little time, and whose names they may not even know. Attending to the relational dimension of the pedagogy is one way to define stewardship.

4.   Learning from and in the Atmosphere

The pedagogy of the MBIs is not so much about delivering information as it is about facilitating transformation. Much of the possibility of transformation is available in the classroom experience. Through the atmosphere that they co-create, participants and teachers help each other to maintain the practice of mindfulness, particularly in its key move of being with/in the experience of the moment, however dire or delightful. As the class develops this capacity together, participants find that it may also be available to them outside the class.

We might express the process as teachers and participants "steeping" in the co-created atmosphere of the MBI classroom, and being transformed. The relational constructionist theorist Gergen (2009) describes this process as the development of a *potential*, which is then a part of the participant's *multi-being*. In other words, the new capacity is a new mode of being that is shaped in specific relationships and can then be accessed in other situations.

A useful perspective on this process again comes from the anthropologist Ingold (2013). He explains that

…it is wrong to think of learning as the *transmission* of a ready-made body of information, prior to its *application* in particular contexts of practice. On the contrary, we *learn by doing*, in the course of carrying out tasks of life. In this the contribution of our teachers is not literally to pass on their knowledge, in the form of a ready-made system of concepts and categories with which to give form to the supposedly inchoate material of sensory experience, but rather to establish the contexts or situations in which we can discover for ourselves much of what they already know, and also perhaps much that they do not. In a word, we grow *into* knowledge rather than having it handed down to us (p. 13, emphasis in original).

Returning to Gergen's (2009) ideas, a valuable way for the teacher to think about the situation and atmosphere is through the idea of *confluence*. In this view, group "participants" are mutually defined in the moment through the unfolding of the class activity. A session of formal meditation, for example, mutually defines meditators who are sitting still and quiet, and a teacher who is speaking words of "guidance." As the confluence of formal meditation ends, a new confluence may form as meditators become dyad partners and speak aloud to one another, likely in the curious and non-judging manner that, through the teacher's guidance, informs the atmosphere. In the confluence of the plenary dialogue that follows, the teacher may inquire of participants' in-the-moment experiences in the same way.

In the view of confluence, there is no causality, that is, nothing *forces* the teacher or participants to do what they do. Likewise, they have no agency, that is, no force from "inside" compels them. Rather, what happens from one moment to the next in the class issues from the confluence of relationships. This confluence provides a useful way to speak of the process of the "co-creation" of mindfulness in the group. What's more, after time steeping in this particular confluence, participants come away with potentials for formal and informal mindfulness practice, including potentials of curiosity and non-judging that can also be accessed in other situations.

In this view, stewardship is the tending of relationships to ensure that the atmosphere teaches; that the confluence is a context for growing into knowledge, for being endowed with new potentials; and that the practice of the pedagogy of the MBIs can be transformative.

Box 1.2: Greater Expressive Resources from a Collective Culture

It is exciting for MBSR pedagogical theory (in English) to have the opportunity become acquainted with the Korean vocabulary, with such terms as *Ahwoollim* and *Shinmyong*, and the different structure and syntax. They support the insights that humans are relational beings and help to counteract the atomistic, individualistic concepts enforced by the dominant academic and medical research paradigm (McCown & Ahn, 2015). *Ahwoolim* refers to a deep resonance among more than two different persons or things in which they may lose their ordinary self-boundaries. *Shinmyong* suggests a powerful emotional experience within a group—a sense of ecstatic aliveness and mutuality of becoming. Both terms are a contribution to MBI theory. With such expanded language resources, modes of expression may be built that can capture the most profound moments of pedagogical practice.

5. Tending the Ethical Space

Recently, the MBI community and its critics have expressed concern about the role of ethics in the content and pedagogy of the interventions (e.g., Lindahl, 2015; McCown, 2013; Monteiro, Musten, & Compton, 2015; Purser, 2015; Van Gordon, Shonin, Griffiths, & Singh, 2015; Williams & Kabat-Zinn, 2013). A key position that has been espoused by the community throughout its history is that MBSR, and by extension the other MBIs, have an implicit ethics. While this position has been considered as controversial (Baer, 2015), such a claim is greatly strengthened within a relational constructionist view, in which the ethical situation is constructed in the moment in the group.

As my colleagues and I (McCown et al., 2017) analyzed the pedagogy of the MBIs, we identified the qualities of the atmosphere that is co-created in the classroom. These qualities are located in both the actions of teaching, and in the unspoken framing of the space, as the teacher and participants come together. This quality may be thought of as the *ethical space* of mindfulness (McCown, 2013), which can be defined by seven specific qualities, distributed across three dimensions.

Although the word *space* is often used in an abstract or metaphorical way in discourse around mindfulness and meditation, the ethical space is not an instance of this same concept. Rather, the ethical space is an actual architectural situation—a place, with furnishings, where people act together in site-specific ways. In the following descriptions of each dimension and its qualities, this will become clearer. Figure 1.1 may help in understanding the relationships and ultimate integration of the dimensions and qualities.

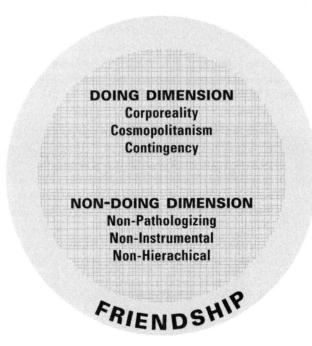

Fig. 1.1 The interweaving (represented by *crosshatched lines*) of the doing and non-doing dimensions is ultimately infused with the quality of friendship—perhaps the best single word description of the atmosphere of the MBI classroom

The Doing Dimension

There are three qualities of action that define the work of the MBI confluence. These qualities are endowed by participation in the pedagogy of mindfulness, the ongoing attempt to turn towards and stay with/in the experience of the present moment.

Corporeality foregrounds the experience of the body. Participants quickly recognize this focus on sensation as different from the typical modes of investigation in mental health interventions. Mindfulness meditation at its foundation is a practice of the *body*. This sense of the body, in sensations of breathing or proprioception, brings participants into intimate contact with their present-moment experience. One cannot feel sensations in the future or in the past—on in the present. This body sense helps make aesthetic and affective experiences available and tolerable for participants. Corporeal experiences are often explored in silence by the participants and may be voiced and explored differently through dialogue.

Contingency deconstructs these experiences, particularly those that are difficult to tolerate. In the formal and informal practices of the class sessions, and in unfinished dialogues and home practice, participants track the arising and subsiding of their body sensations, emotions, and thoughts. Participants can watch how body sensations continually change and pass away. They can encounter and are often able to turn towards and be with/in distressing moments of emotion, opening to the opportunity of observing emotion as body sensation— where, again, the tendency towards change becomes evident. Things may be "worse" or "better" in the moment, but they are constantly moving. It is that kind of experience that helps to deconstruct an emotion—what is it really?— and that opens for participants different possibilities for self-regulation. Finally, they notice the instability of the stream of thought. In such a situation, insight and meaning may arise.

Cosmopolitanism describes the willing acceptance of the meaning that arises in the moment, without a drive to abstract it, reduce it, or fit it into any one system or set of values imposed by the teacher. In other words, meaning is revealed as contingent. This quality is particularly important because mindfulness practice often opens participants to the spiritual dimension of their lives. These dimensions may be widely varied, with specific religious commitments and interpretations, or an ever-shifting but profound curiosity. Although empirical evidence is thin in the literature of the MBIs, a meta-analysis of controlled trials (Chiesa & Serretti, 2009) found five studies that measured aspects of spirituality. Results suggest that MBSR significantly enhances spirituality compared to inactive (but not active) control groups. Two additional studies not included in the meta-analysis (Carmody, Reed, Kristeller, & Merriam, 2008; Greeson et al., 2011) also suggest significant spiritual engagement. Teachers in the MBIs witness much more of this kind of meaning-making than what is captured by researchers. Cosmopolitanism is one way to hold this elusive quality by accepting and allowing the meaning that is created moment to moment, without others' commentary, correction, or critique.

The Non-doing Dimension

In the dimension of *non-doing*, it would be easy to focus on the teacher as the actor establishing the qualities. Yet, as we have seen in our explorations of the pedagogy, the non-doing qualities are actually inherent in the central move of the pedagogy, and become clear in the absence of particular views or actions.

Non-pathologizing refers to that defining perspective so often set in the first class of an MBI, as Kabat-Zinn (1990, p. 2) expressed and countless teachers have reiterated: "as long as you are breathing there is more right with you than there is wrong, no matter how ill or how hopeless you may feel." By taking the focus off pathology, the MBSR gathering re-creates the participants, replacing limited diagnostic identities with unlimited possibilities.

Non-hierarchical refers to the teacher's position of not-knowing when confronted with participants' experiences. It also refers beyond the teacher to describe the "rule" of class dialogue, stating that no one needs to be "fixed" because no one is "broken." One can impose meanings onto one's own ever-changing experiences, yet no one is the expert on the unfolding of the present moment. To phrase it in American vernacular speech, the teacher is as "clueless" as anyone else—and is committed to exploring with participants whatever experience that may be arising. Invoking Ingold (2013) we might say that the teacher does not transmit information, but rather helps shape a context for growing into knowledge.

Non-instrumental is a subtle quality. It is founded on the proposition that the class does not practice the pedagogy of mindfulness in order to be changed or transformed in a particular way—it is not instrumentalized to create a particular outcome. Participants don't practice "because," or "in order to," but rather as an exploration of the unfolding present moment. This quality does not, however, rule out transformation. In fact, transformation may be seen as inherent to the nature of the confluence. Together, participants are observing that all contingent structures of sensation, affect, and thought deconstruct themselves as they unfold within the ethical space and its associated qualities. Participants may indeed come to be endowed with new potentials, guided by the relationships in the moment, and steeping in the experiences of silence and practice, as well as spoken and unspoken dialogue.

The Character of the Confluence

Friendship is a single quality and has its own dimension within the model of the ethical space. Yet it can also be seen as the total character of the confluence of the pedagogy of mindfulness. Friendship is not "held" by the teacher in some way; it is not a choice or action, or "instrument." Rather, friendship is co-created as the pervading essence of the pedagogy. It is the atmosphere of the class. As participants steep in it, they may be endowed with the potential. That potential means that friendship may arise in other confluences, and even in the relationships of participants to themselves—where it might be seen as the care and compassion for self that is a powerful predictor of positive change in individuals in the MBIs (Kuyken et al., 2010).

Ethics in the Ethical Space

The ethical space is co-created through the group or dyad's practice of the MBI pedagogy. It is not something new or extra. Gergen (2009) would say that participants are fully immersed within the "first-order morality" of the MBI, which means that the confluence has defined and may create its own goods that then become potentials for participants. Those in a first-order morality cannot act otherwise than in accordance with the goods defined within it: the confluence, the ethical space, and a first-order morality are identical. However, participants and teacher all have potentials from other first-order moralities as well, which might be defined as allegiances to other communities. Gergen (2009) suggests that such instability of allegiance can be problematic, as conflict arises when first-order moralities contradict each other. At the same time, for MBI teachers, having multiple first-order moralities is useful in maintaining an ethical position.

MBI teachers maintain allegiance to the ethical space of mindfulness when they and the participants are engaged in the pedagogy. When *all* can stay with the key move of turning towards and being with/in the experience of the moment, the situation is inherently ethical. However, should a participant find himself incapable of maintaining the key move of the pedagogy, even with assistance from the teacher, that participant may enact other potentials from other first-order moralities, disturbing the confluence. At this point, the teacher's other first-order moralities, particularly her potentials as psychologist, social worker, nurse, or physician, have great value. She may "step out" of the ethical space of mindfulness and align instead with the ethical code of her particular profession—and those other potentials keep everyone safe.

There also may be moments when the teacher lacks the capacity to maintain the key move of the pedagogy, although the group may be attempting to do so. In this case, her choice to "step out" of the ethical space and actuate the ethical potentials of her specific clinical professional identity is different because her impulse is to protect herself rather than the group. Such reflexive self-protection does also protect the participants—offering pre-established guidelines in an ambiguous situation.

Within the co-created ethical space, the participants steep in the potentials of the confluence. They grow more and more in the capacity to turn towards and be with/in what is arising in the moment. Therefore, the less the participants or teacher "step out" and interrupt that steeping, the more they develop "trust" in the practice—that is, the more they are endowed with valuable potentials. Yet, stepping out is a live option for all, as well. There is safety in both the ethical space and within the alternate first-order moralities of the health care professions. We might say that the ethical space as first-order morality is transparent to participants, and offers a useful, pragmatic situation for teachers.

6. Sensing Sublime Moments

Clinical work with mindfulness is different from teaching mindfulness in educational or organizational settings. There is an aesthetic experience available in clinical settings that is far less easily found in the others. This experience can be described as a form of the sublime.

Imagine a confluence that is well steeped in the central move of the pedagogy, so that the participants find it possible to approach and stay with aversive moments of experience. Imagine, as well, that one particular participant, *Jessica*, who has spoken to the group about her panic attacks, is willing to enter into dialogue with the teacher about an emerging experience:

"How is it with you right now?" the teacher asks. "Is there anxiety here?"
"Yeah, a bit."
"Would you be willing to explore it, just a little, in a mindful way? Maybe there's a way to be with it that's different than what you've been doing. You're in charge, so you can stop any time, OK?"
"OK," says Jessica.
To the group, the teacher says, "While Jessica and I explore her experience, maybe you can find a way—not to watch, exactly, yet to be connected to your own experience. I suspect that quite a few of you may be interested in ways to be with anxiety. Yes?" Hands sprout around the circle. Jessica looks around, maybe settling a little more in her chair.

This move by the teacher to engage the whole group with the spoken dialogue that is beginning (while pointing them to their own unfinished dialogues) is a skill of stewardship—a profound one. Through it, the atmosphere may remain supportive for all involved, the ethical space may be maintained, and many in the group may discover new possibilities and potentials. As the dialogue continues, the teacher's actions nurture both Jessica's unfolding experience and the quality of the atmosphere.

"So, Jessica, are you still noticing some anxiety" the teacher asks.
"Some, yeah," she says quietly.
The teacher asks, also quietly, "If you bring attention to your body right now, can you feel where that anxiety is showing up? Just take your time and feel into it..."
Quickly she answers, "In my back. That's where it's been a lot recently. It sort of moves around..."
The teacher asks, "Can you bring your attention there? And see what you find out about that feeling?"
"That's scary, but I'll try." There is a long pause. "OK, I am... I'm paying attention."
"And what is the feeling like?"
"It's like, constricted... tight."
"Do you know anything more? Like how big the area is, or, maybe, what shape it is..." And the teacher waits quietly, with a curious and patient expression and posture.
With her thumbs and forefingers Jessica makes a long, horizontal oval. "It's a rectangle, about this big, in the center of my back. It's really tight."
"OK," says the teacher. "You're right there with it... I wonder if you can find a way to give it a little room, to open some space around it? Maybe you can use your breath to soften around it..." She looks puzzled, and the teacher elaborates. "Can your breath go to that part of your back when you breathe in? Do you know what I mean?"
"I think so... Yeah."

The teacher pauses a moment to look around the circle to be sure there is some understanding within the whole group. With this look she is reminding participants that they may engage in the exploration too.

"So when you breathe in, letting some space open up around that rectangle...and when you breathe out, letting it stay soft..."

The whole group, as much as they are able, are quiet as they breathe, many with their eyes closed, for thirty seconds or so, which in this atmosphere may feel like a long time. The teacher then checks in; her prompt to Jessica is also acting as a prompt to other participants.

> The teacher asks, *"What more do you know about that spot now? Anything?"*
>
> *"It's gotten smaller,"* Jessica replies. *"Much smaller... It's like the size of my finger, now."*
>
> *"So it changed... You gave it space and it stopped taking up so much space in you. OK. Maybe you want to keep in touch with it, keep breathing and making space,"* the teacher says to Jessica.

After a pause, the teacher then turns to engage the whole group, looking around the circle. She uses the moment to bring forward a teaching point:

> *"That's sometimes what happens. We have no guarantee of a particular outcome. We're not practicing a technique to get rid of something. In Jessica's situation, she was just paying attention to what was there, opening space for it to be, and for herself to see what it was. The important thing was her willingness to be with, and to pay attention to, her experience. Her courage in showing up for what was happening was what really mattered."*

This dialogue was neither easy for Jessica, nor for the other members of the class who watched and listened and perhaps engaged in their own unfinished dialogues. This encounter was not so much of the teacher with a participant as it was an encounter of the class with an affective charge—the question of turning towards and being with/in one's own anxiety. This encounter was an instance of steeping in the deeply human, seriously committed way of being that it is possible to experience in an MBI class. One potential description of such experiences is of the *sublime*.

The term sublime is borrowed from aesthetics and rendered with particular connotations for mindfulness pedagogy. It is beyond the scope of this chapter to enter a detailed discussion of the history of the many uses and interpretations of the sublime (e.g., Shaw, 2006). However, a useful view of the sublime and its activities on the person is described by the eighteenth century English philosopher, Burke (1759/1999). He makes the experience of "terror" a central idea in his definition. The terror to which he refers is found in overwhelming natural phenomena, such as storms at sea or ascents of mountains. The observer cannot express such experiences, and is carried beyond the rational dimension, and ultimately beyond the limited self. The sense of "I," is reduced, and the observer is more open to the experience. In mindfulness pedagogy, then, those moments when participants confront more of the fullness and contingency of human existence—the possibilities of death and madness, to name two extremes—may be considered sublime.

In the classroom dialogue with Jessica, many participants may have had strong affective experiences. The depth and willingness to be present carried in the atmosphere may have opened them to Jessica's experience of anxiety—and their own. As Burke and other theorists note, *the terror of the sublime* may include a paradoxical sense of pleasure, which, Burke suggests, becomes possible when there is space for observation. We can watch a frightening storm at sea from the safety of land. Likewise, we may witness a courageous grappling with emotion from a chair across the room. We may even view our own frightening situation with the clarity of mindfulness practice and support of a silent, caring, resonant group.

The experience of the sublime arises in observing in a clear and spacious way that which may deeply frighten or move us. This experience is also the central move of the pedagogy of mindfulness—the turning towards and being with/in the experience of the moment. The pedagogy, then, makes the experience of the sublime possible for MBI participants.

The sublime has particular value for the teacher in the MBIs. When the atmosphere in the classroom has been sublime for moments at a time, the teacher may presume that the pedagogy is "working," and that participants are steeping—being endowed with potentials for living in more profound and authentic ways. Sublime moments become ways to measure stewardship.

As contrast to the sublime, Burke (1759/1999) proposes the beautiful. Shaw (2006) quotes Burke in making this distinction:

> Where the sublime 'dwells on large objects, and terrible' and is linked to the intense sensations of terror, pain, and awe, the focus of the beautiful, by contrast, is on 'small ones, and pleasing' and appeals mainly to the domestic affections, to love, tenderness, and pity. Crucially, with the sublime 'we submit to what we admire', whereas with the beautiful 'we love what submits to us' (p. 57).

Beauty brings us closer together as we agree on the pleasure of an experience. The sublime also connects us, but through terror, through facing a fearful prospect together. Consider the value of this insight for stewardship. When a class steeps solely in the beautiful, without being interspersed with the sublime, the power of the central move of the pedagogy is not revealed, so participants cannot steep in it. The potentials endowed are restricted.

Clinical situations are rich in possibilities for sublime moments. Fear, madness, and death may not actually appear, but they hover nearby, affecting atmosphere. The stewardship skill is not merely to steer close to the sublime, but also to make certain that the atmosphere is available to the whole class for steeping. Inviting all participants to make the key move of the pedagogy—even when only one person is engaged in spoken dialogue—can bring participants there and help endow powerful potentials.

7.   *Positioning the Self for Teaching*

All of this discussion of steeping and potentials suggests that MBI teacher formation has unique dimensions. It is not limited to learning theories or techniques. It is not best described as following the modeling of an accomplished teacher. It is not ultimately driven by an individual daily practice of meditation. Rather, teacher formation is the endowing of potentials through steeping in the confluence of the classroom, within an ethical space that sometimes achieves the character of the sublime. Teachers, then, are formed by steeping, by being in many MBI classes both as participant and teacher. In this way, a teacher may grow into the potentials of the curriculum and the key move of turning towards and being with/in the moment. The teacher grows into potentials in the classroom with the participants—a teacher is co-created, made of many experiences.

The self of the teacher can best be understood through a first person approach: Somehow, making up my multi-being are potentials for relating in ways that might be identified with corporeality, contingency, and cosmopolitanism; as well, there are potentials for relating in non-pathologizing, non-hierarchical, and non-instrumental ways; and, finally, potentials for friendship. On reflection, I have potentials that help me to steer towards sublime moments. These potentials are continually changing and growing, as I teach, moment to moment in the classroom, and through year after year of classes. But they do not simply lie at the ready, prepared, or pre-cooked; my potentials are available to be grown into, only in the moment, as they are needed. My response to one participant or to all at once is unmediated. I do not debate, dialogue, or choose in the moment what to do, but rather, I act within the entire, populated situation with its unique atmosphere. As a colleague expresses it: "I don't know where it comes from, but it comes." The best description I know is from the painter Philip Guston, as described by his daughter, Mayer (1988, p. 80):

> During the difficult times of the 1970s, when the artworld was busy being shocked and offended by my father's late, figurative work, his shows at the David McKee Gallery were always well attended by young painters and painting students. After the long-standing disappointment of no sales and negative reviews—which persisted for a decade, until shortly before his death—it was heartening for him to see the interest of the younger generation in these strange new images.
>
> Some powerful force had moved through him, he often told these young painters. That was how he had come to see it in those last years. My father refused to claim ownership of this force; he approached it with great humility and trepidation. What he had learned by the end of his life was how to position himself, he told his students, how to make of himself a vessel for what moved through him. "I never feel myself to be more than a trusting accomplice," he said.

There are two ideas here that help describe what happens in the moment in the classroom. First is the idea that I have literally and figuratively learned "how to position" myself. I sit, in my chair or on the floor, oriented to the group and to my interlocutor, in a posture, relaxed and attentive, that is congruent with the confluence. The way I am disposed physically makes evident my emotional and intellectual disposition. The potential of being with/in the experience shows up. This is not metaphor. It's my embodied experience. Second is the idea that, in the moment, I allow all the potentials of multi-being, the years of steeping in the ethical space, to "move through" me. As Guston suggests, I am a vessel for them. My responses in the confluence simply flow when I am making the key move of the MBI pedagogy of turning towards and being with/in the experience.

However, when tension enters the confluence, my access to potentials may be reduced, which reduces access for participants to their own developing potentials. If the situation sets me scrambling for precedents, theories, or models from my own teachers, rather than responding unpremeditatedly from the confluence, something is lost. Whatever I might say or do that comes from weighing thought will fall in the moment like lead and disturb—even disrupt—the class. Then, all of us will have to find our way back into confluence to again achieve the *co-created* flowing disposition.

This situation is why the teacher's so-called personal practice of mindfulness is fundamental. But it is decidedly *not* personal. The teacher's potential for turning towards and being with/in the present moment is inextricably woven into a web of relationships extending from her own teachers, past and present, to current participants in her classes, to those for whom she is preparing. Each relationship, each confluence, or each endowed potential contributes to the co-creation of each moment of the practice of the pedagogy. Each is precious and must be met and cared for with the generosity, hospitality, and friendship that is emblematic of stewardship.

Conclusion

This chapter began with the question "What is it like in the room right now?" Through the discussion that followed, it may have taken on new dimensions, depth, and even power. Now, it may be more clear that asking this question, and responding to the answer from moment to moment, defines the skill sets of stewardship.

These skills are subtle, beyond cognitive learning and stepwise training. They reveal the MBI teacher as more than a technician or clinician. To define the teacher and skills, we need to move beyond the individualistic expectations of professional education to include others, places, things, and spaces. The stewardship skills are potentials that are endowed by steeping in the confluences of MBI classes and may be accessed again in other classes. The MBI teacher, as steward, senses the atmosphere of the classroom and steers the participants, as possible, towards the key move of the pedagogy, turning towards and being with/in the moment. All of the stewardship skills facilitate this navigation, by helping to shape the atmosphere, or to sense its qualities. When the teacher and participants together can maintain an atmosphere of mindfulness over time, they may co-create a safe place and an ethical space in which they may steep and be endowed with new potentials. That is, they may ultimately transform each other.

References

Agazarian, Y. M. (1997). *Systems centered therapy for groups*. New York, NY: Guilford.

Baer, R. (2015). Ethics, values, virtues, and character strengths in mindfulness-based interventions: a psychological science perspective. *Mindfulness, 6*, 956–969. doi:10.1007/s12671-015-0419-2.

Böhme, G. (1993). Atmosphere as the fundamental concept of a new aesthetics. *Thesis Eleven, 36*, 113–126.

Böhme, G. (2011). The art of the stage set as a paradigm for an aesthetics of atmospheres. *Ambiances*. [On line posted February 10, 2013]. Retrieved June 9, 2015, from http://ambiances.revues.org/315

Bollnow, O. F. (2011). *Human space*. London, England: Hyphen Press.

Burke, E. (1999). *A philosophical enquiry into the origins of the sublime and beautiful: And other pre-revolutionary writings*. London, England: Penguin. (Original work published 1759)

Carmody, J., Reed, G., Kristeller, J., & Merriam, P. (2008). Mindfulness, spirituality, and health-related symptoms. *Journal of Psychosomatic Research, 64*, 393–403.

Carr, L., Iacoboni, M., Dubeau, M.-C., Mazziotta, J., & Lenzi, G. (2003). Neural mechanisms of empathy in humans: A relay from neural systems for imitation to limbic areas. *Proceedings of the National Academy of Sciences of the United States of America, 100*, 5497–5502.

Chiesa, A., & Serretti, A. (2009). Mindfulness-based stress reduction for stress management in healthy people: A review and meta-analysis. *Journal of Alternative and Complementary Medicine, 15*(5), 593–600.

Cozolino, L. (2006). *The neuroscience of human relationships*. New York, NY: Norton.

Crane, R. S., Kuyken, W., Hastings, R., Rothwell, N., & Williams, J. M. G. (2010). Training teachers to deliver mindfulness-based interventions: Learning from the UK experience. *Mindfulness, 1*, 74–86.

Crane, R. S., Stanley, S., Rooney, M., Bartley, T., Cooper, L., & Mardula, J. (2014). Disciplined improvisation: Characteristics of inquiry in mindfulness-based teaching. *Mindfulness*. doi: 10.1007/s12671-014-0361-8. [Published online November 29].

Creswell, J. D., Way, B. M., Eisenberger, N. I., & Lieberman, M. D. (2007). Neural correlates of dispositional mindfulness during affect labeling. *Psychosomatic Medicine, 69*, 560–565.

Feldman, C., & Kuyken, W. (2011). Compassion in the landscape of suffering. *Contemporary Buddhism, 12*(1), 143–155.

Gallese, V., Fadiga, L., Fogassi, L., & Rizzolatti, G. (1996). Action recognition in the premotor cortex. *Brain, 119*, 593–609.

Gallese, V., & Goldman, A. (1998). Mirror neurons and the simulation theory of mindreading. *Trends in Cognitive Sciences, 2*(12), 493–501.

Gergen, K. (2009). *Relational being: Beyond self and community*. Oxford, England: Oxford University Press.

Gergen, K. (2015). *An invitation to social construction* (3rd ed.). London, England: Sage.

Greeson, J. M., Webber, D. M., Smoski, M. J., Brantley, J. G., Ekblad, A. G., Suarez, E. C., & Wolever, R. Q. (2011). Changes in spirituality partly explain health-related quality of life outcomes after mindfulness-based stress reduction. *Journal of Behavioral Medicine, 34*(6), 508–518. [Published online March 1].

Hayes, A., & Feldman, G. (2004). Clarifying the construct of mindfulness in the context of emotion regulation and the process of change in therapy. *Clinical Psychology: Science and Practice, 11*(3), 255–262.

Horvath, A., & Bedi, R. (2002). The alliance. In J. Norcross (Ed.), *Psychotherapy relationships that work: Therapist contributions and responsiveness to patients* (pp. 37–70). New York, NY: Oxford University Press.

Imel, Z., Baldwin, S., Bonus, K., & MacCoon, D. (2008). Beyond the individual: Group effects in mindfulness-based stress reduction. *Psychotherapy Research, 18*(6), 735–742.

Ingold, T. (2008). The social child. In A. Fogel, B. J. King & S. G. Shanker (Eds.), Human development in the twenty-first century: Visionary ideas from systems scientists (pp. 112–118). Cambridge, UK: Cambridge University Press.

Ingold, T. (2013). *Making: Anthropology, archeology, art and architecture*. New York, NY: Routledge.

Ingold, T. (2015). *The life of lines*. New York, NY: Routledge.

Kabat-Zinn, J. (1990). *Full catastrophe living*. New York, NY: Delacorte.

Kuyken, W., Watkins, E., Holden, E., White, K., Taylor, R. S., Byford, S., … Dalgleish, T. (2010). How does mindfulness-based cognitive therapy work? *Behaviour Research and Therapy, 48*(11), 1105–1112.

Lieberman, M. D., Eisenberger, N. I., Crockett, M. J., Tom, S. M., Pfeifer, J. H., & Way, B. M. (2007). Putting feelings into words: Affect labeling disrupts amygdala activity in response to affective stimuli. *Psychological Science, 18*(5), 421–427.

Lindahl, J. R. (2015). Why right mindfulness might not be right for mindfulness. *Mindfulness, 6*, 57–62.

Mauss, M. (1973). Techniques of the body. *Economy and Society, 2*(1), 70–88. (Original work published 1934)

Mayer, M. (1988). *Night studio: A memoir of Philip Guston by his daughter Musa Mayer*. New York, NY: Knopf.

McCown, D. (2005). Marketing mindfulness: A dialogue to share insights for program success. In *3rd Annual Conference: Integrating Mindfulness-Based Interventions into Medicine, Health Care, and Society, Worcester, MA, April 1–4*.

McCown, D. (2013). *The ethical space of mindfulness in clinical practice*. London, England: Jessica Kingsley.

McCown, D. (2015, February 27–28). *A mindful campus: Cultivating awareness and connection in a distracted world. Keynote*. Indiana, PA: Indiana University of Pennsylvania.

McCown, D., & Ahn, H. (2015). Dialogical and Eastern perspectives on the self in practice: Teaching mindfulness-based stress reduction in Philadelphia and Seoul. *International Journal for DIalogical Science, 9*(1), 39–74.

McCown, D., Reibel, D., & Micozzi, M. (2017). *Teaching mindfulness: A practical guide for clinicians and educators*. New York, NY: Springer.

McCown, D., & Wiley, S. (2008). Emergent issues in MBSR research and pedagogy: Integrity, fidelity, and how do we decide? In *6th Annual Conference: Integrating Mindfulness-Based Interventions into Medicine, Health Care, and Society, Worcester, MA, April 10–12*.

McCown, D., & Wiley, S. (2009). Thinking the world together: Seeking accord and interdependence in the discourses of mindfulness teaching and research. In *7th Annual Conference: Integrating Mindfulness-Based Interventions into Medicine, Health Care, and Society, Worcester, MA, March 18–22*.

Micozzi, M., & Cassidy, C. (2015). Issues and challenges in integrative medicine. In M. S. Micozzi (Ed.), *Fundamentals of complementary and alternative medicine* (5th ed.). Philadelphia, PA: Elsevier Health Sciences.

Monteiro, L. M., Musten, R. F., & Compton, J. (2015). Traditional and contemporary mindfulness: Finding the middle path in the tangle of concerns. *Mindfulness, 6*, 1–13.

Porges, S. W. (2011). *The polyvagal theory: Neurophysiological foundations of emotions, attachment, communication, and self-regulation*. New York, NY: Norton.

Purser, R. E. (2015). Clearing the muddled path of traditional and contemporary mindfulness: a response to Monteiro, Musten, and Compson. *Mindfulness, 6*, 23–45.

Santorelli, S. (Ed.). (2014). *Mindfulness-based stress reduction (MBSR) standards of practice*. Worcester, MA: UMASS Medical School, Center for Mindfulness in Medicine, Health Care & Society.

Shaw, P. (2006). *The sublime*. New York, NY: Routledge.

Siegel, D. (2007). *The mindful brain*. New York, NY: Norton.

Van Dam, N., Sheppard, S., Forsyth, J., & Earleywine, M. (2011). Self-compassion is a better predictor than mindfulness of symptom severity and quality of life in mixed anxiety and depression. *Journal of Anxiety Disorders, 25*, 123–130.

Van Gordon, W., Shonin, E., Griffiths, M. D., & Singh, N. N. (2015). There is only one mindfulness: Why science and Buddhism need to work together. *Mindfulness, 6*, 49–56.

Williams, M., & Kabat-Zinn, J. (2013). *Mindfulness: Diverse perspectives on its meaning, origins, and applications*. New York, NY: Routledge.

Zimmerman, J., & Coyle, V. (1996). *The way of council*. Las Vegas, NV: Bramble Books.

Chapter 2
Guidance: Refining the Details

Aleezé S. Moss, Diane Reibel, and Donald McCown

Introduction to Theory and Practice

Providing guidance is one of the key pedagogical skills and actions of the teacher in the Mindfulness-Based Interventions (MBIs), along with stewardship, homiletics, and inquiry. These skills are interrelated and each includes and influences the others. Guided meditation, both "live" in class and through recordings, plays a crucial role in the cultivation of mindfulness, a way of being in the world in relationship to self, to others, and to the flow of experience moment by moment.

Guidance is using spoken language and all of the corporeal ("body language") possibilities for communicating in a way to catalyze the pedagogy of mindfulness in the classroom. While the forms of language and other communications differ from teacher to teacher, and context to context, there are some general considerations and guidelines that are helpful to consider. Some of these considerations are more theoretical (for instance, the function of guidance) and some are more practical (say, specific uses

A.S. Moss, Ph.D. (✉)
Mindfulness Institute, Jefferson-Myrna Brind Center of Integrative Medicine, Thomas Jefferson University Hospitals, 1015 Chestnut Street, Suite 1212, Philadelphia, PA 19107, USA
e-mail: aleeze.moss@jefferson.edu

D. Reibel, Ph.D.
Mindfulness Institute, Jefferson-Myrna Brind Center of Integrative Medicine, Thomas Jefferson University Hospitals, 1015 Chestnut Street, Suite 1212, Philadelphia, PA 19107, USA

Emergency Medicine, Sidney Kimmel Medical College, Thomas Jefferson University, Philadelphia, PA 19107, USA
e-mail: diane.reibel@jefferson.edu

D. McCown, Ph.D., M.A.M.S., M.S.S., L.S.W.
Center for Contemplative Studies, West Chester University of Pennsylvania, Sturzebecker Health Sciences Center, #312, West Chester, PA 19383, USA
e-mail: dmccown@wcupa.edu

© Springer International Publishing Switzerland 2016
D. McCown et al., *Resources for Teaching Mindfulness*,
DOI 10.1007/978-3-319-30100-6_2

of language, or vocal tone and volume). Ultimately, the theoretical and the practical understanding and implementation go hand in hand.

In this chapter, we discuss the function of guidance in the MBIs, situating it within a discussion of the concept of co-creation, and describe how the skill can be cultivated. We examine four practical dimensions of guidance, and present a full script for the example of seated yoga practice through which we examine the details.

The Function of Guidance in the MBIs

The intention or function of the guided meditations in the MBIs is to cultivate mindfulness. While there are many ways to talk about mindfulness, Kabat-Zinn's influential definition (e.g., 1990) describes mindfulness as the awareness that develops from paying attention, on purpose, in the present moment, nonjudgmentally. Shapiro and colleagues elaborated on this definition to posit three axioms of mindfulness that are engaged simultaneously in the process of cultivating mindfulness: intention, attention, and attitude (Shapiro, Carlson, Astin, & Freedman, 2006). Guided meditation can catalyze and cultivate all three.

This kind of catalyzing and cultivating is not "just one more method or technique, akin to other familiar techniques and strategies we may find instrumental and effective in one field or another" (Kabat-Zinn, 2010, p. xi). Rather, mindfulness is "a way of being, of seeing, of tapping into the full dimensionality of our humanity, and this way has a critical *non-instrumental* essence inherent in it" (2010, p. xi). It is important to remember that guidance has this non-instrumental essence. Guidance is not about leading towards some preconceived, idealized state. Rather, it facilitates an intentional turning towards and being with/in the present moment flow of ordinary experience, with an attitude of openness, nonjudgment, non-striving, curiosity, and kindness.

There is a particular premise in the pedagogy of the MBIs right from the start. With ubiquitous reassurance that there is "more right with them than there is wrong," participants are directed *away* from acquiescence to the dominant culture of diagnosis, and *towards* taking a new, active role in their own health and well-being. It is assumed that they already have the necessary resources to cultivate mindfulness. Further, teachers often state at the outset that no one in the class needs to be "fixed," because they are not broken. In fact, it easily becomes apparent that participants and teacher alike are "in the same boat," when it comes to the sorrows and joys of being human. It is implied that the teacher is not an expert (although she knows the curriculum and acts as a steward), and that what happens in class is co-created, moment by moment. Opening remarks also suggest that we cannot know how things will unfold from moment to moment, in the class or with each participant. Thus, a certain kind of fearlessness is required—a willingness to not know.

This theoretical basis of mindfulness practice in the MBIs is manifested through the teacher's guidance of meditation and other practices. Language choices, vocal tone and volume, gestures, postures, and the ineffable nuances of the teacher's own mindfulness practice are all influential. Rather than just imparting information or knowledge, we could say that guidance *catalyzes* mindfulness as a way of being, seeing, and sensing.

The Context of Guidance

We suggest that guided meditation is a relational act; an act of co-creation. Although the teacher is guiding, and participants are responding in silence, it is the relationship among them that informs and influences everyone, including the teacher. Because it impacts the practicalities of guidance, it is worth exploring the notion of co-creation in the MBIs. A clear evocation of co-creation comes in Gergen's (2009) description of *confluence*. In the dominant discourse of individualism, participants in a class or dyad are seen as autonomous individuals first, bound up in their chosen identities and only (perhaps even grudgingly) accountable to others. In contrast to that discourse, Gergen's concept of confluence sees participants as relational beings first, with identities shaped in each instant by the unfolding of the shared activities.

For example, in an MBI class, when the curriculum calls for the practice of sitting meditation, participants mutually define meditators who sit quietly and a teacher who "guides" with her voice. Participants know what to do (who they are) in that moment. Then, when the confluence that is formal meditation practice ends, the meditators may be redefined as dyad partners that speak aloud to each other, or as part of the entire group in dialogue. Relationship defines who we are and what we do in any situation (McCown, 2015). This approach defines the activities of teaching and learning mindfulness as an ongoing co-creation, involving and affecting all participants. Each instance of co-creation is unique, arising in the moment, and therefore unrepeatable (McCown, 2013).

Another definition of co-creation is that we are all in a shared space of continually flowing streams of experience, occurring within us and among us. In the view of Shotter (2012, p. 4), expanding the boundaries of social construction, we are sensitive and responsive to the flow of information with others:

> Ephemeral though they may be, the particular sensings [sic] and feelings that we can pick out of the stream are not only crucial in our shaping and guiding our behavior, as we move around within our surroundings, but the ways in which we make sense of them—i.e., orient towards them—are basic to "who" and "what" we take ourselves to be.

As MBI teachers guiding meditation in class, we can be considered as using what Shotter describes as "the spontaneous responsiveness of our living bodies, and our inner sensing of the situation in which we are immersed at the very moment of opening our mouths to speak" (2012, p. 4). This description provides a way of viewing guided meditation as a shared activity, an exchange among all the participants.

Shotter also describes the notion of "joint action" through which we are co-constructing each other as relational beings, within the continuous, chaotic flow of moment-by-moment experiences in which we are embedded. One feature of joint action is that it does not derive from the intentions of particular participants but rather *in the exchanges between and among them*. What arises, then, is not anything that could have been predicted. This unpredictability is extremely relevant in the context of the MBIs. Understandings of confluence, shared space, co-creation, and joint-action provide useful ways of seeing the MBI class. Something happens in this coming together, being together, often in silence, during guided meditations, discussions, and dialogue. The world of the participants (including the teacher) changes with each silence, each word, each motion, and each feeling. Shotter (2011, p. 58, emphasis added) describes it thus:

> But more than simply responding to each other in a sequential manner—that is, instead of one person first acting individually and independently of another, and then the second also by acting individually and independently of the first in his/her reply—the fact is that in such a sphere of spontaneously responsive dialogically structured activity as this, *we all act jointly as a collective-we.*

One way in which guided meditations lead to the co-creation of a "collective-we" is through both interpersonal and intrapersonal resonance, perhaps leading to a sense of "wholeness" that plays a powerful role in the development of new ontological possibilities, i.e., new ways of being.

Four Dimensions of Guidance

The ever-changing context of the shared space of the classroom is important in shaping guidance. It should go without saying (but is worth saying) that one must consider context, whether teaching in Philadelphia, Israel, or Korea; to children or elders; or to specific clinical populations. As we often say to new teachers honing their skills in guidance, context is everything. Context includes not only the "who" and "where" but also "when." Thus, the use of language (and silence) will be different in guiding a practice during the first class, than when guiding that same practice 6 or 7 weeks later.

Accordingly, it is not practical to establish rules of thumb for guidance. Likewise, it is counterproductive to develop a formulaic script for a guided meditation that would be suitable for every who, where, and when. There are, however, many common considerations worth calling out. McCown, Reibel, and Micozzi (2017), have described four interdependent dimensions that a teacher needs to be familiar with for effective guidance. Let's consider, in order, embodying, orienting, languaging, and allowing.

Embodying

This dimension is the most critical for guidance—the connection of the teacher to her own practice while she is speaking. Without embodying, there can be no connection. Guiding a meditation is not just using words to instruct others. Rather, as implied in the role of a "guide," the teacher is engaged with the practice. She is "dropped in" to her own moment-to-moment experience and speaks from that perspective.

The verbal constructions of guidance are rooted in the teacher's personal understanding of the practice and her moment-to-moment experience of the confluence or shared space. It is very difficult, if not impossible, to effectively use language to catalyze mindfulness without simultaneously embodying the practice. However, the teacher cannot be so deeply "dropped in" to her personal experience that she is unaware of what may be happening for other participants. More concretely, she cannot be practicing with her eyes closed the whole time she is guiding. She may not notice the condition of the other participants—shifts of affect, body movements, even leaving the room. All of this important information shapes guidance. Further, it is worth noting that a change in volume and vocal tone as the teacher drops in is a natural effect of embodying the practice. The teacher needs to monitor this effect, to make sure that she continues to project enough volume to be heard, while also allowing her more relaxed vocal tone to become part of the guidance.

Orienting

In one sense, the orientation of all guided meditations is towards the flow of experience in the present moment. Here, again, Shotter brings insight (2012, p. 13):

> …while some of the communications directed towards us can change us simply in our *knowledge*, others—that influence our *orientations*—can change us in our very ways of *being in the world*, in how we express ourselves as *being* in our *ways* of orienting or relating to the others and other-nesses around us.

This orientation, this way of being in the world, can lead towards an open, accepting awareness of whatever is arising, rather than identifying with particular concepts or thoughts about what is happening. The guidance of a meditation practice can facilitate such shifts in consciousness.

It might appear that using a narrative or an organizing concept when guiding a meditation would not support the practice of moment-to-moment awareness. However, in the early classes, it is helpful for participants to sense coherence and direction as they attempt to follow a practice that is so different from their typical experience in the world. Therefore, the teacher may find or adopt an organizing principle. Some practices have an inherent narrative trajectory, such as the body scan, in which we move our attention and experience sensations in and through the body sequentially. Practices of mindful movement also suggest an orderly progress through sequencing of movements. Even sitting meditations—particularly the "expanding awareness" practice of the MBIs—can have a narrative arc, as participants expand attention from the breath to the body, to sound, thoughts, emotions, and finally to choiceless awareness.

On the other hand, a sitting meditation with awareness of the breath, or the practice of open awareness, may seem amorphous to participants at first. The teacher can, nevertheless offer coherence and direction without resorting to narrative. There are at least three strategies that can help teachers guide such meditations in ways that allow participants freedom to explore.

First, the teacher can introduce a simple refrain, a recurring verbal construction that offers some stability in the flow of experience. For example, in choiceless awareness meditation, the repeated question "what are you aware of in the present moment?" can bring participants to their direct experience.

Second, the teacher can introduce and then elaborate a concept, which may blossom in meaning as the practice progresses. For example, in an awareness of breath meditation, the teacher could introduce the principle of nonjudgment and kindness towards oneself, and guide by elaborating the practice of cultivating a caring and kind response to one's mind wandering. Participants are then prompted in an ongoing way to come back gently to the breath, without struggle or self-blame, when their minds wander. The teacher might even weave an elaboration of a second, supportive concept—for example, that the tendency of the mind to wander is not personal. When the participant is aware that her mind is lost in thought, in that moment of noticing, she is already present.

Third, the teacher may ground the practice by incorporating mention of the moment-to-moment events in the environment into the guidance as it progresses. By calling out a momentary event in the environment without predetermining how participants will experience it, the teacher can support an open, curious awareness in the group. In the context of an urban setting or perhaps a large institution, street level sounds (sirens, trash-trucks, jackhammers) or hallway happenings, or even the undependability of heating and air-conditioning, can be noted and offered to the group. Something like, "perhaps noticing what's happening within you as the sound of the siren continues."

These basic strategies can be combined creatively to improve guidance for any specific practice, for any "who, what, when, and where" of a class.

Languaging

What choice of language, what tone or modulation of voice facilitates the cultivation of mindfulness? It is crucial that teachers consider this dimension. In order to support participants' understanding and practice of mindfulness the language used in guiding needs to be invitational rather than directive. In order to be allowing of whatever participants encounter, guidance needs to be inclusive, i.e., including the different possibilities of experiencing all that arises moment by moment.

An important feature of the MBI style of guidance is language intended to reduce the resistance of participants. There are at least three ways in which a teacher can invite participants to practice, rather than directing them. A discursive analysis of a Kabat-Zinn audio recording of the body scan practice for MBSR by Dreeben, Mamberg, and Salmon (2013), identifies three features of language use that are of interest here. What they call "inclusivity" involves use of the first person plural in guidance, rather than second person, implying that all in the group are participating together. Something like "now, *let's* let the focus of *our* attention…." What they call "process over ownership" involves, among other ways of speaking, using the definitive article, rather than first or second person possessive. That is, "Raising *the* left leg," not "*your* left leg," suggesting that the action is already underway and participants may join in, or not. Bringing us to the third feature, which Dreeben et al., call "Action without agency." This feature involves the inevitability represented by the present participle, combined with constructions that diminish the call for doing. It sounds something like "If you're ready, *just raising* the left leg and *perhaps noticing….*" For participants, the impression might be that these actions are taking place right now in the room, and that they are free to notice and choose to join in—or not.

Context, as we noted earlier, is all important. For instance, there are languages in which there is no present participle. In such cases, the teacher will use appropriate constructions that invite rather than direct or command, that are process oriented rather than goal oriented, and that highlight the cultivation of awareness of whatever is happening rather than giving the impression that anything in particular must happen. Even the choice of a definitive article rather than a possessive pronoun can depend on the context. Early in a course, the participants are less likely to be in touch with their bodies, so for a time using the possessive article "raising *your* left leg…" may actually be beneficial. The participant may come to realize through guided practice that she indeed has a left leg, and, over time, can come to inhabit her body. Rather than thinking of one approach to language as being better than another, it is useful to consider the effect of what is chosen in any given context—perhaps even choosing to go back and forth to find a balance. As Kabat-Zinn (2004) advises, too much use of the present participle can become distracting, while too much distancing through the definitive article may result in a "she's not talking to me" reaction. A possible rule of thumb, then, is "Do not hold to rules too tightly."

Allowing

It is all too easy to see this dimension of allowing as being a specific form of languaging. However, it is most clearly seen as a function of the confluence. On a concrete level, the teacher senses whatever arises in the environment—say, hallway sounds of whispered conversations or noisy groups, or squeaky cart wheels—and uses language to guide participants closer to their experience. As the teacher adds detail and specificity participants may find it easier to maintain a connection to the practice. Yet, such guidance still allows each participant to have their own unique experience. And, of course, the teacher's way of being helps to allow an infinite range of possibilities for participants. Ideally, each feels free to have his or her own experience of the moment.

Teachers are challenged to find balance between incorporating specificity and allowing each participant to have their own experience. This balance can be accomplished by offering a range of choices and by couching suggestions in tentative phrases, such as "perhaps you are noticing warmth or coolness." Guiding a body scan, when asking participants to bring their attention to the forehead, for example, the teacher may say: "noticing any tightness or softness in the muscles … perhaps there's tingling, or pressure, or numbness. You may be noticing the sensation of air moving in the room … or maybe there's no sensation available to feel … and that is okay … that's simply your experience in this moment." Using language in this way offers permission for whatever arises, encouragement for exploration beyond habitual responses, and unconditional acceptance of any outcome.

Another feature of language that can be helpful is the interrogative. In guidance, questions do not direct participants to find answers, but rather to catalyze their attention and curiosity. A question such as "can you feel the floor beneath you?" does not so much pull participants into their head as it orients them closer to the direct experience of contact with the floor. A question such as "what is the quality of the breath in this moment?... perhaps long or short, smooth or jagged?" has as many answers as there are listeners, and can often lead to a deepening of attention. Skillful languaging can help participants sense into their moment-by-moment streams of experience, rather than staying at a conceptual level of what they think is or should be happening. It points towards the "flowing, indeterminate, still developing reality."

Yet another potentially flexible way of considering language use that fosters allowing comes from the work of the sociologist Richard Sennett, who in working across two books, *The Craftsman* (2009) and *Together* (2012), approaches an understanding of the very real practices that humans use to foster cooperation. The approaches he notes are used by craftspersons confronted with resistance of their material, and the analogous practices of diplomats working with difficult relations. These approaches can contribute to the work of guiding meditation:

> Applying minimum force is the most effective way to work with resistance. Just as in working with a wood knot, so in a surgical procedure: the less aggressive the effort, the more sensitivity. Vesalius urged the surgeon, feeling the liver more resistant to the scalpel than surrounding tissues, to "stay his hand," to probe tentatively and delicately before cutting further. In practicing music, when confronted by a sour note or a hand-shift gone wrong, the performer gets nowhere by forcing. The mistake has to be treated as an interesting fact; then, the problem will eventually be unlocked (2012, p. 210).

The concept of minimum force may be used to shape the languaging and allowing dimensions of guidance. In applying minimum force to dialogical or collaborative situations, such as the MBI classroom, there are three distinctive insights that Sennett (2013) offers from diplomatic practice, which deserve serious consideration as rules of thumb. First, one may refrain from insisting on one's own ideas and take on another's view of the situation. From whose position are we guiding? Second, one may deploy the *subjunctive mood* in one's language; the "what if…" and "perhaps…" way of talking that opens possibilities for dialogue—that is, as an unfinished dialogue experienced by the participant. Third, is that technique known as *sprezzatura*, recommended by Baldassare Castiglione, in that sixteenth century Italian diplomat's *Book of the Courtier*. Sprezzatura is a lightness of touch, a nonchalance that makes it difficult for others to find offense in what one says. In the MBI classroom, such lightness, such a sense of humor is a powerful unguent. This is not comedy; it is the generation of a welcoming and informal atmosphere. Lightness of touch, use of minimum force, opening to the boundless possibilities—all are invaluable when confronting what is often difficult in the classroom, such as physical and emotional pain, loss and longing, grief and sorrow. It can be incorporated in guidance, through both the choice of language and the tone and modulation of voice. In the co-created space, as we open to the confluence of whatever is arising from moment-to-moment, we may often find a deep joining together when we can laugh and cry at the same time!

Guidance as a Craft

In *The Craftsman* (2009), Sennett notes that "nearly anyone can become a good craftsman." There is assumption that craft abilities are innate and widely distributed, and that when properly stimulated and trained, they allow craftsmen to become knowledgeable public persons. They know how to negotiate between autonomy and authority (as a teacher must in delivering a workshop); how to work not against resistant forces but with them (as did the engineers who first drilled tunnels beneath the Thames); how to complete their tasks using "minimum force" (as do all chefs who must chop vegetables); how to meet people and things with sympathetic imagination (as does the glassblower whose "corporeal anticipation" lets her stay one step ahead of the molten glass); and above all they know how to play. It is in play that we find "the origin of the dialogue the craftsman conducts with materials like clay and glass." All of these concepts are wonderfully applicable to developing the craft of guiding meditation as well as to the teacher's own development.

Sennett notes how the use of minimum force applies to mastering the tools one has—whether to drive a nail, bow a cello, or begin a meditation session. In applying the idea of minimum force to the teacher's honing of her skill in guiding meditation, she can playfully see mistakes (e.g., misspeaking during a "live" guidance for instance) as simply interesting facts to be explored, rather than something to be overcome. Reducing aggression towards oneself as a teacher not only helps the teacher herself but will profoundly shift the environment in the classroom as well. Thinking of guiding meditation as playing, rather than as work to be accomplished, can bring a sense of non-striving, curiosity, and friendliness into the shared space of confluence.

A craft or a skill is developed over time with practice. The subtleties of hammering or bowing cannot be learned conceptually or theoretically but only through enactment. This reality is equally true of guidance. In guiding a meditation, a teacher is not just imparting information but is catalyzing the pedagogy of mindfulness. Skillfulness is required. A teacher would need to be thoroughly familiar with the various meditations she needs to guide, so she would need to have practiced them intensely herself. She would want to experience the guidance of other skilled teachers, so she would attend classes by others and review others' recordings. She would even create scripts for the practices, and rehearse with them many times— ideally in situations where she may get feedback from peers (other teachers in training) and her own teachers. Eventually, when she is ready to guide "live" in a classroom with participants, she would let go of the script—because now she has the depth of skill required to improvise.

Developing and deepening the skill of guiding happens in the actual doing of it; that is, one gets better at guiding meditations by guiding them. The ecological anthropologist, Ingold (2008), suggests that we do not learn by bringing knowledge from "outside" to "inside" us, but rather that we "grow into" knowledge. As he describes, "the minds of novices are not so much 'filled up' with the stuff of culture, as 'tuned up' to the particular circumstances of the environment" (2008, p. 117). He refers to this status not as learning or education, but as "*enskillment*," and provides the example of a child learning to make an omelette. There is no one right way to crack a given egg because each egg is different. The child learns the feel for it from hands that are skilled being placed on or over hers. What is more, this process happens in a particular kitchen, with particular bowls and pans. The knowledge is in the system, not inside the child. Ingold notes that "you only get an omelette from a cook-in-the-kitchen" (2008, p. 116). Similarly, a meditation teacher goes through this (ongoing) process of enskillment. She senses into it and gets a feel for what is required in any given context, over and over. First, with the help of teachers (in person or through teachings), and then on her own.

Applying Craftsmanship

In this section, we explore the specific practical applications of the four dimensions of guidance by commenting upon a sample script for a selected formal practice. We chose a seated yoga script for three reasons.

First, it offers many opportunities for elaboration of the four dimensions with very concrete examples.

Second, the practice itself has broad application—with populations such as elders (Chap. 10), people with disabilities (Chap. 10), employees in office settings, and in any MBI program where classroom space is cramped—yet is rarely presented as a script from which teachers may learn.

Third, in our experience, MBI teachers in training often feel challenged when guiding yoga, and a detailed treatment may be of use. The challenge sometimes arises because the aspiring teacher has no prior background in yoga, and is hesitant to guide such a seemingly complex practice. In this case, the best route to learning yoga is to practice with and learn from more experienced MBI teachers. This is the most direct way towards a clear understanding of what is required in the classroom. Alternatively, the challenge sometimes arises because the aspiring teacher actually has a background in teaching yoga, but has taught in a different style and for different reasons. In this case, a process of "unlearning" may be necessary. For instance, yoga teachers usually are trained to demonstrate the pose as an ideal and then to walk around the class, evaluating their students, sometimes stopping to make physical adjustments to a student's posture. This can imply a goal to strive for, and can instill a sense of self-judgment. To the contrary, in the MBIs, the teacher practices along with the participants, guiding from her own embodied experience of the practice and the sense of the confluence.

What Kabat-Zinn has written about the yoga practice in MBSR is true for both teachers and participants (2003):

> Mindful yoga is a lifetime engagement — not to get somewhere else, but to be where and as we are in this very moment, with this very breath, whether the experience is pleasant, unpleasant, or neutral. Our body will change a lot as we practice, and so will our minds and our hearts and our views. Hopefully, whether a beginner or an old-timer, we are always reminding ourselves in our practice of the value of keeping this beginner's mind.

The intention of mindful yoga practice, then, is to cultivate awareness, rather than to "perform" yoga postures.

There are statements or ideas specific to movement practices that are worth discussing before the script for the practice proper begins. Participants should be reminded to pay attention to the experience of their bodies, to honor any limitations encountered in the moment, and to rely on their body's natural wisdom when it is sensible to adapt the teacher's instructions. They should also be aware that, if they need to refrain from any postures, they can still choose to vividly imagine the body making the movements — not to fill time, but rather as a highly effective alternative physical practice. They may be assured that studies suggest that imagining physical movements can improve motor performance (e.g., Gentili, Han, Schweighofer, & Papaxanthis, 2010).

It is also worth considering the content of the practice. In the MBIs, movement practices are offered as an unfolding exploration of the body. A limited number of yoga poses are taught, so that participants will develop familiarity and ease, and because they are chosen to be accessible to those with physically limiting medical conditions.

The sequence of poses in mindful yoga offers a natural narrative or orientation, which becomes more evident with repetition. It is important for the teacher to decide in advance how she will sequence the movements. (However, sometimes the confluence of the shared space may require her to be flexible.) Will she start at the feet and move upwards? Or start at the region of the face and neck and move downwards? It is not so much that there is a right or wrong way to sequence, but rather that the sequence of poses will influence how participants experience sensations in the body.

When sequencing postures that stretch one side of the body at a time, it is important to work symmetrically — for instance, stretching to the right with the arms raised, and next stretching in the same way to the left.

Poses may be chosen and sequenced for optimum participant engagement, with attention to orienting to the present moment, orienting to gravity, sequencing of poses (to include both sides of the body), duration of poses, and duration of rest between poses — including a final rest pose. For a developing teacher, it may be instructive to read the script and track the flow of postures from the top to the bottom of the body. In fact, it may be of value to do the practice, as sequencing is a subtle skill that may be more accessible to embodied understanding.

The following script for seated yoga offers guidance through words only in the left-hand column, while in the right-hand column we offer comments to clarify and to expand into the deeper dimensions of embodying, orienting, languaging, and allowing.

A Script for Seated Yoga Practice

We are going to be practicing mindful yoga in our chairs. As in other mindfulness practices, with mindful yoga we are cultivating awareness, specifically bringing a curious, kind attention to sensations in the body, moment to moment, as we move into and out of poses	**Languaging: It is helpful for the teacher to start with an introduction, orienting participants to present moment experience, while creating a sense of safety by letting participants know what it is they are going to be doing**
There are no ideal movements we are trying to perform, no right or wrong way to do this. We are not trying to get anywhere. Rather, we are learning to be exactly where and how we are right now	
While the center of our attention is on sensations in the body, there is nothing you have to exclude or push away; you can make space for whatever arises in your awareness	
Starting by sitting upright in the chair and placing both feet on the floor if you are able to. First, simply notice how it feels in the body, as much as possible letting go of judgment and just observing. Feeling the contact of the body with the chair, the feet with the floor. Allowing the chair and floor to support your weight, feeling gravity holding you here	**Orienting: using gravity to ground participants in their chairs**
Being curious about the sensations where the body is making contact, maybe noticing pressure, hardness or softness … bringing attention to the soles of the feet, thighs, and buttocks … If you care to, inviting muscles to soften a bit … noticing that they may soften, or not … simply noticing—as much as possible without expectation or judgment…	**Allowing: any experience is acceptable, and change may be noticed—or not**
From this stable base of the body, feeling the torso lengthening up without any straining or striving … Allowing the spine to find its natural extension, all the way from the tailbone to the base of the skull … Inviting the shoulders to drop as you let the hands rest on your thighs or wherever you find it comfortable	**Orienting: naming specific body parts (*the tailbone to the base of the skull*)** **Allowing: offering alternatives (*or wherever you find it comfortable*)**
How much effort is required to maintain this seated mountain pose?	**Languaging: a question that brings attention into the body**
Perhaps inviting jaw to drop a bit … the shoulders to fall away from the ears … and the belly to soften …. We're inviting the body to move towards rest without demanding that anything has to change. Letting the breath flow freely … and feeling into the sensations of breathing	**Orienting: the sequence of movement is downward through the body**

(continued)

(continued)

Now, on your next out-breath, bringing the chin down *towards* the chest … making this movement as the shoulders are dropped down … breathing and feeling the stretch	**Languaging:** *towards* **reinforces the idea that there is no right way, no goal**
Remember that you can adapt any instructions that I give, and come out of a pose whenever you need to without having to wait for me to say so (Pause)	**Allowing: encouraging participants to give themselves permission to be as they are and to make their own choices; giving plenty of time for exploration**
	Embodying: the teacher's ability to sense into her own body as well as to be aware of what is happening in the shared space will influence the length of the pause in each pose
When you are ready, slowly bringing the head back up as if you were placing each cervical vertebra on top on the one below, and letting the head rest on top … Maybe feeling into the entire body here … how is it with you now? (Pause)	**Languaging: preferring observation over action, encouraging sensing in the body**
Slowly moving the chin up slightly upwards towards the ceiling … perhaps feeling the stretch in the front of the neck and along the jaw as you breathe … (Pause)	**Languaging:** *towards* **and** *perhaps* **offer freedom**
	Allowing: giving participants time for experience
And when it's right for you, slowly bringing the chin down so that the head is once again centered … feeling any sensations, maybe in the region of the neck and the face … (Pause)	
If at any time you notice that the mind has wandered, remembering that mind wandering is not a problem—that's just what the mind does! Each time you notice that you've wandered is a moment of mindfulness … so you can simply acknowledge it and come back—maybe even with a smile—to feeling sensations in the body…	**Allowing: encouraging the use of "minimum force"; the teacher's humor and kindness reinforces this principle**
When you are ready, breathing in … and as you breathe out, bringing the right ear towards the right shoulder, inviting both shoulders to stay relaxed … Breathing and feeling sensations in the body … then, slowly bringing the head back up to center … pausing here for a few breaths (Pause)	**Orienting: having just moved the neck forward and back, now exploring movement from side to side**
Breathing in … and as you breathe out, bringing the left ear *towards* the left shoulder … Are the shoulders are trying to get involved? Can they drop back down? Just breathing here … noticing sensations … Remember, there is no need to force or strain in any way … if you find that straining is happening, is it possible to find some ease? (Pause)	**Embodying: through self-awareness and awareness of the group, holding poses for a suitable amount of time—not too long, but long enough for participants to feel sensations and allow a stretching of the muscles**
Bringing the head back up … and just noticing how it feels throughout the body, as you sit here in seated mountain pose … (Pause)	**Allowing: whatever is happening may be experienced in the pause**

(continued)

When you choose, taking a breath in … and as you breathe out, turning your head to look over the right shoulder … inviting neck and shoulders to stay as relaxed as possible … There is nowhere to be but here and nothing to do but this … Just breathing and feeling sensations in the body … (Pause)	**Orienting: having bent the cervical spine side to side, now exploring a twist in this same region** **Allowing: reminding participants that there is no goal to reach, no way of being that is preferred**
Now, when you breathe in, slowly bringing the head back to center … Pausing here to notice what you notice … Perhaps there's impatience or a sense of "I know what we're doing next" … Maybe you can see if it's possible to just be here, now … (Pause)	**Languaging: using the subjunctive mode:** *perhaps, maybe, see if it's possible*
When you're ready, breathing in … and as you exhale, turning your head to look over your left shoulder … Softening into the pose… breathing and feeling sensations … (Pause for roughly the same length of time as before)	**Languaging:** *when you're ready* **suggests that the group is engaging again, and that individuals nevertheless have choices**
Now, slowly bringing the head back to center, staying with those sensations … breathing in through the nose, opening the mouth, and letting the air out with a gentle sigh … Sensing the entire body … what's here for you now? (Pause)	
Whenever you notice that the mind has been lost in the virtual world of thinking, you are no longer lost … That noticing means you're already present … so you can simply continue bringing your attention to sensations in the body…	**Orienting: reminding participants again to bring a quality of nonjudgment and a light touch**
Bringing attention to the shoulders, now. Moving the shoulders forward … up … back … and down … and continuing to move the shoulders in this circular fashion, without any straining … The movement can be as big or as little as feels right for you … and you can move at your own pace…	**Orienting: moving from the neck to the region of the shoulders; calling out that the movement is circular; making sure to engage both sides** **Allowing:** *as feels right for you, at your own pace*
Really feeling into the shoulder joints as you make this movement … If you care to, using the out-breath to help relieve any strain … And, now, reversing the direction of the movement, and noticing sensations as you move in this new direction … (Pause)	**Orienting:** *giving time for participants to move and feel the sensations of movement*
Coming back into stillness … and just resting now in the seated mountain pose, rooted and uplifted … shoulders dropped, arms just resting by the side of the body, hands on the thighs or lap…	**Embodying: sensing the time needed in between poses to rest and feel sensations**

(continued)

(continued)

When it seems right, without any straining, allowing the spine to be elongated .... Bringing attention to the torso ... aware of the back and front of the body ... aware of the sides of the body ...	**Orienting: having brought attention and movement to neck and shoulders, now bringing attention and movement to spine and torso, including arms**
Now, becoming aware of the arms, and, as you inhale slowly, lifting them out to the sides and bringing them upwards ... noticing sensations moment by moment—perhaps the resistance of gravity as the arms move ... Maybe they come all the way up alongside the ears, maybe they don't ... so just adapting in any way you need to ...	**Note: if there isn't room between participants, having them bring the arms forward and up** **Allowing: use of subjunctive mood, so that this is exploration, not striving**
If the arms are up by the ears, turning the palms so that they face each other ... however they are, inviting the shoulders to relax ... and stretching through the fingertips. Is it possible to feel the stretch all the way from the hips to the fingertips? What are you noticing about how you are? Seeing if there may be a sense of ease even as you stretch in this pose, tuning in to the sensations in the body .... Perhaps the muscles of the face, neck, and shoulders soften as the breath flows ... or perhaps not ... Just knowing what you are feeling in the body (Pause)	**Orienting: reminding participants to let the breath flow; this is important because holding the breath seems to be a default mode, particularly for beginners** **Allowing: in the subjunctive mood; keeping it light and gentle**
With your next exhalation, slowly bringing the arms back down ... paying attention to sensations as you negotiate with gravity ... (Pause)	**Orienting: the returning motions of a pose are as important as the movements to assume it; there is much to be explored in moments that are often discounted**
Feeling the body as you sit here in mountain pose ... During mindful yoga, we are letting the sensations in the body be at the center of the attention ... but there is nothing to push away ... sensations, thoughts, and emotions come and go ... we are simply noticing and making room for it all ... (Pause)	**Allowing: reminder that whatever is in present moment experience is allowed** **Embodying: the pause here is regulated by self-awareness and sense of the confluence**

(continued)

(continued)

Now, as you inhale, bringing the right arm up, if possible, alongside the ear, and turning the palm to face the left … dropping the shoulders as you breathe out … and on another in-breath stretching upwards … and on your out-breath gently bending to the left … can you soften where you don't need tension right now? Maybe checking the muscles of the face, neck, and shoulders … and just breathing and feeling this stretch… If you notice that you're pushing, see if it's possible to ease off a bit … (Pause)	**Note: this next movement could be done with both arms up, moving once towards the right and then towards the left, or using one arm up at a time; context can help determine which to use**
Now, as you inhale, slowly coming back to center, feeling the motions of the body … and on your next out-breath bringing the right arm back down, and tracking those sensations … (Pause)	**Orienting: attending to both directions of the pose; it's all worthy of notice**
Resting here in seated mountain pose …. Noticing whatever sensations are here in the body. Perhaps there is tingling, pulsing, throbbing, or some other sensation … (Pause)	**Languaging: offering possible sensations**
Now, when you are ready, taking a breath in and lifting the left arm up, and turning the palm to face towards the right … on the out-breath, perhaps the shoulders can drop down … and on the in-breath, stretching through the left fingertips … and on the out-breath, gently bending towards the right … feeling the left side of the torso lengthening … Can you feel the sensations of stretching on the left, as well as sensations on the right side of the body? Perhaps you can find areas that don't need to be working, and allow them to soften … (Pause)	**Orienting: symmetrical movements**
As you inhale, slowly sensing your way back to center … and as you exhale, being in touch as the left arm comes back down…	**Embodying: pauses are always regulated by self-awareness and sense of the confluence**
Pausing here and simply noticing sensations, including sensations of the breath moving the body … (Pause)	

(continued)

(continued)

We are going to move now into some gentle twists … So, bringing your right hand behind you—you can choose to place it on arm of the chair, or on the seat behind you, or just grab hold of the side of the chair or wherever it feels right for you … Paying attention to the right shoulder … can it stay dropped down?	**Orienting: having practiced lateral bends, moving now into twisting movement of the spine**
Now, bringing the left hand to the outside of the right knee or thigh … still facing forward—you can look at my version of this pose, if the instructions seem confusing … as you inhale, lengthen through the spine … and as you exhale, slowly start to twist the torso towards the right, beginning from the base of the spine … just breathing and twisting … continuing to feel the twist move up the spine, perhaps even turning your head to look over your right shoulder … (Pause)	**Embodying: *you can look at my version of this pose*—the teacher is not an ideal model, but a helpful reference point**
How is it with you now? What is it like in the region of the face, neck, and shoulders? Is there tightness or softness? There's no way it should be, but it is interesting to know…

On your next out-breath slowly bringing your head back to center, feeling how it is to unwind the body … and when you're unwound, just sitting and breathing … knowing how it is … (Pause) | **Orienting: attending to the entire movement of the pose; sensing what it is to come out of the stretch, to come to center, and only then taking the pause** |
| Now, let's do the other side …. bringing the left hand behind you and placing it wherever it feels right for you in this moment … Keeping that left shoulder dropped down and placing the right hand to the outside of the left knee or thigh, still facing forward—just look at me for the basic idea … Now, without rushing or forcing anything, breathing out slowly, and starting to twist the towards the left … starting at the base of the spine … and on each in-breath pausing to lengthen the spine, while on each out-breath, continuing to feel the twist move up the spine … perhaps even turning the head to look over the left shoulder … (Pause) | **Orienting: using the pose symmetrically**

Embodying: using the teacher as a guide not an ideal |
| Breathing here as you feel the sensations of twisting … What happens if you are able to soften and relax a bit more into the pose? (Pause) | **Languaging: the subjunctive mood, in a question, to encourage exploration without judgment** |
| On your next out-breath, slowly bringing your head back to center, unwinding through the body and just feeling the sensations … when you come to center, noticing how it is as you sit here and breathe … (Pause) | **Embodying: pauses are always regulated by self-awareness and sense of the confluence; perhaps here participants may be ready for a longer pause** |

(continued)

(continued)

Now bringing your attention to the hips and pelvis...feeling the buttocks and how they make contact with the chair...sensing into the legs and feet....As much as possible, letting go of judgment, and simply bringing a curious, kind attention to sensations...	**Orienting: bringing attention and movement to the region of the hips, pelvis, buttocks**
Perhaps lifting the toes and wiggling them around a bit...and as you place the toes back on the floor feeling the sensation of contact that the feet make with the floor...Pressing into the balls of the feet, and letting the heels come off the floor...and then bringing the heels down and letting the front of the foot come off the floor...and returning the feet firmly to the floor....Now, if it feels right, raising your right leg up, extending the leg as much as is comfortable...flexing the foot, stretching through the ball of the foot, while keeping the toes relaxed...And moving back and forth—flexing and pointing the foot and feeling into the sensations here, perhaps in the ankle joint. You may notice the muscles in the back of the leg more as you reach through the heel and the front of the leg more as you reach through the ball of the foot...(Pause)	**Orienting: bringing attention and movement from the feet upwards through the legs** **Embodying: calling out specific possibilities, based on the teacher's experience in the moment**
Now rotating the foot in one direction...	
...and then the other...staying with the sensations of the foot, ankle, and leg...Coming to quiet, and then bringing the sole of the foot back to the floor...(Pause)	
Sensing the body as a whole sitting here. What sensations are you aware of right now?	**Orienting: ensuring symmetry**
[Repeating this set of instructions for the left foot...]	
Now, coming back to seated mountain pose....If you care to, taking the right foot off the floor and placing it across the left thigh just above the knee, flexing the right foot and gently encouraging the right knee to move downwards. Breathing and feeling sensations...	**Embodying: a teacher who is sensitive to the shared space will see if participants are struggling, or if someone is not doing a movement, and can then include such possibilities in the guidance**
Remember, you can adapt any instructions that are given, and if you are refraining from a movement you can imagine the body making the movement...	
[Repeat on other side]	**Orienting: symmetry**

(continued)

(continued)

Coming back to a seated mountain pose, feeling the body as a whole. Taking a breath in and as you exhale, shifting the weight forward, bringing the chest forward towards the thighs, keeping the spine long as we bend forward. Coming only as far forward as is comfortable for you. If you need to, you can rest your forearms on your legs or let them hang alongside the legs … if it is comfortable, allowing the head to move towards the floor, following gravity… Breathing here … perhaps feeling the breath in the back of the body … (Pause) As you're ready, slowly rolling back up, noticing how that movement feels, moment by moment … (Pause)	**Orienting: concluding the sequence of movements with a forward bend** **Allowing: offering alternatives**
Coming back, now, into the seated mountain pose … rooted and uplifted … and inviting the body to be as relaxed as possible in this pose. Just resting now, and feeling sensations throughout the entire body … (Pause)	**Orienting: returning to the starting posture** **Allowing: opening to sensations without judgment** **Embodying: pauses are always regulated by self-awareness and sense of the confluence; each class will need its own time before moving on after a practice is done**

Conclusion

Throughout this chapter, we have tried to make clear the full investment of the teacher that is required in the skill set of guidance. The necessary and thorough discussion of language use, together with the presentation of a complete script may seem to locate the guidance skillset in a cognitive realm of definitions, connotations, phraseology, and other analyzable and potentially controllable features. However, we have strongly suggested that other realms of skill, of perhaps even greater complexity and less open to direct control, are just as important in catalyzing and cultivating mindfulness in the group. It is mindfulness, co-created, that offers the depth, safety, and power of a shared space in which participants and teacher alike may be transformed—endowed with new potentials.

Languaging certainly does matter. There are concepts, techniques, and even words and phrases which a teacher can use skillfully to help cultivate mindfulness. The other three dimensions are far less transparent. Orienting, embodying, and allowing involve the full being of the teacher. Even the best descriptions of all of them together will certainly fail to describe the qualities of an effective teacher guiding mindfulness practice. Yet, before we close, it may be useful to sketch out the possibilities of each.

Orienting has its evident techniques—for example, a narrative arc, or a refrain, as we've noted—but its roots lie in a deeper place. We suggest that the skill of orienting is ultimately affective—it comes from *caring*. Through guidance, the teacher offers each practice in a way that balances the gentleness and comfort of being led along a trail that the guide knows well against the insights and possibilities that arise in moments of being lost and vulnerable. Such balance and such caring require courage—and a total commitment to learning every inch of the territory to be traversed.

Embodying is the skill that most exposes the teacher. As the concept of confluence suggests, each participant—with the teacher the most visible—is continually responding to whatever is happening in the room in the moment. Therefore, the teacher is also the most likely source of others' responses, particularly in the early classes. There is no way out, nowhere to hide, and no time for the teacher to perfect herself. Mindfulness is a co-creation by definition, not by choice. This feature is challenging and yet possibly transformative. For example, as a class "drops in" to a formal mindfulness practice, physiological changes take place. The teacher's expression and posture may shift to reflect greater relaxation, while her vocal qualities of tone and volume may do likewise. Guidance offered in such an embodied situation (when the teacher can maintain volume!) may catalyze and transform the shared practice of the group.

Allowing is a culmination of the guidance skills. Languaging, as it affects the cognitive realm, can make the practice more psychologically available to participants. Orienting draws participants in, through navigation with a caring affect. And embodiment catalyzes the key move of the pedagogy, the capacity for participants and teacher to be with and in their experiences of the moment. That, of course, is the allowing of which we speak. There is no technique to master. There is only the practice to enter. And—this cannot be said often enough—the practice teaches the teacher and participants alike.

References

Dreeben, S. J., Mamberg, M. H., & Salmon, P. (2013). The MBSR Body Scan in Clinical Practice. *Mindfulness, 4*(4), 394–401.

Gentili, R., Han, C. E., Schweighofer, N., & Papaxanthis, C. (2010). Motor learning without doing: Trial-by-trial improvement in motor performance during mental training. *Journal of Neurophysiology, 104*(2), 774–783.

Gergen, K. (2009). *Relational being: Beyond self and community*. Oxford, England: Oxford University Press.

Ingold, T. (2008). The social child. In A. Fogel, B. J. King, & S. G. Shanker (Eds.), *Human development in the twenty-first century: Visionary ideas from systems scientists* (pp. 112–118). Cambridge, England: Cambridge University Press.

Kabat-Zinn, J. (1990). *Full catastrophe living*. New York, NY: Delacorte.

Kabat-Zinn, J. (2003). *Mindful yoga movement & mediation*. Honesdale, PA: Yoga International.

Kabat-Zinn, J. (2004). The uses of language and images in guiding meditation practices in MBSR. In *Audio Recording from 2nd Annual Conference sponsored by the Center for Mindfulness in Medicine, Health Care and Society at the University of Massachusetts Medical School, March 26.*

Kabat-Zinn, J. (2010). Foreword. In D. McCown, D. Reibel, & M. Micozzi (Eds.), *Teaching mindfulness: A practical guide for clinicians and educators* (pp. ix–xxii). New York: Springer.

McCown, D. (2013). *The ethical space of mindfulness in clinical practice.* London, England: Jessica Kingsley.

McCown, D. (2015). Being is relational: Considerations for using mindfulness in clinician-patient settings. In E. Shonin, W. VanGordon, & M. Griffiths (Eds.), *Mindfulness and Buddhist-derived approaches in mental health and addiction.* New York, NY: Springer.

McCown, D., Reibel, D., & Micozzi, M. (2017). *Teaching mindfulness: A practical guide for clinicians and educators.* New York, NY: Springer.

Sennett, R. (2009). *The craftsman.* New Haven, CT: Yale.

Sennett, R. (2013). *Together: The rituals, pleasures and politics of cooperation.* New Haven, CT: Yale.

Shapiro, S., Carlson, L., Astin, J., & Freedman, B. (2006). Mechanisms of mindfulness. *Journal of Clinical Psychology, 62*(3), 373–386.

Shotter, J. (2011). *Getting it: Witness-thinking and the dialogical… in practice.* New York, NY: Hampton Press.

Shotter, J. (2012). Keynote: The transmission of information: An "awful deformation" of what communication really is. *Proceedings of the New York State Communication Association, 2012,* 1–21.

Chapter 3
Remembrance: Dialogue and Inquiry in the MBSR Classroom

Saki F. Santorelli

The Essential Ground of Dialogue and Inquiry

We have a treasure within us. We were born with it. Reclaiming it costs us a lot. Some would say, *everything.* "Everything" has everything to do with leaving behind much of the small, comfortable self all of us have constructed and that, often enough, now functions as our jailer.

We don't have to obliterate or get rid of this self. We just have to discover that there is infinitely more space surrounding what we call "self" than we've ever imagined or been taught to feel and recognize. As we learn to trust and lean into this spaciousness, we come into direct contact with our *bigness,* our vastness. Anytime we feel into how big we actually are—even in what may seem to be the tiniest of moments and the smallest of ways—we transcend our limiting views, ideas, and opinions about who and what we are and, therefore, are capable of. This is called liberation. And liberation is always transformative.

Much of the time, it seems like we have forgotten what we have been endowed with. We walk around as if we are poor while closer to us than our breath is a treasury. This forgetting, and the suffering it generates within us is often the motivation necessary for waking up. Sometimes people touch this remembrance when they are dying. Other times, in wakeful moments across our lifetime, we do have glimpses of our richness. These moments make us happy. This treasure is called by many

---

If I am not in the world simply to adapt to it, but rather transform it, and if it is not possible to change the world without a certain dream or vision for it, I must make use of every possibility there is not only to speak about my utopia, but also to engage in practices consistent with it (Freire, 2004).

S.F. Santorelli, Ed.D., M.A. (✉)
Center for Mindfulness in Medicine, Health Care, and Society, University of Massachusetts Medical School, 222 Maple Avenue, Shrewsbury, MA 01545, USA
e-mail: saki.santorelli@umassmed.edu

© Springer International Publishing Switzerland 2016
D. McCown et al., *Resources for Teaching Mindfulness,*
DOI 10.1007/978-3-319-30100-6_3

47

names. For the purpose of this chapter and within the context of this book about mindfulness-based stress reduction (MBSR), let's call it awareness.

Within the MBSR classroom, the sole purpose of the lively process that has been termed "dialogue and inquiry" is to assist participants in their direct, unmitigated remembrance of this treasure that they actually *are*.

The Real "Work" of an MBSR Teacher

The "how" of assisting people to remember this treasure emerges out of what the MBSR teacher has lived and therefore knows. In a very tangible way, the teacher is the *instrument* through which the entire MBSR program unfolds and, coextensively, the process of dialogue and inquiry. This requires the teacher to be actively and persistently engaged in a range of developmental processes aimed at refining her or his *instrument*. These include psychotherapy or other means of developing a detailed understanding of and a coming to terms with one's personal history, trauma, relational patterns, etc., an ongoing commitment to personal growth and self-development, a regular and sustained personal meditation practice, years of teaching MBSR accompanied by ongoing MBSR teacher mentoring with senior teachers and peers, a direct relationship with a meditation teacher (whenever possible) and consistent silent retreat training all focused on a sustained commitment to investigating the central questions of who and what am I.

The commitment to such deliberate inquiry is a lifetime's work. Treading this path inevitably leads to vulnerability, dissolution, eventual openness, a sense of spaciousness and integration while unavoidably leading to new cycles of dissolution, discovery, and integration. The path is full of surprises and insights that are humbling, deeply revealing and simultaneously healing. While it is not particularly comfortable at times, it is compelling—at least for some. Many discoveries emerge from such a disciplined, nonaggressive, and long-term education and training process. Among them are a clear recognition that (1) the heart/mind can be deliberately trained; (2) the "one" who likes, prefers, dislikes. etc. is amalgamated out of many co-dependent causes and conditions rather than being fixed, "true," and insurmountably solid; (3) the view of who and what I *think* I am is, at best, highly suspect and largely impoverished; (4) the seemingly solid boundary between "self" and "other" is fuzzy and, for the most part, culturally constructed; and, (5) human beings, all of us, are constituted of, have access to, and are capable of inhabiting a spectrum of consciousness ranging from the ordinary to the sublime.

The lively process of dialogue and inquiry that I have called "remembrance" is a straightforward means of knowing directly this "spectrum" and therefore, by extension, supporting participants' experiential discovery of their innate human capacities. As an MBSR teacher becomes more comfortable and at ease living into these insights, what she discovers about herself plays heavily in the dialogue with program participants. This is demanding and delightful simultaneously.

Generally speaking, MBSR is taught within non-sectarian settings. Nevertheless, I find it nothing less than *sacred* because MBSR is an uncompromisingly deep honoring of the nobility and wholeness of a human being. Each MBSR program participant is a unique package with a unique history and "story." Therefore, each participant must be recognized and respected as an individual by the MBSR teacher when attempting to explore with them conditioned habits and patterns accrued across a lifetime and the ways these patterns may be inhibiting their choices and sense of freedom. This is hard work for everyone in the classroom. This is one of the reasons why, in the middle of the MBSR course, participants often say, "Wait a minute. This isn't about stress reduction; this is about my life."

And let's face it, such a reckoning is not the sole domain of the "student" or "participant." It is equally true for the MBSR teacher. All human beings, no matter our role, suffer. We all feel anguish, bear suffering, and are capable of transcending our conditioned proclivities and becoming more open, aware, and at ease. The work of the MBSR teacher is to learn the "how" of leaning into and lingering with the full range of experiences arising out of his humanness and, in parallel, our common humanity. Ultimately, MBSR is a non-dual educational approach that is therapeutic in nature. Here's the British psychiatrist, D.H. Winnicott, commenting on the non-dual nature of the therapeutic relationship:

> A sign of health in the mind is the ability of one individual to enter imaginatively and accurately into the thoughts and feelings, hopes and fears of another person; also to allow the other person to do the same to us… When we are face to face with a man, woman or child in our speciality, we are reduced to two human beings of equal status (Phillips, 1988).

Therefore, the MBSR teacher's capacity for appreciating and cultivating mutually ennobling relationships with participants, for sympathetic resonance, gratitude, warmth, clarity, and flexibility in making moment-by-moment choices in response to class participants' experiences requires them to be firmly committed to a keen and persistent observation of their own experience. And, in turn, to an understanding of the particular temperament, characteristics, tendencies, and life circumstances of program participants when engaging with them in dialogue and inquiry. I'll explore this in greater depth later on in this chapter.

For now, I'll say this much: awareness is the central axis around which the entire process of dialogue and inquiry turns.

Awareness

Awareness is knowing itself: a mirror-like receiving and recognition of whatever passes before the metaphorical glass without preference, evaluation, or the desire to grasp and retain the image encountering this innate reflectivity. Sobering and highly attractive, whether we know it or not, we have all experienced moments of direct, nonconceptual, non-dual awareness. The words of the Indian sage, Nisargadatta Maharaj, capture in lucid detail what he calls "the great work of awareness":

> By being with yourself, by watching yourself in your daily life with alert interest, with the intention to understand rather than to judge, in full acceptance of whatever may emerge, because it is there [here], you encourage the deep to come to the surface and enrich your life and consciousness with its captive energies. This is the great work of awareness; it

removes obstacles and releases energies by understanding the nature of life and mind. Intelligence is the door to freedom and alert attention is the mother of intelligence (Nisargadatta, 1998). [parenthesis mine]

Thankfully, awareness need not be developed. It is complete with no center and no periphery (Kabat-Zinn, 2005). However, our *familiarity* with awareness, in all its dimensionality and unimpeded vastness, can be cultivated. We can remember. We can reclaim our treasure. Mindfulness is one pathway for cultivating this remembrance, this "removing of obstacles and release of energies." This process of cultivation—a fitting agricultural term suggesting the direct, deeply experiential nature of the labor required—is why mindfulness is referred to as a "practice."

MBSR is simply a contemporary expression of a twenty-six hundred-year-old meditation tradition that has at its heart the cultivation of a human being's familiarity with the one awareness that already *is*.

The "Holding Environment" of the MBSR Classroom

Change is constant. Often enough it is downright painful because change alters our way of being and living in the world. And, since change is inevitable and further heightened during specific times in our lives, we all need support for moving from one way of being to another. D.H. Winnicott coined the term "holding environment" as a way to describe an optimal setting for negotiating the inevitability of change (Phillips, 1988; Winnicott, 1964).

In his landmark book, *The Evolving Self*, Robert Kegan explicated and expanded Winnicott's work on the holding environment as a useful way of looking at the whole of human development and therapeutic relationships (Kegan, 1982). Using Winnicott's basic matrix, Kegan posits this holding environment as having three primary characteristics. He suggests that a healthy holding environment *confirms, contradicts,* and offers *continuity* to people as they move along an evolutionary developmental continuum. MBSR was not developed out of either Winnicott's or Kegan's theoretical models. Yet my long-standing clinical and educational work as an MBSR teacher and teacher–trainer suggests to me that these characteristics provide a useful framework for looking at the environment of the MBSR classroom, the primary "work" of the teacher, and the central role of dialogue and inquiry in MBSR.

For Kegan, the holding environment provides two primary functions: supporting individuals in their current developmental stage, and fostering movement to the next stage. He likens the holding environment to an "evolutionary bridge" to the next developmental stage and delineates three processes at play, suggesting that (1) *confirmation* is about "holding on"; (2) *contradiction* is about "letting go"; and (3) *continuity* is about "staying put for reintegration" (Kegan, 1982). Similarly, Phillips suggests that in an effective holding environment people feel *validated* (confirmed/"holding on"), *encouraged* (contradiction/"letting go"), and *supported* (continuity/"staying put") (Phillips, 1988).

I have conceptualized and attempted to place these three processes within the lived context of the MBSR classroom while hopefully retaining the spirit and explanatory nuances of Winnicott, Kegan, and Phillips.

Confirming

The welcoming encounter with a human being, in this case an MBSR participant, however they are at this moment in their life, does validate and offer a safe, trustworthy haven to "hold on" as they begin their journey. The capacity for an MBSR teacher to recognize and actively engage with the innate genius of 25 or 30 participants with a wide range of symptoms and conditions requires an open and warm, curious, and persistently friendly approach. Of course, this begs the question: how can the MBSR teacher stand in relationship to another human being in this way if she is not cultivating the same kind of investigative friendliness, honesty, kindness, and clarity towards herself? In a very real way, within the context of MBSR, this embracing of self and other is the bedrock of a safe and secure learning environment.

Contradiction

As we now know, Kegan's formulation of "contradiction" suggests a developmental process of "letting go." Over and over again, my experience corroborates that contradiction in the right dose and timing creates just enough friction or disequilibrium to fuel learning and growth. Of course, growth always involves a "letting go" of something that may have served us well at some time in our lives and may now be exerting a counter-evolutionary influence on our development. Thus, the skillful introduction of contradiction by the MBSR teacher in the form of questions like — *Is that really so? Are you sure? Is the pain really killing you? Are you saying that all your thoughts are true and therefore believable?*—aid in the interrupting of long-held patterns and views about self, others, and the world that when investigated honestly and openly may catalyze development and greater freedom.

For an MBSR teacher, these are the very questions one would be inquiring into *within oneself* in both the "laboratory" of formal meditation practice and in the midst of everyday life. *What am I noticing in my body at this moment? Is this pain killing me? Is this an accurate thought? What is this feeling of wanting that's gripping me? What am I really craving? Am I capable of refraining from this conditioned impulse? What might happen if I do? Who is the "I" that wants to know?* It is this closely personal and simultaneously impersonal work of the MBSR teacher that is the seedbed from which dialogue and inquiry emerge in the classroom.

Continuity

Likewise, creating a learning environment and process that offers "continuity" is critical. In MBSR, this continuity or "staying put" function may have more to do with *not forcing any kind of movement.* MBSR teachers are not trying to change anyone. We are not shaping people's experience to match a curriculum matrix. We are not "pulling" for emotion or revelation or result. Rather, we are trusting in the nobility and inborn genius of human beings and creating a learning environment in which this nobility and genius might emerge and be known *by them*.

In this way, an MBSR participant learns to become her own "holding environment." The MBSR teacher embodies these "holding" qualities, and the daily engagement in mindfulness *practice* provides participants a practical foundation for a substantive and continuous deepening of clarity, warmth, understanding, and equanimity that can be put to good use in their everyday life far beyond the completion of an 8-week MBSR course.

The dialogue and inquiry that go on between teacher and participants are intended to support all three aspects of the ongoing developmental process of confirming/validating, contradicting/encouraging, and providing continuity/supporting. Likewise, the possible questions we, as MBSR teachers, might ask our program participants are endless. In a very real and absolutely alive manner, the questions arising in a moment of exchange and inquiry will not be found in a book. They are awaiting discovery within the MBSR teacher. The American novelist, Herman Melville, points to this reality with great brevity and directness (Melville, 1922):

> It wasn't down on any map; true places never are.
> —Herman Melville

In the spirit of Melville, our work as MBSR teachers is to discover these questions and explore their landscapes within ourselves. This is our "true place." Committing ourselves to just such an odyssey will develop a firm inner foundation for our work in the classroom. In turn, out of such a foundational commitment and intra-empirical discovery, studying the variety and use of questions that may be used in the highly therapeutic, educational context of the MBSR classroom can be salutary and tremendously helpful to the MBSR teacher.

The Value of Questions

The Socratic Method

As we are beginning to see, the use of questions plays heavily in the dialogue and inquiry process in MBSR. As an educator and MBSR teacher, I have studied with keen and enduring interest the uses, types, and values of questions in the learning process within and outside of the MBSR classroom. While our western world has a deep tradition of question asking, most notably through the lineage of Socrates, the vector of modern educational practice has too often fostered learning environments in which answers take precedence over questions. Yet, in very real terms, isn't it the unanswered questions that activate and animate our intention to learn? It seems to me that what makes learning compelling are questions about what I don't know and want to know or never thought about before. It is within this "not knowing" that my curiosity and thirst for understanding unfurl, gaining depth and breadth and detail through the exploration of the unexamined and unanswered. In parallel, aren't the real and yet unresolved problems we are facing in our everyday lives the kindling and fuel that fire the quest for learning and understanding? This is the very nature of *praxis*—the active learning and problem solving catalyzed by real-life situations that compel a person to learn—as described by Paulo Freire in his emancipatory educational work in San Paolo, Brazil.

> *Education makes sense because women and men learn that through learning they can make and remake themselves, because women and men are able to take responsibility for themselves as beings capable of knowing—of knowing that they know and knowing that they don't.* (Freire, 2004)
>   *For apart from inquiry, apart from the praxis, individuals cannot be truly human. Knowledge emerges only through invention and re-invention, through the restless, impatient, continuing, hopeful inquiry human beings pursue in the world, with the world, and with each other* (Freire, 1968).

Not surprisingly, the open admission by a human being that my life is "not quite right" is a powerful admission and a potential catalyst. Such self-honesty, coupled with a desire to do something about it by rolling up ones' proverbial sleeves, is the fertile ground, the primary reason people enroll in an MBSR program and for the experiential learning central to MBSR. All of the potential learning is ignited by unanswered questions: Can I handle the stress and strain in my life more effectively? Will I have to live with this anxiety all of my life? How can I deal with this cancer? Am I fated by my diagnosis? Is there something I can do for myself along with the help I'm receiving from my physician? Can I begin to change my relationship with my children or my body or my image of "me?" And more frequently these days, "How can I learn to change my mind?"

MBSR participants are asking themselves these questions and they are asking us as their teachers. Therefore, as teachers, our work is to engage program participants in these questions and through such inquiry invite them into a process in which the distinct possibility of "revealing oneself to oneself" might emerge (Phillips, 1988). Questions, if asked honestly and openly, have a way of opening up the space in a human being and in the larger MBSR learning community for this self-revealing to naturally unfold.

However, asking people questions that are designed to produce the answer that we as teachers want is fundamentally dishonest. Nearly 20 years ago, I first recall hearing my medical students call this approach "pimping." During an end of semester feedback session, they told my teaching colleague, Dr. Ilia Shlimak, and me that we were not "pimping" them. They told us that they abhorred this behavior in their teachers. They said that it turned them right off because they felt used and demeaned; it conveyed to them the feeling that their teachers were not really interested in what they thought or were wondering about. Instead, it relayed the sense from the teacher that "I am far more interested in what I think and supposedly know." This way of relating to students *closes* the space. Anyone who teaches knows that it is hard work to keep the space open. I have learned about this hard work by failing miserably and, as a consequence, asking myself nearly continuously what it really means to be a teacher and *practice* the art of teaching. Over the years, my students have been patient with me and generous in their commitment to learning. Through them, I have learned that more than simply asking good questions, keeping the space open requires us to respect our students, plan well for our classes, understand and explicate the learning objectives embedded in our curricula, refrain from our tendency to be at the center of the conversation, become a part of rather than separate from the learning and discovery process and hold in high esteem the innate and emergent wisdom of each human being inhabiting the larger learning community.

Keeping the space open has been a central feature of dialogue and inquiry in the MBSR classroom since its earliest inception (Santorelli, 1999). Over the years, my colleagues and I have had endlessly fruitful conversations about this approach and how it is the very expression of meditation practice embodied in an individual and a communal learning experience. Not surprisingly, Parker Palmer, one of the great educators of our time, has written extensively about "open space and skillful means":

> *Of course, the skill of asking questions goes beyond asking the right kinds of questions to asking them in a manner that is neither threatening nor demeaning—and receiving responses in the same open and invitational way. Every good teacher knows how easy it is to respond with the right words but dismissive nonverbal judgments—and how quickly this will freeze the conversation. When learning to ask good questions, we discover that yet another competence is needed: the ability to turn a question-and-answer session between the teacher and individual students into a complex communal dialogue that bounces all around the room* (Palmer, 1998).

Yet, I suspect that the Socratic method is risky for many of us who teach because it moves us from "professors" of a subject or topic to something more akin to mid-wives or coaches and *learners*. This means that as teachers we are charged with *creating space* for discoveries to emerge within and be expressed by students rather than *filling space* with our own voices and defaulting back to delivering answers to them. This makes teaching a risky, dynamic, and highly improvisational process even as we remain fundamentally true to the structure, objectives, and units of study a curriculum or syllabus represents.

With all of this in mind, it may now be helpful to take a closer look at the typology of Socratic questions and, in turn, their potential integration into the MBSR learning environment (ChangingMinds.org). These include:

Questions that wonder about *assumptions*:

- In what ways have these views shaped your life?
- Have your assumptions about a person or situation always been accurate?
- What if you discovered evidence of another possibility?

Questions that probe *rationale and evidence*:

- Is this always the case in your life?
- How do you know this?
- Are you absolutely sure?

Questions that explore *conceptual clarification*:

- Can you say exactly what you mean?
- How is this for you?
- What do you already know about this?

Questions *about questions*:

- What do you make of this?
- Does this make sense to you?
- If so, how so?
- What is it within you that is generating this question?

Questions that challenge *viewpoints and perspectives*:

- Do you benefit from this view?
- What if you looked through another set of lenses?

Questions that probe *implications and consequences*:

- What might happen if?
- How does this view about yourself (or others) inform your life?

Together, these constitute a broad palette of questions suitable to many contexts and situations. As teachers, they ask a lot of us. If we are willing to live with and into these questions, we may then have license to ask them to our students. This is the inner, non-dual demand of good teaching: we are required to embrace within ourselves what we are asking others to examine and embrace within themselves. In parallel, as we move back and forth between asking questions to individuals and asking the same questions to the entire community of learners, we enter into a rich environment that challenges MBSR teachers to become educators rather than technicians.

The Buddha's Approach to Questions

It is said that the historical Buddha treated questions four ways. Here is a direct quote about this approach from Walpola Rahula's book "What the Buddha Taught":

> *1) Some should be answered directly; 2) others should be answered by way of analyzing them; 3) yet others should be answered by counter-questions; and 4) there are some questions that should be put aside* (Rahula, 1959).

Not surprisingly, they mirror closely Socrates' method. In my experience, the treatment of questions as elucidated by the historical Buddha is naturally employed within the MBSR classroom, not because the Buddha said so but because these are commonsensical ways of being in relationship to people, their questions, and their comments. Of course, within MBSR the specificity and depth of questions we ask needs to take fully into account the human being to whom we are asking such questions. As we learn more about our program participants, our questions can evolve in specificity, precision, and depth by taking more fully into account the current developmental stage and tasks, medical and/or psychological conditions, idiosyncrasies, penchants, curiosity, and depth of mindfulness practice of individual participants.

The Heart of the Matter

Clearly, a hallmark of MBSR is the lively dialogue that takes place between the MBSR teacher and class participants. This back and forth exchange between student and teacher is ancient, embedded in the very fabric of any good learning process and a foundational characteristic of what happens between student and teacher in the meditative and contemplative traditions found everywhere on this planet. This latter point is essential to understand from the outset.

Moments of dialogue and inquiry in the MBSR classroom are an expression of student and teacher co-investigating and co-cultivating what I have called *remembrance*. I consider these moments to be nothing less and nothing more than real conversation among human beings. And since it is a very human conversation, there is no special technique; there are no prescribed steps to be followed, and no algorithm to be mastered. Of course, these moments of exchange often change over the span of an 8-week course. Learning is not a singular event; it does not have a beginning, middle, and end. When we allow it to, it just keeps going…

So let's examine inquiry and dialogue as it actually unfolds within MBSR. I'll begin with some brief background comments: The dialogue that follows took place in my MBSR courses. Weekly classes were recorded in audio and/or video with advanced permission from all participants. In what follows, there is no commentary or interpretation by me regarding these "conversations." They are spontaneous moments of conversation between my class participants and me. *These examples are not intended to be reproducible models or formulas for engaging in inquiry.* In fact, any attempts to do so would be less than adequate because all such attempts would be grounded in the past, in memory, rather than in the living reality arising at a specific moment, in a specific class, with a specific person.

One more comment before looking more directly into these classroom exchanges: In the course of this chapter, when describing aspects of inquiry and dialogue, I repeatedly use the word "conversation." I am speaking about a particular kind of conversation, one that Sufis refer to as "sobhet" [*so-bet*]. Sobhet is the intimate conversation between Sufi teachers and students about being human that ranges from the seemingly commonplace to the most serious of matters. (Note: I have never used the word *sobhet* in the classroom; it is jargon, has no relevance to what's taking place in that setting and there is no accurate rendering of the word in English.)

This kind of intimate conversation is not unique to Sufi teachers and their students. I have had such conversations with teachers from many contemplative traditions, with patients at their bedsides and participants in my MBSR classes. Likewise, I have borne witness to such conversations within the context of the everyday medical practice of my physician/provider colleagues. Three decades of experience in the sacred yet non-sectarian setting of the MBSR classroom tells me that sobhet is alive and well in contemporary healthcare.

Based upon experience, it seems to me that adult MBSR program participants across a wide racial, ethnic, socioeconomic, and geographic strata have a longing for the same kinds of conversations. Over time, most become full participants in the conversation about what it means to be human while actively engaging in learning how to actualize innately available reserves for coping and thriving, discovery, and resiliency while facing into a host of disruptive, disquieting, unforeseen, and unsatisfying conditions and situations. In fact, the longing for this is so compelling that often enough, weeks before the completion of an MBSR program, participants sometimes express great concern about their anticipation of no longer having such a learning environment available to them. They say things like, "I've never been in such a program"; "I've never spoken with people like this"; "I'm not sure what I'm going to do when this is over."

So let's begin. Here's an exchange took place in Class 2. The entire class was having a conversation about the *Body Scan Meditation* we had just practiced together for 45 minutes and that we'd been practicing at home, 45 minutes a day for six of the last seven days. In the exchange below, "D" is Dawn. "S" is Saki.

D: So, as soon as I lay down to begin the *Body Scan* my left knee was throbbing because I had a knee replacement 3 months ago.

S: This happened today?

D: Yes. So I said to myself, it's throbbing. I'll just deal with it … and then, all of a sudden what happened is that my knee wasn't hurting for about 20 minutes. As soon as I became aware of this, it started throbbing again. But for 20 minutes, it didn't hurt. That's weird.

S: Did you say, "That's weird?"

D: Yes. That never happened before. Maybe I was so concentrated on other parts of my body. That was *really* weird [emphasis Dawn's].

S: So one way or another what you are saying is that you have a strong, steady sense of throbbing in your left knee. But today, for 15 or 20 minutes, you weren't aware of it.

D: Right. I wasn't aware of it.

S: And you said that was really weird.

D: Yeah. For months it has been constantly throbbing.

S: What do you make of all this?

D: That my mind was just somewhere else … or maybe I'm just paying too much attention to it [the knee].

S: Well, who knows? This is an interesting experiment, isn't it? You do know one thing for sure: for some period of time, the sensations you associate with the left knee were not here.

D: Right. They weren't registering.

S: You know that the sensations you are usually aware of weren't registering. But you were awake?

D: I was awake…

S: And throughout the *Body Scan* you followed [attended to] the other parts of the body is what you said?

D: Yes. And then I said to myself, "my knee is not throbbing." And then it began throbbing.

S: Okay. So this is interesting. [Long pause]… So let's be clear. You had an experience. And you might just hold this openly and wonder: isn't this curious? Isn't this interesting that maybe what I call pain or strong sensations in my left knee have more variability than I know? Because what we tend to do is create a monolithic experience called [in this case] "knee pain." But maybe you noticed it [knee pain] isn't so monolithic, not so solid. In fact, you absolutely did notice this because you reported that for 15–20 minutes the left knee wasn't the way it usually is. For now, I'd suggest that you just be interested in that. I wouldn't try to reproduce it. I'd just try to be curious about it and know that this was your experience.

For decades, I have witnessed new MBSR teachers flounder with these conversations asking, "What are the steps for dialogue." "How do you 'do' inquiry?" While these are fair questions, I cannot say exactly because I don't experience it as having steps or being expressed via an algorithm or hierarchy of questions. Someone says something in class and sometimes I ask a question or wonder aloud with that person. Sometimes, the process begins with someone asking me a question or making a statement.

Here's a dialogue with the entire class of 40 participants that went on for 34 minutes. I have included a short section of this very long and dynamic exchange to give you a sense of the process. Here's some context: this conversation took place in Class 4, in the second hour of a 2.5 hour class. Leading up to this exchange we'd practiced Standing Yoga for 20 minutes and Sitting meditation for 30 minutes. During the 2 weeks prior to Class 4, participants had been systematically exploring their experience of *Pleasant Events* (between weeks 2 and 3) and *Unpleasant Events* (between weeks 3 and 4) through the use of weekly calendars that on a daily basis asks them to become aware of and record their responses to four questions: What was the event? What bodily sensations were occurring? What thoughts and emotions? What is it like right now to recall this event? (Kabat-Zinn, 1990, 2013).

The following dialogue began after people described with enthusiasm and great detail bodily sensations, thoughts, and emotions associated with a *Pleasant Event*. I almost always repeat their descriptions verbatim. For the sake of brevity, I've left these mirroring comments out of the text. In this dialogue, "P" stands for Participant (in this case, many participants); "S" is for Saki.

S: So, we know something about the bodily sensations, we know something about the thoughts, and we know something about the emotions arising in a pleasant moment. So, I'd like to ask you a question and ask you to reflect on it for a moment and then pop out an answer. So, here's an image…. If you want to make a necklace and you have a bunch of stones or pearls or beads on a table, what do you need to make a necklace?

P: String.

P: String.

S: Right. You need a string. You need something that ties all the stones or beads or pearls together. Okay, so what's the "string" that runs through all of those experiences that you had during your week that caused you to label them "pleasant?"

P: Stress.

S: Was it? How could it be "stress" if you labeled it pleasant?

P: The contrast .... Not feeling stressed.

S: Okay ... so the absence of stress was your string.

P: Being awake....

P: Other people being involved.

P: Focused on what I'm doing right now.

P: Awareness.

S: Awareness?

P: Yes, the awareness of now.

P: Beauty.

S: You say, beauty? So here is an example where it isn't absence of something but the presence of something identifiable — in this case, beauty.

P: Feeling, "in the moment"....

S: Someone else.

P: Laughter.

S: Okay, someone else.

P: I'm thinking as I listen that for me it might be appreciation. Not only am I "in it" but I'm also knowing how good it feels....

S: Okay. Let's continue this exploration. So here's another question. I'll repeat it twice. If I let go of wanting anything to be different, if I let go of wanting the pleasant event to remain forever, what might happen? What could I see? What might I learn? What could I lose? (I repeated the question again)

P: I might not be so frustrated.

P: I might see another pleasant moment.

P: I'd stay connected.

P: I'd lose anxiety.

P: There might be other pleasant moments.

P: I'd open myself to the next possibility.

S: What else? (I repeat the question)

P: I might see the truth.

P: I might be in harmony with life

P: I'd lose the fear that it won't come back...

S: Okay ... Let's go on and look at Unpleasant moments.

Note: We then "unpacked" the bodily sensations, thoughts, and emotions associated with unpleasant moments that they logged into their Unpleasant Event Calendars. This took between 8 and 10 minutes of non-stop "popcorn-ing"—people spontaneously calling out aspects of their experience. Here is a brief sample:

S: So what were some of the bodily sensations associated with unpleasant moments?
P: Aloneness.
P: Nausea.
P: Tension.
P: Sinking feeling.
P: Tightness.
P: Out of breath.
P: Sweating.
P: Restriction.
P: Smallness.
P: Shakiness.
P: Pressure.
P: Increased heart rate.
P: Flushing.
P: My head was spinning.
P: Blurred vision.
S: What were the thoughts associated with an unpleasant moment?
P: I never should have trusted this guy?
P: Why are you doing that?
P: Not this again.
P: I have my response ready this time.
S: What else? Thoughts associated with an Unpleasant moment...
P: Man, I should've known better.
P: I should've done this myself.
P: I wish I had paused and didn't say that.
P: It might not bother me so much.
P: I might learn something.
P: I might not be so compelled to try and make it go away.
P: It might not take up all my energy
P: My fears of the future might diminish.
P: I might be able to see something more clearly
S: Alright ... Let's take a moment to digest what we heard ourselves and others in the room say (long pause).... So what does this have to do with stress? What's this have to do with learning to meet the challenges we are facing in our lives in new ways?

And on it went....

As you can readily see, this awareness-familiarity can happen through words, in exchanges ranging from the seemingly benign to the zesty, brief or extended, provocative to laughable and to moments of great tenderness and heartbreak. And, they are omnidirectional.

Here's another exchange that took place in Class 5 between me and, for the most part, one other person. "K" is Kurt; "S" is Saki.

K: I've noticed some change in the acute stressors where, you know, it's a very specific limited thing.

S: Yes?

K: The pausing and the breathing and so on. The reason I'm here is because I'm dealing with a much more of a chronic issue and I'm having a hard time and wondering how I should be changing my relationship to be more productive. This has been going on for years now. I've dealt with it sort of by being fearful of it, and I know that's not ideal....

S: But it's what you're saying and what you are doing at this time, that's the truth of it, right now.

K: Yeah. And so you say, well, I should sort of turn towards it, and I don't really want to turn towards something that scares me.

S: Yes, of course.

K: So I guess my comment... and this may be more of a question, is how do you change your relationship to a stressor that, you know, I don't think this will go on forever, but while it's happening, it's, scary?

S: Yes. Thank you, Kurt. And so just to be clear, I've never said that we should do anything.

Another P: You should do what?

S: I've never said we should do anything. The operational word here is *should*.

What I was describing a couple of weeks ago and last week in a bit more detail is two of the ways that we are coping, two very powerful strategies, right? Really, we talked about three ways....

K: Mm-hm.

S: We talked about knowing that we can fight, we can flee—and denial is part of this—and we can freeze. And we've now been exploring this fourth way, this other possibility that is also built in to our human capability, which is that we could turn towards it. We have that capability.

K: Is that the acknowledgement, just acknowledging that it's there?

S: That's part of it and it may be, at least for a while this is exactly where you land—acknowledging it and seeing it clearly. You just named it incredibly clearly to 40 people. "It's a place where I feel fear. And I don't want to turn towards where I feel fear." This is a deep and direct acknowledging that is a huge step forward. Or maybe not even forward, it's just a huge step for us as human beings to say: this is the way it is. Because mostly we don't want to say: this is the way it is. And, we don't really recognize often that unless we get to the point of being able to name a situation or experience the way it is, there's no chance of actually relating to it differently. Because we actually haven't put our finger on it; we haven't seen it clearly. We haven't actually named the problem, or the situation, as it actually is. So your saying this is a big movement right there.

K: So, what do I do now? [laughs].

S: Well, the simplest thing to do ... I think that the most direct answer I can say is, I don't know. Because something will come out of your willingness to live with this knowing. Something will come out of your paying attention in this way and I don't mean this in some mysterious way. So let's explore this in the context of what we are learning about in the practice. What's the first instruction, the most fundamental element of instruction in the practice? And all of these practices have the same fundamental instruction. So, let's say we can pull from any one of them. Let's take "sitting" here for a second. So here you are, you're "sitting." What's the most fundamental instruction?

K: Breathe.

P2: Breathe.

S: The breathing?

P3: Awareness?

P4: Be attentive.

S: To be attentive to what's here, right? Okay? Because you have a choice about the breath ... and you could be attending to sound, you could be attending to thoughts and emotions. So the most fundamental instruction is to attend and open to what is actually here, right? And we often choose a particular object. So, in this case, fear comes down the line. You know it. If you thought about that instruction in relationship to fear, then the work would be to acknowledge: here is fear. You could then notice and ask, for instance, what's happening in my body? What do you notice in your body when you feel fear, Kurt?

K: I feel ... you know, I feel a lump in my stomach. I can feel that now. Sometimes there is more of, sort of a buzz up here [points to his head].

S: Then it's up here? [I point to my head mirroring K]

K: Yeah. It's really mostly in my head in fact, it seems.

S: So you have some sense of what it feels like viscerally. The body sensation is down in here (stomach)?

K: Yeah.

S: Okay.

K: Yeah.

S: Can you describe it?

K: Sickness, nausea.

S: Nausea?

K: Yeah.

S: Okay. Is it here now?

K: No.

S: Okay. And then you have this buzz up in the head.

K: Yeah.

S: And do you notice that there are thoughts, and emotions associated with that buzz?

K: I get angry. I get frustrated. I get more scared maybe.

S: Okay. So it has a kind of cycle?

K: Yeah.

S: Nausea, anger, fear, frustration, and maybe more?

K: Yeah, then I have sensations and thoughts about having those sensations, like why is this? I'm in this difficult legal situation and my livelihood kind of depends on how I deal with this ... and I've never been in this situation before ... never really controlled by other people to this extent and it's scary.

S: Yes.

K: And so, then I'm angry, because I'm angry about this and I have so many other things going for me.

S: Do you mean that since you have so many good things going you shouldn't be angry?

K: Yeah.

S: And do you mean, I've got so much else going for me why should I put all my attention on this?

K: Yeah.

S: Well, how come?

K: I'm conditioned, that's why. My wife says, "Look at all these great things we have." And she's right but still, I think we all want our independence and the ability to think that we have control.

S: So you want your independence?

K: Yes, my independence. I don't like it when I feel like people are controlling me. But the problem is, they are.

S: Yes?

K: Yes. It's a legal issue.

S: And what's the fear about? Usually fear is about, what's the worst, what's the worst that can happen.

K: By the way, now I sweat, too. [laughs]

S: Thank you. Thank you so much for your honesty, because what you're really, I don't even want to say, sharing .... What you are relating directly to, in yourself and to us is happening right now. So this mind-body connection is not a myth.

K: Mm-hm.

S: You know, these people who you say are controlling you are not in the room but, of course you are sweating, you are having bodily sensations. So, here you are in the laboratory [of your life] right now. That's what it is. This is not a metaphor. You're actually telling us about what's happening in your laboratory. And look how much detail you were able to tell us about it because you know something about it very intimately. And you're telling us what you want is control or at least you don't want to be controlled.

K: That's right.

S: Right and you feel like you are [being controlled].

K: Yeah and for me, that's the fear.

S: Yes. So then here's a question and it is not esoteric, Kurt. Everything that you're describing to us is a product of your awareness. You already *are* aware. You already know this, yes? So is the awareness itself fearful?

K: That's a good question. And it's, it's, well it's, it's interesting.

S: Is the awareness itself fearful?

K: I don't know. [laughs]

S: You don't know?

K: I'm not sure.

S: So, find out right now. Is the part of you that knows "fear," fearful?

K: Yeah, a little bit.

S: How can awareness be fearful?

K: Well, it's a little scary seeing the body react, and I don't want to sweat, but like I'm sweating, you know? And like, I don't want my heart rate to start going up.

S: Right. But is your awareness sweating?

K: No.

S: No?

K: No.

S: No? Okay. So your awareness is simply like a mirror. It's actually revealing to you what's so. What's so in your body and in the mind but it itself is not holding the fear.

K: Yeah.

S: See if you can attend to that much for a moment.

K: I'm sorry ... I didn't mean to take up all this time.

S: You know, you're not taking up all this time. You are talking about *us*. While the content may be different, we've all had this kind of situation. If you ask me if I've had situations in my life where I'm fearful .... If you ask me if I've had situations in my life where I feel like some external force is controlling me....

P5: Of course.

S: Yes. Of course, this is a human situation.

K: So the goal is to be with the awareness of the bodily reaction and of what's going on in my head?

S: Right, and also to recognize and ask yourself: Do "they" really have control of me?

K: Well, cognitively, I know the answer's no. I know that, yet it still has the grasp on me.

S: Yeah. So there you go. You see, you just actually teased something apart here, Kurt. Cognitively or intellectually you're saying something like, "I know they don't have control of me, at least not the whole of my life. But, there is this place that is very sticky—a place where I do feel like I'm not free."

K: So I need to engage the cognition a little more?

S: Well, maybe.

K: Maybe?

S: Maybe not. Maybe it's much more useful to engage with your awareness itself, with this capacity that knows. Here's an example because I don't want to get at all obtuse. Have you ever had a situation, where most of your day went really well and you had 20 or 30 minutes or even an hour of the day that really sucked? [laughter in class] And then, when you came home and saw someone that you live with—if you live with anyone—or you had a phone call with somebody that you know and they asked you how your day was and you said, "It sucked." Have you ever had that experience?

P6: Sure.

P7: Sure.

S: And if you looked back at the entire day, did it?

P8: No.

S: Really, it was that hour, right?

K: Right

S: So, so I only used that example, because your wife is pointing at something important … Things are generally good and this situation is not so good. But this kind of cognitive knowing is not enough. It is just not enough. If it were enough, you'd walk out of here and you wouldn't have to come back next week. Right? So you're right on the cutting edge here, or on the evolving edge here, because what you're really asking about is, here I am in an adverse situation that's not to my liking and highly challenging to me.

K: So there's no reason not to feel fear?

S: No reason at all not to feel fear … maybe lots of reasons to feel fear because in some way you wonder if your survival, in the most fundamental sense of the word, in the most primal sense of the word, is at stake. Because this [situation] is a threat, right?

K: Yeah.

S: Yes. It's a threat.

K: Mm-hm.

S: Isn't this exactly what we've been talking about? So no pretending, here. No "I'll work more hard on the cognitive side" is going to get rid of that, and it need not. This is a perceived threat in your life. So the invitation here—and that's why I asked you about the awareness itself—is what if for the next week you just experimented with: what if I keep bringing my attention to the feelings of fear in the body. Noticing how they show up, the sensations in the body, the thoughts and emotions in the mind, whenever they come up, without trying to make them nice … and begin to ask, 'How am I standing in relationship with them? And how can I bring elements of this practice of mindfulness into this situation?' Okay? Just that much … and you still have a body, you still have your breath, you still have lots of ways of stabilizing yourself as you turn towards whatever is here just as it is and let it teach you something rather than you having to operate on it. That's not easy.

K: Mm-hm. That is not easy.

S: That's not easy because you're a person of action. We all are. We want to *do* something about it.

K: Thank you.

S: You are welcome. Your awareness is big enough to live with how much is good in your life … And how much this situation is taxing you because it's not going to go away and there's no magic to make it go away. But you're asking a really fundamental set of questions, Kurt, about something that we're going to continue to unpack today.

Clearly, the provocation of awareness can come from the MBSR participant towards the teacher, from the teacher towards the participant, from participant to participant and, for that matter from a glimpse of the sky or shaft of light entering the classroom window. Often enough, this waking up occurs in silence or in those moments that spontaneously arise unforeseen. I have witnessed this countlessly in MBSR classes. Everything just stops; all the stuff floating at the surface of life just falls away. It may only last a few moments but everybody knows something has happened, something out of the ordinary has transpired behind what appears, even if what just happened can't be described. Such moments are ordinary and magical all at once. Like opening the treasure chest I was talking about.

In fact, this is just what happens. The treasure in the chest is opened. The heart, or what we might call love, is felt and known directly. Every one of us, despite what we say or think, is mad for love, pulled by the force of love, and when we get comfortable with this *pull* we can actually learn how to lean into the feeling of love, how to linger in love, how to fall open into what we actually are—and know it beyond knowing itself. Even for the briefest of moments. When this happens, we can't go back to sleep. Ever. We can and do doze and nap and become forgetful but not in the same way as before because we have glimpsed through our pores our fullness—the fullness that is our treasure, our birthright. When we experience a moment like this everything changes. As Emily Dickinson puts it, we begin to "dwell in possibility" (Franklin, 1999).

The Ethos of MBSR and Some Guiding Principles About Inquiry and Dialogue

Based on my experience in the MBSR classroom, here are seven foundational pillars of MBSR and 21 guiding principles of dialogue and inquiry. Together, in a very tangible way, they comprise the *ethos* of MBSR and, therefore, the "work" of an MBSR teacher. For additional details, see *MBSR Standards of Practice* (Santorelli, 2014).

Seven foundational pillars of MBSR:

- Non-harming (*primum non nocere*) is the primary mandate of an MBSR teacher.
- The MBSR teacher's capacity to vouchsafe the safety of every program participant is paramount.
- MBSR rests in the view that the essential nature of human beings is luminous and unimpeded. While this essential nature is often obscured, nonetheless, it is absolutely available to people facing a wide range of conditions and circumstances and may have substantively salutary effects on their health as they learn to be in wiser relationship to these conditions and circumstances.
- MBSR, while therapeutic and substantively researched, is *not* a therapy; it is a way of being (Kabat-Zinn, 2006).
- MBSR teachers are not providing psychotherapy.* They are not group facilitators. They are meditation teachers and educators. Their subject is mindfulness. As educators, their aim is assist program participants to learn how to experientially explore and directly understand their own human terrain and begin integrating that learning into everyday life.
- Ask others to do only what you do. To honestly ask program participants to formally practice mindfulness meditation 45–60 minutes per day, requires the

MBSR teacher to be formally practicing at least this much and, preferably, considerably more than the course participants.

- Teach only what you know; only what you have actually lived through.

Note: At the Center for Mindfulness in Medicine, Health Care, and Society at the University of Massachusetts Medical School, we have enormous respect for psychotherapy. We see psychotherapy as a specialized process aimed at treating mental health challenges or problems. We sometimes ask potential MBSR candidates to engage in psychotherapy before participating in an MBSR program and, as well, often refer participants to psychotherapy after completing an 8-week MBSR course. Sometimes MBSR program participants engage in these two modalities simultaneously.

Founded on these seven foundational pillars, the following 21 guiding principles express the spirit of the dialogue and inquiry process within MBSR:

1. Dialogue and inquiry is an expression and reflection of mindfulness meditation practice.
2. Dialogue and inquiry is grounded in the body.
3. Dialogue and inquiry is grounded in present centered awareness.
4. Dialogue and inquiry is respectful.
5. Dialogue and inquiry is an expression of awareness. Awareness illuminates and, in turn, seems to be further illuminated and enriched by the new knowing discovered through the process.
6. Dialogue and inquiry is directed towards inner growth and the implications of this learning and growth in everyday life.
7. Dialogue and inquiry is an expression of the dignity, nobility, and multidimensionality of a human being.
8. Dialogue and inquiry is non-goal oriented.
9. Dialogue and inquiry is for the benefit of the participant, not for the teacher (although the teacher and other program participants may benefit enormously from being in this kind of relationship with another).
10. Dialogue and inquiry is intimate.
11. Dialogue and inquiry is not directed towards changing or fixing anyone or anything.
12. Dialogue and inquiry is about discovering and cultivating greater understanding.
13. Dialogue and inquiry, even when painful, is always oriented towards the principle of ennobling.
14. Dialogue and inquiry is founded upon the sovereignty of every human being. Permission is always asked before proceeding with inquiry.
15. Dialogue and inquiry both provokes and educates through direct experience the possibility of a person learning to "turn towards" the difficult and/or unwanted in service of discovering innate capabilities obscured by what is conditioned and habitual.
16. Within MBSR dialogue and inquiry often occurs in community.
17. In the presence of dialogue and inquiry, the community does not give advice.

18. In the presence of dialogue and inquiry, the community learns to bear witness to the self-revealing of another.
19. In the presence of dialogue and inquiry, one of the great gifts of an MBSR program community is their capacity to listen and "sit" with one another in solidarity and silence.
20. What happens in dialogue and inquiry is not fair game for any other member of the community to speak about without first seeking permission from the person who spoke about their experience.
21. What is revealed by and about oneself in dialogue and inquiry may become a treasury for the many.

Closing Comments

This is neither the first, most definitive or final word about dialogue and inquiry in MBSR. A lot more could be said about this subject. My hope is that you now have more questions about this process than when you began this chapter. Our willingness to live with and into these questions without relying too heavily on premature answers or incomplete maps is the wellspring from which compelling, insight-provoking, and potentially transforming conversations stream forth as remembrance.

References

Changing Minds.org. *Socratic questions.* Retrieved March 31, 2015, from http:changingminds.org/techniques/socratic_questions.htm
Franklin, R. W. (Ed.). (1999). *The poems of Emily Dickinson.* Cambridge, MA: Harvard University Press.
Freire, P. (1968). *Pedagogy of the oppressed.* New York, NY: Seabury Press.
Freire, P. (2004). *Pedagogy of indignation.* Boulder, CO: Paradigm.
Kabat-Zinn, J. (1990). *Full catastrophe living: Using the wisdom of your body and mind to face stress, pain, and illness.* New York, NY: Delacorte.
Kabat-Zinn, J. (2005). *Coming to our senses: Healing ourselves and the world through mindfulness.* New York, NY: Hyperion.
Kabat-Zinn, J. (2013). *Full catastrophe living: Using the wisdom of your body and mind to face stress, pain, and illness* (Rev. ed.). New York, NY: Random House.
Kegan, R. (1982). *The evolving self.* Cambridge, MA: Harvard University Press.
Melville, H. (1922). *Moby-dick; or the whale.* London, England: Constable.
Nisargadatta, M. (1998). *I am that.* Bangalore, India: Nesma Books.
Palmer, P. (1998). *The courage to teach.* San Francisco, CA: Josey-Bass.
Phillips, A. (1988). *Winnicott.* Cambridge, MA: Harvard University Press.
Rahula, W. (1959). *What the Buddha taught.* New York, NY: Grove.
Santorelli, S. F. (1999). *Heal thy self.* New York, NY: Random House.
Santorelli, S. F. (Ed.) (2014). *MBSR standards of practice* (Rev. ed.). Worcester, MA: Center for Mindfulness in Medicine, Health Care and Society.
Winnicott, D. W. (1964). *The child, the family, and the outside world.* Reading, MA: Addison-Wesley.

Chapter 4
Interpersonal Practices: A Transformational Force in the MBIs

Florence Meleo-Meyer

MBSR participants begin the program primarily as strangers. Over time, they become a vibrant community that discovers together each one's uniqueness, commonality, and potential for transformation. As one participant stated: "This class is more than stress reduction—this class is about being human! And there are not many learning situations like this."

This skillful engagement with one's own life is known as *participatory medicine* (Kabat-Zinn, 2013). It involves accessing innate resources to share the responsibility of supporting health and wellness in concert with one's healthcare provider. The program requires a commitment from participants to engage fully and wholeheartedly by attending each of the eight classes and practicing meditation daily. The group develops a sense of mutuality, intimacy, and support as they return to class weekly and share experiences and questions from engaging with their mindfulness meditation practices in class and at home.

After the orientation meeting, participants appear for the first MBSR class and meet the members of their group. They will all become co-learners for the next 8 weeks. After reviewing the underlying intention, structure, and guidelines of the MBSR program and experiencing "the raisin exercise" (a mindfulness practice that offers a direct and normalizing experience of paying attention with intention and curiosity), participants are invited to introduce themselves. Sitting most often in a circle, the group members share in a council-like fashion, one by one, the unique reason each has chosen to take this class. Individuals express stories of loss, dissatisfaction, resistance, suffering, illness, and medical and emotional, as well as curiosity, intentions, and hope to participate in creating a better quality of life. Individual stories often revolve around self-worth, aging, family, relationships,

F. Meleo-Meyer, M.S., M.A. (✉)
Train-the-Trainer Program, Oasis Institute for Mindfulness-based Professional Education and Training, Center for Mindfulness, University of Massachusetts Medical School,
38 Dragon Hill Road, Shelburne Falls, MA 01370, USA
e-mail: florence.meyer@umassmed.edu

© Springer International Publishing Switzerland 2016
D. McCown et al., *Resources for Teaching Mindfulness*,
DOI 10.1007/978-3-319-30100-6_4

changes with work, finances, and expectations. People talk about what life once was—and what it could be. As each person shares, participants listen with interest and, in the listening, begin to identify similarities to their own reasons for attending. They often enter the program feeling isolated and strongly identifying with their suffering. By the end of the course, many have cultivated more skillful ways to relate to their problems, gaining a sense that all people have a share of suffering as well as the innate capacity to be awake with life's sunshine and shadows.

Often, with the launch of the first class, there is a budding sense of empowerment simply from having shown up. Each person has made the choice to engage in a life training that involves practicing mindfulness with others who are similarly willing to engage in this venture. As such, the MBSR class participants join and co-create a proactive learning community. They are each willing to take on the discipline needed to mobilize innate capacities of awareness and compassion in order to engage more fully and skillfully in life's unfolding. Over the next 8 weeks, with continuing development of formal and informal meditation practices and dialogue, this learning community will progressively and synergistically become a supportive and powerful source of personal transformation.

MBSR is essentially about intimacy and relationship. As participants engage with meditation practices, their innate capacity for awareness is highlighted as they become more deeply familiar with the conditions that contribute to the moment-to-moment experience of life. This shift includes becoming more sensitive to acknowledging bodily cues and developing more fluency in the sensory language of the body. Through their awareness of thoughts and emotions, participants become more alert to the constrictive and, at times, destructive effects of strong identification with opinions, feelings, assumptions, habits, judgments, assessments, conceptualizations, and projections.

The primary quality and style in the teaching of MBSR is dialogic with a particular emphasis on the evocation and exploration of participants' experiences and reflections as a result of engaging with formal and informal meditation practices. The MBSR teacher's engaged interest and curiosity encourage participants to "look again" at their experiences and possibly gain insight into the ways they relate to their daily lives. Focus is on the *process* of the experience rather than the content or history. Several sources influence this methodology, including Zen koans, Socratic, and Bohmian dialogue, as well as practices from Judaism, Christianity, and Sufism. Through a mindful dialogue with classmates or inquiry with the teacher, the MBSR participants receive affirmation about their individual practices and also may be challenged about old self-limiting opinions of themselves and their pasts. Following each in-class meditation practice, there is time in small and large groups to share experiences and to ask questions. These periods of dialogue and inquiry allow integration of the meditation experience through clarifying questions and exploration of the shared realities that come with being alive. Intrinsic to the essence of MBSR is potential wondering about, and investigation into, being human and waking to natural capacities of openness, warmth, and presence. Indeed, after completing the MBSR program, one participant reported saying, "I am not worried about stress now, but I have another question: 'Who Am I?'" This question points to the deepest level of being rather than the surface of personality or the closed system of self.

Deepening curiosity in relation to one's direct experience through the practice of mindfulness and engaging in the mutuality of practice with classmates can support inner and outer attunement. The possibility of expanding this sense of attunement from self to others, to direct moments of experience, may emerge as the experience and definition of self becomes less a rigid narrative than an emergent process. Joanna Macy writes about the potential "to be awakened by all things" in this way:

> The way we define and delimit the self is arbitrary. We can place it between our ears and have it looking out from our eyes, or we can widen it to include the air we breathe, or at other moments we can cast its boundaries farther to include the oxygen-giving trees and plankton, our external lungs, and beyond them the web of life in which they are sustained. (Macy, 2007)

Boldly put, the heart of the MBSR experience cultivates and reveals love: love for oneself, love for others, love as one's core presence, and love in relationship with all life. All of the sources of wisdom that underpin the philosophy of MBSR are expressions of love. They penetrate the form and delivery intrinsically while not being explicitly or overtly taught. Being made aware of choices creates a foundation for authoring one's own life and claiming innate sovereignty. Choosing to inhabit one's life fully through times, filled either with challenges or awesome beauty, means choosing to steer one's life in beneficial ways.

The intensive and rigorous training in mindfulness meditation cultivates access to what is already present as innate awareness, insight, intuitive intelligence, and compassion. It also builds bridges to one's common humanity and, in so doing, widens an individual's sense of self as being larger than previously known, allowed, or experienced. Maya Angelou expresses this definition of love: "By love I mean that the condition in the human spirit so profound, it encourages us to develop courage and build bridges, and then to trust those bridges and cross the bridges in attempts to reach other human beings (Angelou, 2014)."

Intimacy, Intention, and Independence

The experience of engaging in the MBSR program calls forth a strong intention from the individual, which is held in the context of a group. While one enters the MBSR class with others, it is only as an individual that one can make a commitment to fully engage, to be a learner, and to be proactive about one's health and quality of life. It is the individual who will choose to attend class, who will develop the discipline and take time each day to practice, who will be curious about identifying and possibly challenging automatic, habitual patterns of reactivity, and who will look deeply at what nourishes and creates value in life. It is only the individual who will choose a way to live with more clarity, skill, and kindness. It is a personal journey toward making wise choices that leads to living with greater sovereignty. A paradox is that individual development of intimacy with the direct, present experience of being alive has the potential to ripple and extend to others. In the shared experience, there lies inspiration to witness the journeys of others on the same path.

In the first MBSR class, the group reflects and reports on their individual intentions to participate. The teacher poses a central question: "What brings you here?" There are many ways that this process may unfold. Some teachers guide a reflection using an image that allows the question to deepen. At times, the contemplation may be framed as if one were following the question like a stone falling deeper into a well: "What brings me here? What is it I want or hope from taking this class?" As the stone drops deeper, more subtlety may emerge. Some teachers support this deepening process with a repetition of the same question: "What really, really brings me here?" The question allows for one's innate wisdom to emerge with a response that is individually true.

Embedded in the reflection and inquiry are a number of values: each individual has a source of wisdom that can be tapped; the approach is nonjudgmental and the process of deeper curiosity is invited. Answers to the question may arrive as words, images, bodily sensations, and/or nothing specific. With this first inquiry, key attitudes of mindfulness are evoked: beginner's mind, nonjudging, patience, nonstriving, acceptance, and trust. And, in the shared experience, there is the inspiration to hear the multiplicity and familiarity of what drew others to this program.

Often people will report their reflections in layers, saying:
"When I first heard the question, I heard myself say, 'because I am stressed!'"
"I have a challenging situation with my daughter and I am angry all the time."
"I was just diagnosed with cancer. I need to help myself."
Then the question came a second time.
"I have been living by the side of the stream, and I don't want to come to the end of my life and feel I missed being fully here."
"I need guidance on how to connect better with myself."
"I saw an image of a tree; it seemed steady… I want to be more like that."
And the third time? "I felt in my whole body, a shiver that I don't know who I am and I want to find out."
"The third time, I just was silent, still."
"I was surprised to hear myself say, 'I want to be happy.'"

The motivations that bring participants to an MBSR class are as unique as each individual in the circumference of the circle. Honoring the life narratives and the stories that have motivated attendance is essential. It is the launch pad for further investigation. As each participant is invited to share the reason for choosing to attend the MBSR class, all listen attentively. Life stories filled with challenges and inequities unfold in the space of the circle. In the speaking and listening, the group supports the individual with a collective intention to participate in this MBSR process. This learning contract affirms one's willingness to be a participant in one's own health and to make a genuine effort to fully engage with the program.

Intimacy, Intention, and Interdependence

"It's better for everybody when it gets better for everybody."
Eleanor Roosevelt (Albion, 2013)

It is an individual choice to participate in the MBSR program, and it takes individual intention to show up for all classes as well as to initiate and maintain a daily practice. However, the individual's learning is embedded in the structure and context of a group. Individuals who are mostly strangers to one another are united weekly with the unfolding development of the program. It is here that the group itself becomes an essential element of the learning process. Understanding is deepened and extended as individuals pose questions and share experiences.

This process is particularly evident as participants share experiences about their implementation of meditation practices in class and at home, waking up to automatic, habitual patterns of reactivity, gaining a fresh view, and choosing new options to respond to conditioned circumstances. One voice is likely to express the experience of several, and the "group process" becomes a deep well of collective wisdom from which all can draw. As one person embraces the discipline of daily practice and shares her/his learning, others might be inspired to amplify their own weaker resolve.

The program invites and cultivates awareness of one's relationship to all the facets of life. The small blessings and gifts in daily life that may have been formerly taken for granted now become recognized and appreciated. Investigation into stress reactivity and response invites a deep engagement with how one perceives and relates to challenges, whether in health, work, and/or relationships. The MBSR program is a crucible; along with the meditation practice, discipline building, and class themes, the relational and group dynamics contribute to the heat that can lead to transformation.

Stories move in circles.
They don't go in straight lines. So it helps if you listen in circles.
There are stories inside stories and stories between stories,
and finding your way through them is as easy and as hard as
finding your way home.
And part of the finding is the getting lost.
And when you're lost, you start to look around
and to listen.
Deena Metzger (1992)

On the most basic level of human organization, we are relational creatures. The structures of the body and brain are designed with relational elements (Siegel, 2007). Human survival once closely depended on the presence, care, protection, and support of others. Earliest people gathered in nuclear families, extended families, and kinship communities in order to procure food, maintain warmth and safety, and share bounty. Humans could not have survived alone, and we continue to have exquisite sensitivity to each other. Human beings are finely attuned to subtle messages. Just a glance offers significant information. A grimace, turn of the head, raise of an eyebrow, and a sideway look all carry potential meanings.

Relationships resonate with the complexity of earlier influences and conditioning. There are many well-worn grooves of patterns and behaviors with those closest and most familiar, such as family members and work colleagues. Below the surface of any interaction may be tremendous activity, indicating complex feelings and associations. Feelings of ease, connection, fear, and wanting may drive the tenor of an exchange but often are not conscious. As mindfulness deepens and strengthens through the MBSR program, patterns that drive reactivity begin to be known.

The Buddha identified the source of reactive patterns as profoundly deep desires or cravings (Walpola, 1959). The word *tanha* in Pali is translated as "hunger," signifying an urgency to fulfill an impulse that is profoundly evocative and deep, as if one had been hungry or thirsty for days and urgently fixated on quelling the need for food or water. The hungers identified by the Buddha are for sensual pleasure, to exist, and not to exist. These cravings may also be understood as interpersonal: the hunger for pleasure in relationship and the urge to escape loneliness, the hunger to be seen and to know that one exists, and the hunger not to be seen and to escape intimacy or engagement with others. It seems natural to enjoy social contact and to feel the pleasure of company with others and to enjoy being appreciated and recognized. It seems natural as well to savor solitude and silence. The interpersonal hungers point to urges that are profoundly deep and compulsive. They are organized around escape. The very essence of stress reactivity is present with the urges to flee or to fight. When the hungers are very activated, stress increases. When this hunger emerges interpersonally, other people become objects to alleviate the press of the wanting. In this storm of tension and desire, other people are not appreciated for who they are as unique and whole beings, but as a means to escape what is directly experienced and is uncomfortable.

Mindfulness allows one to work more skillfully with the suffering that comes with intense resistance to the way life is right now. While these forces and patterns are always going on without awareness, it is possible to wake up to this pulling away from life. Practice with others allows mindfulness to be cultivated both inwardly and outwardly, and being a member of a learning community sets the stage for sharpening this possibility.

Awareness is progressively developed through the MBSR classes, beginning with awareness of the bodily sensations, what is perceived as pleasant and unpleasant, and then of thoughts and emotions. With this initial foundation, awareness of social patterns of how one gets caught in difficult conversations or relationships can be more clearly seen. Recognizing reactivity and stuck patterns is the key to gradual release and opening to more freedom—if even to a small degree. Stepping back from identifications with… shyness, cleverness, being inarticulate or not interesting, taking too much space, not being good with others…can provide powerful moments of greater ease in the presence of long-held frozen and fixed grooves of self-perception.

The class establishes the practice of mindfulness in and throughout the dialogue and group sharing, and the naturalness of meditation practice is established. The potential for challenging old patterns and embracing new ways of being may then be supported in the presence of one another. When people choose to be awake together and offer to infuse discussion with mindfulness and kindness, it builds mutual support to be awake. The interconnectivity can blossom into an easing of the suffering that intrinsically rises with the sense of being separate. As Thich Nhat Hanh writes: "To be is to inter-be. You cannot just *be* by yourself alone. You have to inter-be with every other thing (Thich Nhat, 2012)." In the shared space of mutual practice, a sense of oneness can arise, and with it a sense of sacredness as wholeness meeting wholeness. Martin Buber refers to this presence as a movement from I-It to I-Thou (Buber, 1970).

Relational Practices in MBSR

Throughout the MBSR program, mindfulness is invited into all moments of one's life and strengthened with formal and informal meditations. Intrapersonal and interpersonal mindfulness is engaged in all classes. While the value of sharing experiences is recognized and employed throughout the entire program, the experience of self and other is the highlight of class 6. The specific exploration of awareness in relationship is featured after weeks of cultivating greater regularity and stability with meditation. It follows the investigation of habitual, automatic stress reactivity (class 4) and mindfulness-mediated stress response (class 5). From this base of understanding, the class is invited to explore internal and external communication, stress, longing, and development of greater ease. There are several practices, exercises, and reflections which create pathways of deeper understanding. Below are a few used in classes at the University of Massachusetts Medical School Center for Mindfulness. Each teacher needs to employ flexibility in choosing what methods serve the needs of the group.

1. *Listening: A Body Awareness Practice*

This MBSR group reflection reveals the shared human sense of suffering that comes with feeling separate and the possible ease of longing when being met, listened to, and seen.

The class is invited to stand and establish the *mountain pose*. Feet are firmly connected with the solid base below; the body is aligned, hips over feet, shoulders over the hips, and shoulder blades gently flattened.

The invitation is offered to balance the neck and head, allowing the arms and hands to rest at the sides of the torso. While participants are breathing and sensing the grounded and upright, stable, and elevated posture, a reflection is introduced:

"Call to mind a time in your life when you had something you longed to share with another. This might be a joyful news, something confusing, or troubling. There was a feeling of wanting to connect and be heard. For whatever reason, the person you chose would not be present for and with you. Perhaps they were busy, or not interested, or threatened by your request. With this memory recalled, allow your body to express the way this felt for you. Let yourself exaggerate."

People often collapse with this invitation; as a group, the upright mountain posture collapses into looking down, folding hands and arms over the chest, and bending forward.

Holding this posture, they are asked to name any thoughts that have emerged from this experience. They might say: "Why don't you listen to me?" "I must not be important to you." "This hurts." "Why did I even try?" "I am angry." "I am not loved."

Still holding the pose and reflection, they are asked to name emotions that may be present. Sadness, grief, anger, hopelessness, despair, frustration, and self-blame are voiced. At this time, the group is invited to return to the mountain pose and bring awareness to the feeling of moving from the contracted posture to full, upright standing. Many literally shake their bodies as if to shake off an unwanted presence.

A second phase of the reflection is offered:

"Now, recall a time when you had something you longed to share and someone was there for you. They might have been busy, but they paused and focused on you. They gave you full attention."

The invitation to express this memory physically is repeated. At this time, the group often reaches arms high; chests are open and exposed. Some people tenderly place hands over their hearts. With the request for thoughts to be named, the room fills with: "Thank you." "I am so grateful." "I matter." "You care about me." "Finally!" "I am loved." They name emotions that include safety, gratitude, relief, comfort, refuge, and love.

I have seen this reflection repeat in the very same pattern in groups of different sizes across the world. Almost always, with this reflection of being offered attention, someone will say: "I am loved."

It is essential to state that every one of us has played both of these roles at different times in our lives. Unbeknown to us, we may have hurt another in a moment of distraction, self-involvement, or sheer insensitivity. At the same time, we have generously offered another attention and care, even at times when it was not always easy to do.

But something universal is established in this group reflection. We all have the power to gift ourselves with deep listening and to offer this gift to another. Witnessing the power and collective agreement with this practice is stunning. From this shared experience, the invitation to practice mindful dialogue has a base of common ground regarding the human longing to connect, to be seen, and to be heard. This sensitivity can then be strengthened in the dialogue practice.

2. *Passive, Aggressive, and Assertive Patterns and Practices*

Through formal and informal practice, pleasant and unpleasant experiences continue to be investigated in group dialogue. The class participants often report increased sensitivity to their abilities to identify impulses of pulling away with aversion, rushing toward with grasping, clinging, and, at times, sensing neither. "I could feel my body tense when I read an upsetting email." "I wanted to run and felt scared. I paused and really felt it. It was hard, but it started to ease up, a bit." "I felt the warmth and thought." "I want this to stay just like this…I wish this wouldn't end." "I see how much I feel bored…I just tune out. I see how much real-time life I am missing!"

These insights lead naturally to an investigation of emotional, cognitive, sensory, and behavioral patterns of passive, aggressive, and assertive modalities. The intention of these physical practices is to engage the class in an experiential contemplation of habitual ways of meeting challenges. The intention is to clarify—not to judge one modality as better than another. In unique situations, each has utility and skill that can lead to wise action.

Each activity is led as a meditation, as well as a learning rubric, that highlights the possibility of engaging experience with wisdom. Passive, aggressive, and assertive communication patterns are investigated as ways of separating or being with experience internally and externally. Following each activity, the group engages in a discussion highlighting one's perception of threat, the thoughts, emotions, and body postures that automatically accompany that perception and the possibility to pause, turn toward with awareness, and respond with wisdom. The MBSR teacher might find these practices a useful way of encouraging participants to both embody and reflect upon their dominant styles and explore what it *feels like* to deliberately embody styles with which they are all too familiar, or that are foreign to their experiences.

Practice: Sculpting

Passive
- The participants are invited:

    - Into the mountain pose while standing in a circle.
    - To allow the body to express a posture of passivity.
    - To identify what was noticed? What is noticed with the hands, face, posture, and gaze? Any feelings or thoughts? Responses are called out.
    - To listen as the teacher reads some key features of passivity:

    "Allows others to choose for them; value self below others; slumped, leaning body language; possible feelings of fear and hurt."
    "I will only survive if I have other's approval."

The teacher acknowledges that there are times when choosing to step back or not act may be for reasons of safety. If a dangerous situation can be avoided, this response may be most skillful. A woman once asked: "Is it possible to be a doormat all one's life?" The teacher asked her, "How does this question relate to your life?" She responded that in her years working as a bank teller, she had been a victim of three bank robberies. When asked if she might share more, she said as a young child she had learned to avoid conflict by backing away. This way of coping had served her to keep as safe as she could as a child with little power in a home with an abusive parent. As she grew, though, she met most situations by emotionally disengaging and allowing others to make choices for her. As she worked in therapy on the trauma from the robberies, the older pattern of avoidance and self-negation rose in awareness. Engaging with these patterns physically allowed greater connection with the felt sense of the early patterns. She began to open to the possibility of exploring more assertive behaviors.

- The group is invited to return to the mountain pose and feel the transition. Inquiry and group discussion follow.

Aggressive

- The exploration of aggressive behavior follows the same pattern of naming details of the body posture, identifying thoughts and emotions, and expressing these in the group.
- Aggressive behavior is highlighted, with the balanced perspective that it can be a wise use of power, like the force of a spring flower pushing up through the earth to the sunlight.
- Participants are invited to physically feel and express aggressiveness and listen to the reading of some key features:

  - Chooses for others; value self over others; inappropriately close body language; possible feelings of righteousness and vulnerability.

    "I will only survive if I am invulnerable and able to control others."
    The group is invited to return to the mountain pose and feel the transition.

Assertive

As people are invited into an assertive posture, they often say, "It is the mountain pose!" Some widen their arms, open, and curious. Here too, some key features are highlighted:

- Chooses for self and negotiates; value self equal to others; "I messages"; attentive listening; erect body stance; possible feelings of confidence and self-respect.
- "I want to get and give respect, ask for fair play, compromise."

The group is invited to return to the mountain pose and feel the transition. Some say "I hardly shifted position!"

The whole group engages in a reflective dialogue about their experience with this practice, how mindfulness informs wise choices, and the possibility to cultivate a greater range of responses.

Another practice that can be used to demonstrate these three dispositions is found in the Resources section, it is titled Life Space: Demonstrating passive aggressive and assertive dispositions.

Practice: Aikido Postures

Aikido is a Japanese martial art developed by Morihei Ueshiba (Stevens, 1987) as a way for practitioners to protect themselves while they also protected the attacker from injury. It is often translated as "the way of unifying with life energy." The movements in aikido consist of meeting the energy or movements that are approaching and redirecting in a way that diffuses an attack while creating greater harmony. While the art of Aikido involves extensive training and practice, the series of physically interactive exercises offer a teaching that illuminates the values and practices that have been cultivated throughout the entire MBSR program. The movements demonstrate possible ways of meeting interpersonal challenges as well as challenges within oneself. *It is important for the teacher to practice these exercises with friends until she feels confident in being able to offer the demonstrations, hold the entire group, and describe how to apply the teachings to daily life. Difficult memories may be stimulated. It is essential for the teacher to establish safety and leave time for group discussion.*

Below is a description of a process employing the aikido movements. The teacher first introduces this to the group and asks the group to form a circle in the room and describes the process of demonstrating a number of ways of meeting challenges — whether internal or external. Then she invites the whole group to participate with close awareness of the body as if they were practicing the body scan. *Finally, she* chooses a person in the group who is willing and physically able to function as a partner. "It will involve engaging movements a number of times and also involves making physical contact with me. This is OK with me."

First interaction: The teacher invites the partner to stand opposite her. "You will be aggressive, so, holding your arms outstretched towards me, and keeping your elbows locked, come toward me with some energy — make contact with your hands at my shoulders."

As the person does this, the teacher is often knocked slightly off balance. As they come back to the center of the circle, the teacher engages a dialogue with the partner, "What did you notice as we did that?" The response is often: "I didn't want to hit you! It felt odd." The teacher shares: "I knew it was coming, but still did not like getting knocked off balance." The teacher then checks in with the group: "What were you aware of?" Participants respond: "I gasped, this is too reminiscent of my past." "I was surprised, and felt my stomach tighten." "I felt angry." The teacher can help the participants to reflect on how their automatic reactions are shaped by their personal stories and habits of thought and emotion.

Second interaction: The teacher invites the partner: "Let's try this again. Please come toward me once more, keeping your arms outstretched and elbows locked and palms facing towards me." This time, as the "aggressor" approaches, the teacher steps quickly out of the way. The teacher asks how the partner feels: "I didn't like it." I felt duped, surprised, and out of control." The teacher adds, "And this time, I didn't get hit." Checking in with the group, the teacher may hear: "I was relieved that you got out of the way, but I was concerned for the other person, too." "I wanted to laugh."

Third interaction: The teacher repeats the stepping away, but this time also drops to the floor saying: "It is all my fault. I am sorry. I shouldn't have done that." She then dialogues with the "aggressor" and asks how he or she feels. "I find that I feel angry." "All this self-blame, just makes me mad. It makes me feel helpless."

The teacher says, "This time, I got out of your way, and I took all the blame. The problem is still here." The teacher checks in with the group and asks what they are noticing in their body and mind. The teacher may help them reflect on their experiences, noting that "This is a passive approach which denies one's own rights.

Stepping away by taking full responsibility is a way to try to appease the situation as quickly as possible in order to stay safe. The teacher can also normalize times of needing to deny or avoid saying: "If you were a young child in an untenable situation, denial is what you had, but as you grow older, it can become a pattern and a burden and not a help. You can cultivate more ways to meet challenges."

Fourth interaction: The teacher asks the partner to approach once more aggressively. This time, the teacher engages by gripping the partner's hands or arms. The two exert force toward one another moving in circles. The teacher asks the group: "Does this look familiar?" Then she and the partner add words, saying "I'm right!" "No, I'm right!" over and over again.

Inviting discussion about the experience, the teacher asks, "How familiar was this? Trying to have your way, pushing against? How effective was this?" It is clear to see—it ends in going in circles! She then clarifies and normalizes the times one needs to fight injustice and push against what may not be wholesome attitudes and behaviors in relationships and society. The teacher invites the group to share their reflections.

Final scenario: The teacher asks the "aggressor" to approach once more. This time, however, the teacher maintains eye contact while stepping slightly to the side. With her right hand, the teacher takes hold of the partner's right wrist with the thumb and forefinger and leans in slightly, using the momentum of the partner's forward movement to turn with him or her, walking now side by side in the same direction. It is also then possible to turn the aggressor in a different direction— showing the teacher's "point of view."

The teacher then dialogues with the "aggressor" and asks how he or she feels and invites the group to share their experiences with this scenario. The teacher notes that by stepping to the side, she did not get knocked down by the oncoming force, and by making eye contact she was able to see clearly while connecting and was able to harness the oncoming energy to redirect the movement. She asks of the group, "How might this way of meeting and working with challenges manifest in our daily lives? For example, you have a project you need to prepare. You can deny and procrastinate; resist and fight making time to do what is needed. Or, you can acknowledge it, "lean into" the actual problem needing attention, the emotions and meaning associated with it. This is turning toward. From this, one can decide with a step-by-step process how best to complete the task. On an emotional level, when grief, sadness, hurt, and confusion, are allowed and acknowledged, a clearer resolution may be found."

Practice: Verbal Aikido

Class members at times have said: "This is helpful, but how would this be in a difficult conversation? They request a verbal demonstration of this aikido process. Below is an example of applying the aikido principles in a scenario between the teacher and a volunteer.

After preparing the group to bring awareness to bodily sensations, thoughts, and emotions as they experience this practice, the teacher asks the volunteer to express some dissatisfaction or displeasure, anger or frustration toward the teacher.

A. Participant: "I am so mad that you are not more available."
  Teacher: "Oh"

This is "taking the hit."

B. Participant: "I am so mad that you are not more available."
  Teacher: "Did you hear the news today? The weather is going to be very cold."

This is avoiding, denying, stepping away from the issue.

C. Participant: "I am so mad that you are not more available."
  Teacher: "You're mad! You have no idea how mad I am…how you are so demanding and don't understand."

This is opposing what is presented. Aggression is met with aggression.

D. Participant: "I am so mad that you are not more available."
  Teacher: "Wow, you're really angry. You wish we could have more time together."
  "I wish that too. Maybe we can check for times that are ok for both of us."

This is meeting the other, acknowledging the emotions and situation and working together toward resolution. It is aikido—the way of unifying. Many people express a sigh of recognition as they are shown these different scenarios.
MBSR teaching invites and cultivates the possibility to be aware of what is happening as it is happening without judgment. The aikido exercises are teachings about how one can strengthen being with the lived experience, meeting challenges wisely and discovering nondual solutions that may be beneficial to all.

Insight Dialogue and Interpersonal Mindfulness Program

Cultivation of mindfulness alone, and with others, is done both formally and informally throughout the entire MBSR program. As a response to participants' wanting more interpersonal practice, a graduate class has been developed with the key focus on relational meditation practice. The Interpersonal Mindfulness Program (IMP) has been developed to support the deepening of MBSR participant's ongoing meditation practices. The IMP is an 8-week protocol based upon Insight Dialogue guidelines (Kramer, 2007) and an MBSR framework. The course is designed to help participants cultivate and establish mindfulness in moments of sensory and relational contact. It provides a format and container for exploring the shared human experience. It offers a mindfulness practice (drawn from the foundation of Insight Dialogue), developed to take place in relationships, and an interpersonal understanding of the stress that arises in relation to others. The course offers the opportunity to observe and release habitual ways of relating and to experience being with other people outside of that conditioning. It allows participants to deepen their understanding of stress reactivity and their potential to respond. Both the Interpersonal Mindfulness Program and the broader framework of Insight Dialogue utilize the same meditation guidelines and the relational meditation form based on the meditation practice of Insight Dialogue developed by Vipassana meditation teacher, Gregory Kramer, Ph.D.

What Is Insight Dialogue?

Insight Dialogue (Kramer, 2007) (ID) is an innovative, structured interpersonal meditation practice aimed at cultivating freedom individually and collectively. It extends mindfulness and tranquility of silent meditation to interactions with others. The practice seamlessly weaves the three domains of meditation, wisdom, and relationship as a whole life path. It has its roots in the specific dispensation of the Buddha's early teachings and invites study, contemplation, and embodied action rooted in this practice interface.

The inspiration for Insight Dialogue emerged as Greg Kramer discovered (although he ardently practiced and studied the Dharma) that he returned home from attending multiple long silent retreats only to find the same repetitive and binding patterns in his relationships with his family. He became interested in the possibility of closing the gap and supporting a pathway that led to potential awakening in and through relationship and kinship.

Insight Dialogue responds to the inquiry of what it might be to meet another with mindfulness and greater steadiness. With *mindfulness and dialogue*, each of the two participants, through choosing to be present and in relationship, supports the other to awaken the mind's great potential for awareness and freedom. In this practice, the individual has the opportunity to explore how innate wisdom manifests within relationships when the separate "I" is more spacious. The structure establishes the practice as meditation. Distinct from improving communication effectiveness as a "communication exercise," this practice invites participants into relational practice through the progressive engagement of meditation *guidelines*. As the practice unfolds with guidance from the teacher, individuals speak and listen to one another, pausing with awareness, incorporating presence, silence, and spaciousness into dialogue.

The focus of the dialogue is a topic of reflection or *contemplation* that has the potential to evoke and deepen wisdom. Contemplations may focus on human realities, such as aging, illness and death, roles, judgments, generosity, and gratitude. Feelings of being separate are illuminated and investigated through the dialogue practice as people explore their identification with their personal historical life circumstances, opinions, and with the raw explication of comparisons: feeling better than, worse than, or the same as others. Each contemplation has the potential to illuminate the root causes of human suffering. The guidelines and the contemplations work together inviting investigation of direct experience.

The guidelines offer support for awakening while engaged in relationship. The challenges of human contact are met with the meditative qualities evoked by each guideline. All of the guidelines compliment each other and cultivate a capacity for balanced receptivity and presence in relationship.

Pause calls forth mindfulness; *relax*, tranquility and acceptance; *open*, relational availability and spaciousness; *trust emergence*, flexibility and letting go; *listen deeply*, receptivity and attunement; and *speak the truth*, integrity and care.

Awakening to the shared human condition through relationship manifests in this dynamic process of engaging in an intentional dialogue practice.

Patience and focus are strengthened in this process. In this experience of mutuality emerges recognition of the innate wholeness, genius, and spaciousness inherent in both/all people. The rigid and frozen sense of a separate, fixed self, a solid *I, me, mine,* can ease with greater compassion. A co-created fluidity of experience within the sharing ignites awareness of constant change, highlighting impermanence. As each individual shares personal views, struggles, and challenges, a growing sense of the unifying truth of suffering emerges. Moreover, in the vitality of the dialogue practice, one's relationship with suffering can transform into greater freedom.

Interpersonal Mindfulness in MBSR

With the time boundaries of each MBSR class session, an interpersonal meditation practice is adapted while offering a taste of the potential to practice the longer dialogue sequence. The key focus is applying mindfulness, mental stability, and the interruption of habitual stress reaction patterns in relationship. By incorporating awareness into social contacts, the participant grows more able to respond to the perceptions, longings, and aversions that can manifest in relationship with others.

Interpersonal Mindfulness Dialogue Practice

People are asked to find a partner, preferably someone whom they do not know well. This direction is intended to give the participants more freedom from a history of fixed relational views and associations, although those connections can arise in an instant of contact. Emphasizing the importance and impact of the gift each person has the potential to offer with full presence to the other, the teacher introduces the dialogue practice as a meditation. The group often expresses surprise and shifts posture with the invitation to engage in a dialogue practice as meditation. Speaking occurs only during the dialogue, and silence is maintained during pausing and between each phase of practice. As participants find partners and sit facing one another on chairs or cushions, the teacher notes that the practice has several levels of focus and will take time. One person will be speaking while the other is listening, and they will each have a turn. The meditation guideline, *pause,* is introduced as well as the direction to slow down speech and interaction to allow mindfulness to strengthen. One is invited to pause when pulled away from being fully present by distraction, judgment, impatience, strong emotions, or desires, whether one is speaking or listening. Engaging the practice of pausing allows connecting with the body, the breath, and the moment.

The teacher offers guidance about how very sensitive we are as human beings and that sitting with another with direct eye contact may be strongly stimulating. It is important to normalize this reaction and give permission to look down or away and not stare at the partner. It is suggested that people do not keep eyes closed throughout the dialogue practice. When reactions occur they can be known and met with kindness. A bell will ring to invite the speaker into silence.

After a brief pause of stillness, the listener offers what s/he heard through the partner's words and voice tone and what was seen as the speaker expressed with movements of the eyes, face, hands, and gestures.

First Dialogue

Guideline: a focus on the guideline *pause*
   Contemplation: an experience in one's current life where one experiences a challenge
   Dialogue: One speaker/one listener
   Speaker: 4 minutes
   Listener: offers back what was heard through words, voice tone, and speed and what was seen through bodily expression. (4 minutes) Partners reverse

Second Dialogue

This dialogue does not have separate speakers. It is an open, interactive practice with the invitation for both people to rest in the moment of change, speak what is true in this moment, and to listen deeply internally and to one another. It might be expressed as speaking and listening from the heart, from presence. The teacher invites the participants to pause often to strengthen mindfulness and allow the speaking to emerge from this awareness.

A bell rings to begin and end the interactive dialogue practice. The dyad partners briefly share their experiences of the practice together.

The whole class opens a discussion about learnings and challenges as they engaged with the practice.

Insight Dialogue Meditation Guidelines

The six Insight Dialogue Meditation guidelines are as follows:

- Pause: From reactivity to mindfulness.
- Relax: Allow what is perceived internally/externally in the present.
- Open: Widen the lens of awareness; wake up to the experience interconnectivity.

- Trust emergence: Abide and attend with the experience of constant change.
- Listen deeply: Recognize how meaning is carried through words, body language, and most of all, presence.
- Speak the truth: Say what is true from investigating the experience of the body, mind, and heart.

Exploring the Guidelines in MBSR

- *Pause*

The guideline *pause* is of central importance. It is the initial suggestion to step out of habit and bring mindful awareness to the moment. It is an invitation to wake up. As mindfulness, it opens the door to the present moment, to a movement from grasping to non-grasping. It interrupts the habitual pressure of pushing forward and away from what is alive in present moment experience. In Class 6 and throughout the MBSR program, this pausing and choosing to be present is encouraged. In MBSR, it is often expressed with the symbol STOP:

S: Stop and pause.
T: Take a breath; come to bodily sensations.
O: Open—widen the focus of attending; observe nonjudgmentally what is happening internally and externally.
P: Proceed, or pause again.

In the Mindfulness-Based Cognitive Therapy (MBCT) Program the guidance through the *three-minute* or *three-step breathing space* encourages this pausing into awareness and offers a spacious, nonjudgmental brief practice to reconnect with the present moment.

- *Relax*

The guideline *relax* must be held with delicacy in teaching MBSR as it often is encountered as a hoped for *outcome* of the meditation practices by class participants. Teachers clarify it is awareness that is cultivated. Within that knowing, tension, restlessness,

> **Three-Minute Breathing Space (Segal, Williams, Teasdale, 2002)**
>
> Awareness
>
> Bringing yourself into the present moment, adopting an alert yet comfortable posture, close your eyes if this is comfortable and bring your attention inward. Becoming aware of your body and the surface upon which you are sitting, draw your focus to the spine, each vertebra stacked upon the other from sacrum to skull.
>
> Now, turning your attention to your thoughts and feelings, ask "What thoughts and feelings are present right now? What bodily sensations are present?" Acknowledge your experience in this moment, even if it is unwanted.
>
> Gathering
>
> Now, gently direct your awareness to your breathing, following each inbreath and each outbreath.
>
> Expanding
>
> Now, expanding your awareness to the whole body, imagine that you are breathing with the body as a whole, including your posture and facial expression. When you're ready, open your eyes and return to your activities.

pleasant, and unpleasantness may be perceived. Teachers can then underscore that ease and relaxation may be an effect or by-product of the practice, but clinging tightly to the *wish* for relaxation is counterproductive. The Insight Dialogue guideline *relax* points to the ability to allow what is present as one becomes aware of what is experienced. Within the pause, agitation is often revealed, a desire for life to be different from the way it is in the moment, and resistance may be felt in the body and mind. With the guidance of *relax*, support is offered to dwell with what is. Greater tranquility, kindness, and steadiness to tolerate reactivity are cultivated with the guideline, *relax*. The words of poet Danna Faulds express this practice powerfully.

Allow
There is no controlling life.
Try corralling a lightning bolt,
containing a tornado. Dam a
stream and it will create a new
channel. Resist, and the tide
will sweep you off your feet.
Allow, and grace will carry
you to higher ground. The only
safety lies in letting it all in –
the wild and the weak; fear,
fantasies, failures and success.
When loss rips off the doors of
the heart, or sadness veils your
vision with despair, practice
becomes simply bearing the truth.
In the choice to let go of your
Known way of being, the whole
world is revealed to your new eyes.
                              Danna Faulds 2002

• *Open*

Pause and *relax* establish mindfulness and tranquility. In *pause,* the freshness of the beginner's mind is welcomed as awareness of the body, emotions, and thoughts are met with curiosity. *Relax* cultivates acceptance, receptivity, and kindness. The guideline *open* relates to a flexibility of the scope of focus: opening awareness internally and externally and widening to others and to the spaciousness available within the breath, the whole body, and environment. This opening can deepen acceptance and the ability to hold discomfort in a wider field without rejecting the unwanted. This guidance strengthens a pliable mind state vital in all meditation practice. Within interpersonal meditation practice, the guideline, *open*, can be liberating, as it softens the rigid definitions and boundaries between self and others. This process is beautifully expressed in the poem by Wendy Egyoku Nakao (1992):

May we open to a deeper understanding
And a genuine love and caring
For the multitude of faces
Who are none other than ourself.

- *Trust Emergence*

This guideline reveals the ever-changing moment; in fact, it directly explores impermanence. In the moment of interpersonal contact, much is vibrating with constant change. Thoughts, emotions, and bodily sensations are streaming, if not expressed. Here, impermanence becomes the object of practice. Creativity flourishes in the flow of not knowing, surprise, and change. The courage to pause and trust the reality of emergence allows greater ease and the ability to step out the habit-driven pulse to keep talking, say something clever, predict what the other will say, or plan our response. Change is reliable! It can be rested in and known directly with this meditation guideline.

- *Listen Deeply*

Meditation itself has been referred to as deep listening—an attuning with one's direct experience. With the guideline *listen deeply*, the ability to cultivate tranquility while being present with one's self and another creates conditions for the generosity of offering full attentiveness to what is being expressed internally and externally. The listener pauses into steady presence, absorbing the details of the exchange. *Listen deeply* encourages a listening with the ears and eyes. One becomes aware of the nuances of communication as the body expresses through facial and hand movements, and words are used to explicate experience.

- *Speak the Truth*

This guideline takes the support of all the others, to pause in awareness, and allow what is known: to open to the space of mutuality and trust the emergence of constant change as well as the practice of listening deeply to oneself and others. To speak the truth, one must pause and connect with one's experience, feel into the body, and sense what is emerging as true expression. Qualities of wise speech are pillars of this guideline: truthfulness, sensitivity, patience, courage, non-harming, and trust all offer support. To speak the truth, one must connect deeply to know what is the subjective truth in the moment. Clarity is needed to select words that express the meaning one wants to convey.

Insight Dialogue invites the meditator to pause and allow words to rise from greater silence. The Indian philosophy, Kashmir Shaivism (Brooks et al., 1997), describes speech as existing on multiple levels of expression. The levels are as follows:

- *Vaikharī vāk*—spoken word, exterior
- *Madhyamā vāk*—mental speech, interior
- *Paśyantī vāk*—pure intuition, pre-speech
- *Parāvāk*—silence, unity, freedom

This articulation of levels of speech offers another framework to engage with the invitation to "meditate together, speak from silence." Engaging the guidance of speaking the truth, pausing allows a deeper inquiry into listening deeply to the emergence of words, thoughts, and body sense as well as the presence of stillness while with another person.

Beyond the MBSR Course: Extended Insight Dialogue and Interpersonal Mindfulness Practice

A sample of a longer practice is described below to express the larger context of the depth and intention of the ID/IMP practice. It is strongly suggested that teachers regularly attend Insight Dialogue retreats to fully experience and comprehend the potential freedom of the practice.

- Guidelines: All have been introduced; all are engaged in the practice.
- Contemplation: The hungers
- Speaker/Listener
- 5 minutes each and 5 minutes shared dialogue with each other.

After people have settled in with their partners, the teacher introduces the contemplation, expressing that choosing to be awake in life involves recognizing the difficulty, challenge, and stress present in all lives. Interpersonally, stress manifests with the unpleasant aspects of every relationship; the cause of such stress is wanting the relationship to be different from the way it is. There is a push to have control, to "have it our way," which causes tension, resistance, and pain. The wanting can manifest in three main ways:

- The hunger for interpersonal pleasure and the avoidance of interpersonal pain
- The hunger to be seen or acknowledged interpersonally
- The hunger to escape, to be invisible, not to engage with others, or to avoid intimacy

With introduction of the exploration of these hungers, it is important to include balance. These hungers are not to be judged, but are known simply as the dynamics of being human. They may have natural, wholesome expressions as well as be a cause of pain and stress. Acknowledging the experience of these patterns offers a deeper sense of self-knowing that can provide access to greater ease.

First Contemplation: The Interpersonal Hunger for Pleasure and the Avoidance of Pain

Teacher: "Where do you experience this longing for interpersonal pleasure in your life? How does it manifest? As you explore these questions, you may become aware of the longing for interpersonal pleasure with your partner, right now. You can meet this longing with gentle awareness. It is normal for us to enjoy one another's company. But, perhaps you have noticed times when you felt lonely and kept trying to reach a friend—any friend—with whom to talk. At these times, something else is going on. We are using this longing as a strategy to escape the unpleasant experience of being alone. Many people check Facebook several times a day to see whether people have responded to their recent posts. Allow yourself to take the support of the practice and your meditation partner. *Engage the guidelines: Pause, Relax, Open, Trust Emergence, Listen Deeply, Speak the Truth.*"

Speaker and listener reverse roles.
Intersperse each dialogue with a pause invited with a bell.
Dyad engages in open dialogue.
Pause into silence.

Second Contemplation: The Hunger to Be Seen

Teacher: "The hunger to be seen, acknowledged, and approved of, is natural, and yet it can compel our actions. To depend on approval from others is a way to fill a need to feel valued from outside our selves. Where do you long for this approval? How do you recognize this at home, with your family and at work? Do you hope for this approval from your community?"

"Some of our activities hinge on this longing to be approved of, to be appreciated and admired. It is the drive beneath the actions that traps us. A teenager who acted in every high school play said that she was really longing to be seen by her parents. Since this goal did not happen at home, she performed so that they would applaud with the others in the audience. This longing is a hunger to be seen. Some people may make donations as long as large plaques with their names are prominently displayed. The actual action may be beneficial, but the urge for recognition comes from a sense of separation. As you engage in practice now, approach with gentleness, and rest in the meditation guidelines: *Pause, Relax, Open, Trust Emergence, Listen Deeply, Speak the Truth.*"

Speaker and listener reverse roles.
Intersperse each dialogue with a pause invited with a bell.
Dyad engages in open dialogue.
Pause into silence.

Third Contemplation: The Hunger Not to Be Seen

Teacher: "This is the hunger to disappear, to escape interaction and engagement with others. It manifests in all of the ways we hide. Feelings of shame, unworthiness, and addictive withdrawal are ways of not being seen. There are times we choose to be alone, to have the solace of solitude. This is not that, but a driven desire to get out, to not be and to be invisible. There was a Broadway play called: 'Stop the World, I want to Get Off.' This expresses this longing to get out and avoid contact with others. With gentleness and care, explore the ways you want to hide and to avoid intimacy and intensity with others in your family and at work. Speak your truth and listen deeply, resting in the guidelines of *pausing, allowing, opening and trusting emergence.* "

Speaker and listener reverse roles.
Intersperse each dialogue with a pause invited with a bell.
Dyad engages in open dialogue.
Pause into silence.

Closing Interpersonal Meditation Practice

The whole group engages in dialogue about their experience of the practice reflecting on the guidelines, the contemplations, the hungers, compassion, and meeting the moment as it arises. People share that they identified the desires for being seen from wearing flashy clothes, to being the joker in school. They share becoming more awake to their craving to not be alone by joining several community projects or the desire to escape interactions with others through isolation. Pausing allows more awareness, and allowing gives the strength to be with the urges as they manifest. Opening creates space and invites a larger sense of being. The group engages in the dialogue with stillness and spontaneity.

Close with a loving kindness meditation.

Immensity, Intimacy, and Immediacy

The whole of MBSR may be seen as a vehicle with the potential to support a person in becoming more intimate with one's immediate unfolding life, and in so doing, perhaps touch the radiant immensity that interpenetrates and is far beyond the contracted construction of "me." Through relationship "me" is most firmly defined. Through relationship and kinship of community, the limited separateness of "me" can begin to unbind. MBSR is a relationship-based learning that encourages knowing oneself in relationship with one's body, opinions, thoughts, emotions, pain and suffering, values and ethics, and ease and connection. This wonder of *being with* extends to being with others. In this process, one can discover the be-longing to being human and the collective wisdom that is available in mutuality. Through the 8-week program, the intimacy with self expands to intimacy with others. People who would not imagine being friends socially, become strong meditation partners. Truths are spoken within a structure of practice that cultivates safety. In this way, intimacy is constructed over the 8 weeks, from shared time, learning, and discipline; it is also unconstructed, with anonymity and the freedom of rarely having historical views of classmates, as well as the ongoing cultivation of freshness of the beginner's mind. The MBSR program has the potential to develop into a transformational field as the group deepens with regular mindfulness practice. Alone and together, participants grow and refine their enthusiasm and energy to engage mindfulness, concentration, investigation, equanimity, joy, and compassion. Aware relationship becomes a force of resonance and freedom. The Buddha taught that good friends are essential to waking up and engaging with the path to freedom (Ghosa Suttas: Voice (AN 2.125-126), translated from the Pali by Thanissaro Bhikkhu. Access to Insight (Legacy Edition), & 30 November, 2013). He named two elements essential in establishing clear seeing or right view: the voice of another and wise attention. Throughout the fabric of the experience of the MBSR program, these two elements form the warp and weave.

References

Albion, M. W. (2013). *The quotable Eleanor Roosevelt*. Orlando, FL: University of Florida Press.

Angelou, M. (2014). *Interview in 1985*. Time Magazine.

Brooks, D., et al. (1997). *Meditation revolution: A history and theology of the Siddha yoga lineage*. New York: Agama Press.

Buber, M. (1970). *I and thou* (p. 15). New York, NY: Charles Scribner's Sons.

Danna, F. (2002). *Go in and in*. Greenville, VA: Peaceable Kingdom Books.

Egyo, W. (1992). The ten directions, Zen Center of Los Angeles Journal.

Ghosa Suttas: Voice (AN 2.125-126), translated from the Pali by Thanissaro Bhikkhu. Access to Insight (Legacy Edition), 30 November 2013. Retrieved from http://www.accesstoinsight.org/tipitaka/an/an02/an02.125-126.than.html.

Kabat-Zinn, J. (2013). *Full catastrophe living: Using the wisdom of your body and mind to face stress, pain and illness* (2nd ed., p. 171). New York: Bantam Books—A Penguin Random Company.

Kramer, G. (2007). *Insight dialogue, the interpersonal path to freedom*. Boston: Shambala.

Macy, J. (2007). *World as lover, world as self*. Berkeley: Parallax Press.

Metzger, D. (1992). *Writing for your life—A guide and companion to the inner worlds*. New York, NY: Harper Collins.

Segal, Z. V., Williams, J. M. G., & Teasdale, J. D. (2002). *Mindfulness-based cognitive therapy for depression: A new approach to preventing relapse*. New York: Guilford Press.

Siegel, D. (2007). *The mindful brain-reflection and attunement in the cultivation of well-being* (p. 129). New York, NY: W.W. Norton & Co.

Stevens, J. (1987). *Abundant peace, the biography of Morihei Ueshiba*. Boston: Shambala.

Thich Nhat Hahn (2012). M. McLeod (Ed.). *The pocket Thich Nhat Hahn*. Boston: Shambala.

Walpola, R. (1959). *What the Buddha taught*. New York: Grove Press.

Chapter 5
Scientific Literacy as a Foundational Competency for Teachers of Mindfulness-based Interventions

Willoughby B. Britton

Introduction: Standards of Excellence

Maintaining the highest standards of excellence among MBI teachers is one of the most pressing issues of the field (McCown, Reibel, & Micozzi, 2017). Well-delineated MBI teacher excellence criteria include sustained and ongoing personal mindfulness practices, knowledge of Buddhist maps, and a wide range of definitions and discourses about mindfulness (Kabat-Zinn, 2011a, 2011b; Kabat-Zinn et al., 2014; McCown et al., 2010). This chapter addresses another dimension of teacher excellence, a foundational scientific literacy for MBI teachers which includes:

- An understanding of the interdependence of MBIs and scientific research
- A foundational knowledge of the science of meditation
- Practical methods to integrate science-based didactic material into the MBI curriculum
- Skills for evaluating the ever-changing evidence base of scientific research
- Evidence-based practice beyond the classroom

W.B. Britton, Ph.D. (✉)
Department of Psychiatry and Human Behavior, Brown University Medical School, Providence, RI 02906, USA

Department of Behavioral and Social Sciences, Brown University School of Public Health, 185 Brown Street, Providence, RI 02906, USA
e-mail: willoughby_britton@brown.edu

© Springer International Publishing Switzerland 2016   93
D. McCown et al., *Resources for Teaching Mindfulness*,
DOI 10.1007/978-3-319-30100-6_5

The Interdependence of MBIs and Scientific Research

The success of MBIs in gaining a foothold in mainstream medicine has been largely due to the close coupling of MBIs with scientific research and the establishment of MBSR as an "evidence-based treatment" (Dryden & Still, 2006). The continued success of MBIs in maintaining credibility and continued traction with public institutions will depend in part on the ongoing partnership with scientific and empirical investigation. One side of this partnership includes academic scientists who conduct research on the effects of meditative practices, which help establish MBIs as evidence-based treatments. On the other side of the partnership are the MBI teachers—clinicians and educators. MBI teachers uphold their end of the partnership by engaging in evidence-based practice (EBP) (Spring, 2007), which includes ongoing knowledge and implementation of the scientific research in the field. Scientific literacy and EBP are especially important for MBI teachers as "stewards" or protectors of MBI longevity. Teacher literacy can protect against the formation of a "scientist–practitioner gap," which is a well-known prognostic indicator of loss of public trust in a treatment (Tavris, 2003). MBI teachers are key in maintaining public trust, as they have the most direct interface with the public and are therefore the most immediate representatives of MBIs.

Basic Foundations in the Science of Meditation

Science-Based Homiletics in MBIs

As a general principle, MBI teachers draw from a deep well of experience and knowledge to weave teaching points into participants' ongoing experiences. An equally deep, lived, and embodied experiential understanding of the various scientific concepts, models, and research findings allows MBI teachers to weave the scientific or didactic pieces seamlessly into the curriculum. These models are essentially about experience and about the very topics that are explored in practice: attention and distraction, thinking, emotions, and motivations. Didactic material can be sprinkled throughout the curriculum in many forms, ranging from handouts, videos, slides, and exercises to spontaneous responses to participants' ongoing experience. But again, when these models are ingrained in the teachers' understanding of experience, the information flows naturally. Of course, as with depth of practice, or knowledge of maps, scientific literacy is a lifelong learning skill and requires commitment as well as guidance and support, of which this chapter and book provide first steps.

Weaving science into the MBI curriculum serves the multilayered purpose of creating a universal language and framework of understanding and enhancing credibility, confidence, and trust in the programs, which in turn translates into enhancing motivation to practice.

The chapter addresses these topics roughly in the order that they might appear in an 8-week program, accompanied by supplemental material that can be found at the end of this chapter.

Science as a universal language. Since the people receiving MBIs represent a range of worldviews, religions, cultures, and subcultures with different languages and metaphors, finding a common framework is a central challenge. Since the practice of science is an international endeavor with some common language, the language of science, particularly biology and neuroscience, can serve as a unifying framework to describe experience. Indeed, once scientific language is introduced, participants readily adapt it to describe their experiences, for example, "the sympathetic nervous system is on overdrive today," or "the amygdala is causing a negative bias in both attention and memory."

Neuroplasticity. Experience-dependent neuroplasticity means that our brains change with experience and practice, which has radical and inspiring implications for MBI participants. Rather than being fixed entities with unchangeable traits and behaviors, our brains and psychological tendencies are actually quite malleable. Just as exercise and training strengthens physical muscles, mental habits construct and become entrenched in corresponding brain networks. For example, neural networks related to spatial processing grow in taxi drivers as they develop interior maps of city streets (Maguire, Woollett, & Spiers, 2006). Other corresponding networks change in response to playing music (Rodrigues, Loureiro, & Paulo Caramelli, 2010) or juggling (Draganski et al., 2004). Whether we know it or not, we are *always* practicing something, so *choosing* what qualities or abilities to cultivate and which ones to weaken or abandon is a fundamental principle of contemplative practices.

This principle of intentional neuroplasticity is worth bringing up in the first class, as a "meta-framework" for the entire course. It may be as simple as just saying "you get good at what you practice" and then asking, "What are you practicing or cultivating? Is that something you want to grow and strengthen?" This kind of inquiry can bring awareness to participants' intentions and values, while simultaneously generating motivation to notice and stop actively reinforcing unskillful habits.

Resources for Neuroplasticity

TED Talk; http://www.ted.com/tedx/events/2672

Motivation to practice: mindfulness as an investment. Participant motivations and expectations are addressed explicitly in the first class under the question of "What brought you here?" Expectations and motivations to practice are inextricably tied, but not always beneficially. If participants have high hopes for fast results, violations of these expectations may undermine their confidence and lead to drop out (Sears & Stanton, 2001). Of course, fast effects are unlikely, and premature attrition can be thwarted by orienting toward mindfulness practice as a form of self-care and an investment in well-being. For example, the teacher might say:

> When you go to the gym to lose weight or build muscle, we don't do a couple pushups or sit-ups, then immediately check to see if our arms are bigger, or our bellies are flatter. We know that it takes time and repetition. We may not feel anything right away, but that doesn't mean that it's not changing us. Mindfulness is the same way. It's fine to have hopes and goals of what benefits the practice might have, but I recommend checking in with those hopes at the end of the program and not to gauge your progress by how you feel during each meditation session. Sitting on the cushion once a day is like doing your push ups: you do it for long-term benefits.

Motivation to practice: frequency and duration. By the second class, many MBSR/CT participants report difficulty fitting in the 45 minutes per day of home practice into their busy lives. They ask if they can split up the meditations into smaller bits rather than one 45-minutes block to better fit into their schedules. The truth is that *no one knows what pattern of practice will yield the best outcomes*. However, there is some evidence that practicing less than the prescribed 45 minutes per day can still yield psychological benefits (Jain et al., 2007; Reibel, Greeson, Brainard, & Rosenzweig, 2001) and even changes in physiology (Davidson, Irwin, Anderle, & Kalin, 2003, Davidson et al., 2003). In addition, another study in drug-abusing adolescents found that more frequent short sessions were more powerful than the same total duration in a single session (Britton et al., 2010). Teens who practiced as little as 5–10 minutes per day 2–3 days per week increased their total sleep time by more than an hour per night compared to teens that just came to class but did not practice at home. Furthermore, the frequency, but *not* the duration, of practice was correlated with improvements in sleep. Participants report that knowing that even 5 minutes could make a difference encouraged them to practice every day, so I make sure to report this study on the second class, in the handouts, and also mention that "daily practice is more important than finishing the recording" at the beginning of each meditation recording.

Stress Physiology and Neurobiological Models of Meditation

MBIs typically include educating participants about stress physiology as well as the various neurobiological models of how meditation may be helpful to their specific conditions. There are many neurobiological models of how meditation might work to alleviate distress and promote well-being. Many Buddhist (Goleman, 1984; Grabovac, Lau, & Willet, 2011) and Hindu (Travis, 2014) models of meditation are in use, and many participants may be open to them. But they may also be unpalatable to the 90 % of Americans or Europeans who currently identify as either Christian or nonreligious (Lugo, 2012), as well as to the mainstream scientific establishment and public institutions that legally cannot support activities which promote religious frameworks (Wilson & Drakeman, 2003). Thus, in order to be consistent with both EBP and a "wholly secular" approach recommended by the Center for Mindfulness (Kabat-Zinn et al., 2014), MBI teachers can use biological models that are not only universally palatable but also empirically supported by, and in active use, within mainstream neuroscience and medicine.

Considering the above concerns, the hypo-frontality model can be a good choice when teaching MBSR/CT because it (1) is fairly easy to understand and weave into the ongoing experience of the participants, (2) can be delivered in a short amount of time, (3) has broad applicability to a wide range of different populations with different complaints, and (4) is well-supported by ongoing mainstream clinical neuroscience research, i.e., it is consistent with evidence-based practice.

The hypo-frontality model. Very simply put, the hypo-frontality model posits that a wide range of psychological and physiological symptoms can result from an underactive prefrontal cortex (PFC), and that these symptoms can be addressed through strengthening the PFC. The metaphors of "brain training" or "mental fitness" or other references to weight lifting, or going to the gym, can bridge both the principle of neuroplasticity and the hypo-frontality model.

Hypofrontality and the Neuroanatomy of Suffering

The prefrontal cortex. The PFC is an area of the brain, located just behind the forehead, that underlies a wide range of complex functions, including thinking, planning, and control of behavior (Miller & Cohen, 2001). One of the most commonly discussed functions of the PFC is executive functioning (EF) which includes different aspects of types of self-control and self-regulation, especially around attention and action (Wood & Smith, 2008).

As part of its regulatory role, the PFC is responsible for modulating three other brain systems: the limbic system, the default mode network (DMN), and the brain reward system. If the PFC is underactive, then the system that it is supposed to regulate becomes "disinhibited" or out of control, leading to a number of different problems, including depression (Baxter et al., 1989; Bench, Friston, Brown, Frackowiak, & Dolan, 1993), bipolar disorder (Blumberg et al., 2004; Clark, Iversen, & Goodwin, 2002; Meyer et al., 2004), obsessive compulsive disorder (van den Heuvel et al., 2005), schizophrenia (Carter et al., 1998; MacDonald et al., 2005), and addiction (Goldstein et al., 2009; Hester & Garavan, 2004).

The limbic system. The limbic system is a set of interconnected brain areas that include the hippocampus, amygdala, and nucleus accumbens (NAC) (among others). These areas are involved in memory, emotion, motivation, and reward (Morgane, Galler, & Mokler, 2005). The amygdala, which is involved in detecting emotional salience, particularly threat, is tightly coupled with the endocrine and sympathetic nervous systems involved in the "fight or flight" response and therefore is often associated with the bodily expression of emotional reactions (Davidson, Jackson, & Kalin, 2000). A pounding heart, a sinking feeling, a rush of anger, a feeling of being frozen with fear, all of these common expressions are examples of the limbic and sympathetic nervous systems activating.

The PFC exerts inhibitory control on limbic structures such as the amygdala (Davidson et al., 2000; Ochsner & Gross, 2005). Lack of such inhibitory control results in a hyperactive amygdala (Siegle, Steinhauer, Thase, Stenger, & Carter, 2002; Siegle, Thompson, Carter, Steinhauer, & Thase, 2007) and an associated increase in emotional reactivity and sympathetic hyperarousal commonly seen in anxiety, depression, and other kinds of disorders with high levels of negative emotions (Baxter et al., 1989; Clark et al., 2002; Mayberg et al., 1999). Participants will be experientially very familiar and probably quite distressed with signs and symptoms of both acute and chronic sympathetic nervous system hyperactivity (see handout at end of chapter), so reframing these experiences as the impersonal consequences of the stress response can be a relief.

The default mode network. The DMN is a network of midline brain structures that are active during "rest" or when the brain is not otherwise engaged and is thought to be involved in self-referential thought and mind wandering (Qin & Northoff, 2011). The DMN is responsible for a self-narrative, "the story of me" (Gallagher, 2000), and other forms of social cognition, like imagining what other people are thinking or feeling (Schilbach, Eickhoff, Rotarska-Jagiela, Fink, & Vogeley, 2008). While some degree of self-narrative and social cognition promotes cohesion and functioning, often the stories we tell about ourselves or imagine that other people are telling about us are excessively critical, negative, or excessive. Therefore, a default mode that is overactive because it is insufficiently regulated by the PFC can be associated with distress, anxiety, rumination, and depression (Buckner & Vincent, 2007; Farb et al., 2007; Gentili et al., 2009; Hamilton et al., 2011; Sheline et al., 2009; Whitfield-Gabrieli et al., 2009). The handout "Two Arrows" (found at end of chapter) shows the difference between simple pain or loss (i.e., first arrow) and the default mode's contribution of unnecessary, negative, evaluative, self-referential rumination, or worry about the first arrow (i.e., the second arrow).

The brain reward system and addiction. Structures in the limbic system, DMN, and the mesolimbic dopamine system including the ventral tegmental area (VTA) and NAC together comprise the brain reward system, which is also regulated by the PFC (Feil et al., 2010). Poor prefrontal control over the brain reward system is associated with a number of features of addiction, including impulsivity, compulsivity, risk taking, impaired self-monitoring, "denial" of illness, and attentional biases toward substance or reward-related stimuli (Goldstein & Volkow, 2011).

Cognitive and emotional biases. Poor prefrontal control and an overactive amygdala can cause biases in attention and memory away from positive stimuli and toward negative stimuli which are a common feature of both anxiety and depression (Disner, Beevers, Haigh, & Beck, 2011). Conversely, poor PFC control over the brain reward system is associated with biases toward positive or rewarding stimuli that are linked to compulsive action and addictions (Garland, Froeliger, Passik, & Howard, 2013). Similar to the computerized therapy called "Cognitive Bias Modification" (Hoppitt, Mathews, Yiend, & Mackintosh, 2010), a few studies suggest that mindfulness training may improve distress by decreasing cognitive biases and contributing toward a more "evenhanded attention" (Alberts & Thewissen, 2011; Roberts-Wolfe, Sacchet, Hastings, Roth, & Britton, 2012; Vago & Nakamura, 2011).

Everyone has cognitive biases and may be unaware, although consistently "half-full" or "half-empty" tendencies may be very apparent to others. Because unconscious attentional biases occur early in sensory processing, they are not always addressed by instructions to attend to "whatever is happening." Exercises that deliberately investigate cognitive biases empower participants to identify their own patterns of biases and to tailor their practices toward a more balanced and evenhanded awareness. For example, individuals with a negative bias may benefit from learning to notice pleasant events and sensations, while individuals with a positive bias may benefit from touching into unpleasant or painful parts of experience that have been avoided. The topic of cognitive biases arises naturally when discussing the pleasant and unpleasant event calendars, or in group discussions of experiences arising out of MBI meditation practices more generally.

Evidence Base for MBIs

Rationale for cognitive training of the PFC. Positive responses to both pharmacological and behavioral treatments involve restoration of PFC functioning (Davidson, Irwin, et al., 2003, Davidson, Kabat-Zinn, et al., 2003; Hugdahl et al., 2007; Liotti & Mayberg, 2001; Liotti, Mayberg, McGinnis, Brannan, & Jerabek, 2002). In adults, restoration of the PFC can be achieved through cognitive training. Many clinical neuroscientists use neurocognitive exercises derived from neuropsychological tasks to strengthen the PFC and subsequently improve emotion regulation and dysfunction that are associated with PFC impairment. For example, Penades et al. (2006) employed multicomponent attention training in schizophrenic patients and found improved performance on PFC-dependent tasks and decreased hypo-frontality and psychological distress. Similarly, Siegle, Ghinassi, and Thase (2007) used two types of focused attention tasks to increase prefrontal functioning and mood disturbance in unipolar depression. Papageorgiou and Wells (2000) found that PFC-dependent attention training improved depressive symptomatology, emotion regulation, and normalized hypoactivation of the PFC and hyperactivation of the amygdala.

Meditation strengthens the PFC. The heterogeneous family of mental training techniques known as collectively as "meditation" can be viewed as neurocognitive training that is aimed at increasing prefrontal cognitive control and increasing affective regulation and emotional well-being. Many studies in adults have found that meditation practices increase activation of the PFC; decrease limbic and default mode activity; improve attention, emotional reactivity, and rumination; and help to alleviate addiction and mood disorders. Buddhist-derived meditation practices have been found to be associated with increased activity in the dorsolateral PFC (Allen et al., 2012; Baerentsen, 2001; Baron Short et al., 2010; Brefczynski-Lewis, Lutz, Schaefer, Levinson, & Davidson, 2007; Farb et al., 2007, 2010; Hasenkamp, Wilson-Mendenhall, Duncan, & Barsalou, 2012; Ritskes, Ritskes-Hoitinga, Stodkilde-Jorgensen, Baerntsen, & Hartman, 2003) and larger frontal gray matter volumes (Holzel et al., 2008; Lazar et al., 2005; Luders, Toga, Lepore, & Gaser, 2009).

Attention and executive function. More than a dozen controlled studies have assessed the effects of MBIs on objectively measured cognitive abilities such as attention and memory (Chiesa, Calati, & Serretti, 2011). Most RCTs found positive effects of MBIs on PFC-mediated cognitive abilities (Hargus, Crane, Barnhofer, &

Williams, 2010; Ortner, Kilner, & Zelazo, 2007; Wenk-Sormaz, 2005; Williams, Teasdale, Segal, & Soulsby, 2000), while a few found no improvements (Anderson, Lau, Segal, & Bishop, 2007; MacCoon, MacLean, Davidson, Saron, & Lutz, 2014). Similar (mixed) conclusions can be found in recent reviews of meditation for improving cognition in aging (Gard, Holzel, & Lazar, 2014) or cognitive decline in the context of neurodegenerative conditions (Marciniak et al., 2014).

Amygdala. A number of studies have found decreased amygdala response or activation following different forms of meditation (Brefczynski-Lewis et al., 2007; Desbordes et al., 2012; Farb et al., 2007; Holzel et al., 2010; Taylor et al., 2011).

Default mode network. Multiple studies have found that various forms of meditation training are associated with decreased DMN activity (Baerentsen, 2001; Baerentsen et al., 2009; Berkovich-Ohana, Glicksohn, & Goldstein, 2012; Brewer et al., 2011; Farb et al., 2007, 2010; Goldin, Ramel, & Gross, 2009; Hasenkamp et al., 2012; Taylor et al., 2011; Travis et al., 2010), although other studies have found increased DMN activity (Goldin & Gross, 2010; Goldin et al., 2009, Goldin, Ziv, Jazaieri, & Gross, 2012; Hölzel et al., 2011).

Sympathetic nervous system hyperarousal. A number of studies using various meditation practices have found decreased sympathetic hyperarousal in meditators (Barnes, Treiber, & Davis, 2001; Carlson, Speca, Faris, & Patel, 2007; Maclean et al., 1994; Ortner et al., 2007; Sudsuang, Chentanez, & Veluvan, 1991; Tang et al., 2007), but increases in arousal have also been reported (Britton, Haynes, Fridel, & Bootzin, 2010; Creswell, Pacilio, Lindsay, & Brown, 2014; Holmes, 1984).

Emotional reactivity. In adults, a number of studies have suggested a relationship between mindfulness and reduced emotional and stress reactivity, including attenuated emotional responses to threatening situations or faster recovery from transient negative affect (Arch & Craske, 2006; Brewer et al., 2009; Britton, Shahar, Szepsenwol, & Jacobs, 2012; Broderick, 2005; Campbell-Sills, Barlow, Brown, & Hofmann, 2006; Erisman & Roemer, 2010; Goldin & Gross, 2010; Kuehner, Huffziger, & Liebsch, 2009; Ortner et al., 2007).

Anxiety and depression. Several meta-analyses of mindfulness meditation in adults have found overall support for the claim that mindfulness training can lead to decreased levels of negative affect, anxiety, and depression (Goyal et al., 2014; Hofmann, Sawyer, Witt, & Oh, 2010), with similar (medium) effect sizes to other treatments (AHRQ, 2012). For individuals with clinically diagnosed anxiety or depression, one recent meta-analysis found that MBIs, particularly MBCT, could be beneficial for major depression, but cautioned against using MBIs as a first-line treatment for anxiety disorders (Strauss, Cavanagh, Oliver, & Pettman, 2014).

Addiction. Findings that mindfulness may enhance prefrontal control over the limbic system, DMN and reward systems have strong implications for the use of mindfulness to treat addictions (Brewer, Elwafi, & Davis, 2013; Witkiewitz et al., 2014). However, as recently as 2009, conclusive data for mindfulness as a treatment for addiction was deemed "lacking" (Zgierska et al., 2009). A more recent meta-analysis of a handful of randomized controlled trials yielded slightly more positive results and suggested that MBIs that are specifically tailored for use in addictions are superior to nonspecific programs. For example, mindfulness-based relapse prevention (MBPRP) was found to perform as well or better than standard treatments or 12-step programs (Bowen et al., 2014), while MBSR can sometimes be equivalent to no treatment (Alterman, Koppenhaver, Mulholland, Ladden, & Baime, 2004) or "be slightly less efficacious in comparison with established treatments such as CBT" (Chiesa & Serretti, 2014, p. 506). Chiesa and Serretti (2014) also note that "it is unclear, however, to what extent these null findings are related to the ineffectiveness of the intervention for the condition under investigation, or simply to methodological shortcomings" (p. 506).

Making Your Own Evidence-Based Models

The hypo-frontality model and related exercises comprise just one example of many possible evidence-based models (Brown, Creswell, & Ryan, 2015; Holzel et al., 2011). MBI teachers can use the scientific research base in any number of ways that may serve as a foundation for both their didactic material specifically and their EBP more generally. However, the prospect of engaging with the science of meditation can be daunting. An endless procession of studies reports a dizzying array of findings and claims, some circulated and often exaggerated in the media and others overlooked but important. How can we possibly evaluate the validity of these claims? Where do we even start? The next section is aimed at developing skills for evaluating scientific research, so that all dimensions of practice are both informed and evidence based.

Reliable and unreliable sources of information. Not all sources of information are reliable. Popular press articles, magazines, newspapers, and webpages are not valid sources of information. Trade books or book chapters are not peer reviewed and are generally not considered empirical sources, unless they are aggregations of referenced, peer-reviewed journal articles. However, there are many scholarly books and handbooks that can be reliable sources of information. Look for edited volumes, especially by academic presses, or look in the Appendix for a list of recommendations. In general, valid claims are accompanied by a reference to the original peer-reviewed journal article, so readers (or participants) can always check for themselves.

Types of research studies. There are many different types of meditation studies, and different types of studies are associated with different levels of evidence. The following section describes each type of study and the corresponding level of evidence or types of claims that can be supported by each.

Cross-sectional studies. When meditators are compared to non-meditators on a given outcome like attention or well-being, the study design is called "cross-sectional" or "case–control." The meditators already know how to meditate, so meditation training is not part of the study, nor can these studies be "blinded" in the traditional sense. Instead, this type of design assumes that whatever differences are found between the meditators and non-meditators are due to meditation. These types of studies are easy and less expensive to employ because they don't require multi-week classes or repeated measurements. While cross-sectional studies can often provide exciting initial hypotheses about potential effects of meditation, these studies are considered low in terms of evidence. It is impossible to know whether the differences between groups are really due to meditation, rather than some other associated factor that happens to be different between meditators and non-meditators. For example, if a study found that meditators were generally healthier than non-meditators, were less obese, and had lower blood pressure, it would be tempting to conclude that meditation makes people healthy. But it may also be what epidemiologists call the "healthy volunteer effect," that health-conscious people tend to eat more vegetables, exercise more, and better manage stress with meditation; therefore the effects are really due to a preexisting health conscientiousness rather than the meditation practice per se. Thus, when you see claims from a cross-sectional study, take them with several grains of salt.

A second issue with cross-sectional studies is that they often involve differences that may not generalize to the effects of MBIs. For example, many cross-sectional studies involve experienced meditators with more than 10 or 20 years of experience. Research suggests that the effects of meditation practice may differ dramatically depending on the stage and type of practice (Britton, Lindahl, Cahn, Davis, & Goldman, 2014), and caution should be exercised in implying that such effects are generally readily available to all MBI participants. For example, while studies of experienced meditators have found positive effects on experimentally induced pain intensity (Grant, 2014), MBIs have not been found to improve pain ratings (Chiesa & Serretti, 2011; Rajguru et al., 2014). Furthermore, expert practitioners in cross-sectional studies are often trained in contemplative systems that differ substantially from MBIs. In the past, it has been a common practice to draw from a wide range of available research on contemplative practices to promote the scientific credibility of MBIs. Citations often included interchangeable references to Hindu-based meditations like TM and the Relaxation Response, Zen, Vipassana, yoga, Qigong and Tai chi, mindfulness self-report scales, and the effects of a brief (20 minutes) mindfulness session. However, the research has progressed enough to begin to differentiate these different approaches, allowing us to be more precise and accurate in both our knowledge base and our pedagogy.

Mindfulness scales and correlation studies. Mindfulness self-report questionnaires are purported to reflect changes associated with formal meditation practices. However, one may find studies that claim "mindfulness is associated with …" greater well-being, brain changes, empathy, or any number of scientific findings. But if you look more closely at the method sections of such papers, you might discover that the study did not actually investigate any type of meditation practice at all. Instead, a group of people, often college students, completed a paper and pencil scale and their score on that survey is called "mindfulness." While there are many different "mindfulness" scales, they are often measuring different constructs that are not correlated with each other or consistently correlated with meditation practice (Bergomi, Tschacher, & Kupper, 2013). Beware of making any statements about the effects of mindfulness meditation based on "mindfulness" studies that use mindfulness scales without any associated meditation practice.

Longitudinal studies. A better but more burdensome alternative is a longitudinal study, which takes measures both before and after a set of individuals learns to meditate. There are many different types of longitudinal studies, each with its own level of rigor or ability to provide evidence.

Pre-post designs. These studies assess the effects of a meditation course, like MBSR, by comparing the score a person has before they start meditating to the one they have at the end of the class. This approach seems like a straightforward way to assess the effect of meditation, but it isn't. Just deciding (intending) to do something, *anything*, about one's stress or anxiety can cause a person's score to change. Think back to the moment when you first signed up for your first mindfulness class or retreat. Just in that moment, without meditating, you may have felt a sense of hope and optimism, a brief break in what may have been a long stretch of depression, anxiety, or other distress. Even just filling out the questionnaires without doing anything else can cause a person's scores to change. Although it looks like meditation is having the effect, pre-post studies are not necessarily evidence of a specific effect of meditation.

Control groups. In order to control for a person's hopes, expectations, the effect of filling out questionnaires, or simply the passage of time, more rigorous studies use control groups, which can also vary in quality or "rigor."

Randomized controlled trials. While many types of studies may have control groups, it is important that they are "randomized controlled trials" (RCT), which means that neither the participants nor the researchers get to choose what treatment each participant received. Randomization helps ensure that the participants in the meditation group and control group are roughly equal, which helps protect against bias.

Waitlist controls. In a waitlist controlled study, half of the participants are randomized to a meditation class, and half are put on the waitlist. Both groups are measured at the beginning and at the end of the meditation class or waitlist period, in order to control for the effects of time and completing questionnaires. However, the waitlist group does not receive anything, so the effects of the treatment could be due to any number of factors that are part of the treatment but are not necessarily meditation. For example, individuals in the meditation group get to take a 3-hour break from their lives, work, and children once a week. They meet people who have similar symptoms of anxiety and depression and therefore feel less alone and deficient. They also meet an inspiring teacher that also once suffered from anxiety and depression but has learned techniques that have helped her.

These factors inspire hope and decrease depression, but they are not meditation. Thus, while waitlist controls are better than no control group, they are easy to "beat," and they are essentially comparing the meditation group and all that it entails to doing nothing.

Active control groups. The only way to determine if the meditation practice itself is the active ingredient, above and beyond any hope or expectation or social support, is to control for all of those factors with an active control group. There are three general types of active controls: those designed to be more passive, like "health education"; well-established treatments, like pharmacotherapy or cognitive behavioral therapy (CBT); or controls tailor-made to match the intervention. To control for the effects of meditation, the tailor-made matched control condition should have all the same factors as the meditation group except the meditation. For example, the control group meets for 8 weeks, for 2.5 hour, and has daily homework, handouts, and an inspiring teacher who believes in her (non-meditation) treatment. In reality, very few active control studies go to these lengths, and the ones that have (MacCoon et al., 2012; Williams et al., 2014) tend to find little difference between groups. Similarly, meditation tends to be superior to most inert active controls and comparable to standard therapies like CBT or SSRIs (Goyal et al., 2014).

Meta-analyses. Meta-analyses compile the results of many research studies and evaluate the cumulative outcome across all studies. Meta-analyses review the quality of each study and take that into account when evaluating the evidence. Meta-analyses are the best available way to assess the strength of evidence as they should provide a systematic (unbiased) review of all studies, many of which are hard to find. Because the evidence base keeps changing, recent meta-analyses are preferable to older ones (Eberth & Sedlmeier, 2012; Fox et al., 2014; Goyal et al., 2014; Khoury et al., 2013; Sedlmeier et al., 2012).

Some Useful Tips for Evaluating Research

In addition to types of studies, there are other ways to evaluate the strength of the evidence.

Significance and effect size. There are two sets of numbers in the result section that deserve special attention, the p-value and the effect size. The *p*-value confers a "significant" positive finding if it is less than .05 (i.e., the chance of the positive finding happening by chance alone is 1 out of 20), but is considered "nonsignificant" or a non-finding if it is greater than .05. While *p*-value-based significance testing is a common practice, it is actually quite problematic and is being phased out in favor of other metrics (Cumming, 2014). A better estimate of whether meditation "works" is the effect size, which is often called "Cohen's d" (also "Hegde's g"). Effect sizes range from small to large, with corresponding values for small ($d=0.2$), medium ($d=0.5$),

Table 5.1 Types of research studies and levels of evidence

Type of study	Description	Level of evidence
Meta-analyses	Analysis of many studies together	Very high
RCT active control	MBI vs. CBT or health education	High
RCT waitlist	MBI compared to waitlist	Medium
Controlled study	Has control group but not randomized	Low
Pre-post	Measuring outcome before and after an MBI; no control group	Low
Cross-sectional/case–control	Experienced meditators vs non-meditators at a single time point	Low
Mindfulness scale correlational studies	Score on "mindfulness" self-report scale correlated with another outcome	Very low

and large ($d=0.7$). Meditation tends to have a medium effect size for anxiety and depression symptoms, which is similar to most other treatments (Goyal et al., 2014).

Post hoc or subgroup analysis. Sometimes, when researchers find no difference between the meditation and control group, instead of just concluding that, they do more analyses until they find an effect. For example, they may divide the sample into "subgroups" such as males and females, or people who attended a certain number of meditation classes, or have a certain baseline score. According to the Consolidated Standards of Reporting Trials (CONSORT) guidelines, these types of "post hoc" or after-the-fact subset analyses lack credibility (Moher et al., 2010), so beware of conclusions that are based on subgroup analyses.

Study limitation section. Most research papers include a section at the end about the limitations of the study, which can help you determine the rigor of the study and how much weight to put into the findings. All studies have flaws and limitations, so a good metric of honest and thorough disclosure is the presence and extent of the section on study limitations.

Methodological quality. The most common criticism of meditation research is poor "methodological quality," but what does that mean exactly? The CONSORT guidelines describe the expected standards of clinical trials (Moher et al., 2010) and the Jadad score is a numerical metric of study quality (Jadad et al., 1996).

Evidence-Based Practice Beyond the Classroom

Understanding the different types of research and corresponding levels of evidence empowers MBI teachers to create their own evidence-based models for use in class. But the application of the scientific research base in MBIs extends well beyond the in-class didactic material into all aspects of EBP, informing ethical and clinical decision-making that maximizes benefits and minimizes harm (McCown, 2013; Nutely, Walters, & Davies, 2007). The process of informed consent, decisions about inclusion and exclusion criteria, suitability, and risk all depend on an MBI teacher's scientific literacy.

Informed Consent

Scientific literacy is the foundation of an ethical dimension of the teacher–participant relationship known as "informed consent." Informed consent extends beyond the legal right of the patient to be provided with sufficient information to make informed decisions about engaging in an MBI. The process of informed consent is an embodiment of friendship, which includes a respect for a participant's autonomy and right to self-determination, as well as the highest wishes for their well-being. In order to honor this friendship, the MBI teacher provides honest and thorough information about the potential benefits and potential harms of the MBI they are offering and any alternative treatments that might be more suitable (Berg, Appelbaum, Lidz, & Parker, 2001). The elements of informed consent are listed on a legal document called a consent form, which the participant reads and signs before treatment. The informed consent process is also ongoing, beginning with the initial MBI advertisements on websites or brochures and continuing throughout the treatment.

Thorough and honest disclosure. Thorough and honest disclosure includes descriptions of the nature, probability, and magnitude of both benefits and harms. Because these potentials differ among different participants with different conditions, thorough disclosure often requires a face-to-face consultation tailored to each participant. For any given ailment, the available evidence base varies, so providing accurate information about the nature, likelihood, and magnitude of benefit for a specific ailment can be challenging. In terms of harm prevention, the disclosure of potential harms or lack of benefits is more important than benefits. This may simply involve being forthright about the early and mixed nature of the scientific evidence base, the possibility of a "less-than-complete cure," and the simple fact that MBIs may not benefit everyone or may even be contraindicated (Dobkin, Irving, & Amar, 2012).

Avoiding harm. Keeping abreast of the scientific literature is a Herculean task that can only be aspirational and a lifelong learning goal. Rather than focusing on a wide breadth of knowledge, it is more important to focus efforts on not causing harm (Kabat-Zinn, 2011a, 2011b). According to directors of the National Center for Complementary and Alternative Medicine (NCCAM) at the National Institutes of Health (NIH), the biggest potentials for harm are "unjustified claims of benefit, possible adverse effects,… and the possibility that vulnerable patients with serious diseases may be misled" (Briggs & Killen, 2013). For example, a patient may fail to receive appropriate treatment because of the belief that mindfulness is a viable alternative to standard medical or psychological treatment. Being forthright about the uses and limits of MBIs can protect against potential harm. For example, The Center for Mindfulness clearly states in their advertising brochures that MBSR is not a replacement for standard treatments, "MBSR is not offered as an alternative to traditional medical and psychological treatments, but as a complement to these treatments" (Santorelli & Kabat-Zinn, 2014).

Languaging. The way that scientific research is "languaged" is also a dimension of ethical responsibility and integrity. Small changes in our choice of words can make the difference between "unjustified claims" that are "misleading" and fulfillment of honest and thorough disclosure. The scientific evidence for the effects of meditation is far from established, "confirmed," or "proven." Instead, the state of the research may best be described as "promising but inconclusive, tentative, or suggestive" at this stage. In addition to issues of honesty and accuracy, certain word choices are likely to evoke resistance, especially from skeptics who are wary of exaggerated claims. For example, words like "proof" or "proven" can feel more like an attempt to persuade than to inform and will likely have the effects of inflating rather than deflating skepticism. Skeptics can actually be our greatest allies in this respect, as they keep us mindful of unconscious agendas that may manifest in our speech. Table 5.2 lists some examples of more reified vs. flexible language choices.

Resources for assessing potential benefits and harms. Scientific literacy informs decisions about the potential benefits and harms of MBIs, including what type of person is most or least suitable for an MBI. In addition to ongoing research, the assessment of suitability and risk can also be informed by the existing evidence-based guidelines for MBI inclusion and exclusion. For example, current exclusion criteria for both MBSR and MBCT include most psychiatric diagnoses, including acute depression, substance abuse, suicidality, PTSD, psychosis, and some forms of anxiety (Kuyken, Crane, & Williams, 2012; Santorelli, 2014). Of course, as the evidence base changes, these guidelines also change, both becoming more and less inclusive. For example, MBCT is currently only approved for individuals who have had three or more prior episodes of depression but are currently in remission (NICE, 2009). However, new evidence suggests that MBCT may be helpful for individuals with residual depression symptoms (Geschwind, Peeters, Huibers, van Os, & Wichers, 2012; van Aalderen et al., 2012). Alternatively, recent meta-analyses have

Table 5.2 Reifying vs. flexible language

Over-general, reifying language	Open-ended, flexible, and specific language
Proof, proven, proves	Suggests
Heals, cures, fixes, gets rid of, works	May help; may decrease
Demonstrates, shows, confirms	May indicate; is associated with
Example: *Science has proven that meditation works*	*Scientific studies suggest that some kinds of meditation may be helpful for anxiety and depression*
We know from science that…	*Scientific studies suggest that…*

reported that MBIs have not been found to be helpful for relieving the primary diagnosis of anxiety disorders (Strauss et al., 2014), or chronic pain (Chiesa & Serretti, 2011; Rajguru et al., 2014), so being informed about these potential limitations helps participants and their healthcare providers make informed decisions about their care. Integrity around the possible limitations of MBIs may also mean respecting a participant's autonomy in decision-making and honoring their doubt as a manifestation of their own wisdom instead of "doubting the doubt" (Sears et al., 2011).

Adverse effects. The concern that meditation may be contraindicated under certain conditions has been raised repeatedly by the American Psychiatric Association (Shapiro, 1982), the NIH (NCCAM/NIH, 2014), and leading researchers in the field (Dobkin et al., 2012; Greenberg & Harris, 2012; Lustyk, Chawla, Nolan, & Marlatt, 2009). Indeed there have been more than a dozen articles reporting serious adverse effects of meditation including psychosis, depersonalization, mania, and other forms of psychological deterioration (see Lustyk et al., 2009 for a review). Participant risks such as increased depression, suicidality, and meditation-induced flashbacks are listed in MBCT teacher resources (Kuyken et al., 2012). Potential adverse effects are typically conveyed to participants in more general terms such as "you might find that taking the course is challenging for a number of different reasons" (Segal, Williams, & Teasdale, 2011). The degree of disclosure that constitutes adequate informed consent is still a matter of debate, especially since there is a lack of research about the nature, likelihood, and magnitude of MBI-related adverse effects. At the very least, inaccurate, misleading statements that meditation "is 100 % safe" or "has no side effects" should be avoided.

Conclusion and Further Resources

Scientific literacy is a basic MBI teacher competency and is the foundation of all aspects of EBP and pedagogy. Scientific literacy informs our ethical and clinical decision-making, extending to inclusion and exclusion criteria, assessment of risk, and the ongoing process of informed consent, in order to maximize benefits and minimize harm. This chapter has provided some basic foundations of scientific literacy, including the evidence base for some neurobiological models of meditation, as well as skills for evaluating scientific research. This chapter only provides an early step in a much larger commitment to lifelong learning. A number of resources are provided for further self-development, including a resource page of books, articles, and websites for further reading (see section below). A self-inquiry practice provides an experiential aspect of scientific literacy. Similar to the "investigation of cognitive biases in attention and memory" exercises that are provided to participants, the self-inquiry investigates a specific type of bias that impairs EBP called "confirmation bias" (Lilienfeld, Ritschel, Lynn, Cautin, & Latzman, 2013). (see Part IV Chapter 24A).

Resources and Further Reading

Scientific Models of Mindfulness

Holzel, B. K., et al. (2011). How does mindfulness meditation work? Proposing mechanisms of action from a conceptual and neural perspective. *Perspectives on Psychological Science, 8*(6), 537–559.
Note: Models include effects on attention and emotion regulation, body awareness, and change in perspective on the self, and is recommended for further inquiry or a reference for participants.

Brown, K. W., Creswell, J. D., & Ryan, R. M. (Eds.). (2015). *Handbook of mindfulness: Theory, research, and practice.* New York, NY: Guilford.
Note: A survey of basic research from neurobiological, cognitive, emotion/affective, and interpersonal perspectives of MBIs for behavioral and emotion dysregulation disorders, depression, anxiety, addictions, and physical health conditions.

Shapiro, S. L., & Carlson, L. E. (2009). *The art and science of mindfulness: Integrating mindfulness in psychology and the helping professions.* Washington, DC: American Psychological Association.
Note: Contains reviews of MBI research for physical and mental conditions, possible mechanisms of action. Includes a section on clinician self-care.

Willoughby Britton TEDTALK. http://www.ted.com/tedx/events/2672 (video)
Note: 15 minute overview of neuroplasticity, hypofrontality and the effects of meditation.

Evidenced-Based MBI Resources (online)

Mindful experience.org
Note: Provides reviews and meta-analyses of MBI evidence base, a list of MBI research centers and providers, and a monthly newsletter about new MBI articles and trials.

http://mbct.co.uk/about-mbct/
http://www.bangor.ac.uk/mindfulness/

Skills to Evaluate Scientific Evidence for Treatment Effects

Lilienfeld, S., Ruscio, J., & Lynn, S. J. (Eds.). (2008). *Navigating the mindfield: A guide to separating science from pseudoscience in mental health.* New York, NY: Prometheus.
Note: A practical guide for evaluating mental health treatments. Exposes common misconceptions.

Sears, S. R., Kraus, S., Carlough, K., & Treat, E. (2011). Perceived Benefits and Doubts of Participants in a Weekly Meditation Study. *Mindfulness, 2,* 167–174.

Handouts

HANDOUT: Key Brain Areas in the Hypofrontality Model

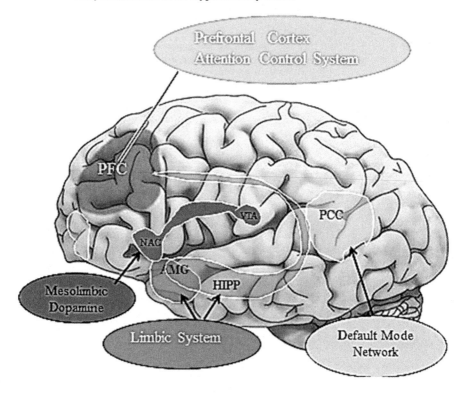

	Affective	Cognitive	Conative
Domain	Body + emotions	Thinking	Reward/motivation/action
Brain areas	Limbic system	Default mode network	Brain reward system
	Amygdala (AMG)	Cortical midline structures	Mesolimbic dopamine
	Hippocampus	Medial PFC	Ventral tegmental area (VTA)
	Sympathetic nervous system	Posterior cingulate (PCC)	Nucleus accumbens (NAC)
			Striatum
			DMN, limbic system
Experience when overactive or poorly regulated	High negative affect	Self-referential processing	Craving
	Emotional reactivity	Mind wandering	Rumination
	Stress sensitivity	Craving	Self-thought-affect fusion
		Rumination	Impulsivity
		Social cognition	Poor self-regulation
Disorders	PTSD	Schizophrenia, OCD	All addictions, ADHD
	Anxiety, panic	Social anxiety	Bipolar disorder
	Depression	Depression	Borderline PD

HANDOUT: Two Arrows

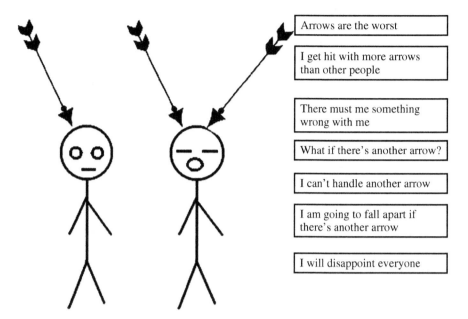

Arrows are the worst

I get hit with more arrows than other people

There must me something wrong with me

What if there's another arrow?

I can't handle another arrow

I am going to fall apart if there's another arrow

I will disappoint everyone

References

AHRQ. (2012). *Meditation programs for stress and well-being: Evidence report.* Agency for Healthcare Research and Quality, U.S. Department of Health and Human Services.

Alberts, H. J., & Thewissen, R. (2011). The effect of a brief mindfulness intervention on memory for positively and negatively valenced stimuli. *Mindfulness, 2*, 73–77.

Allen, M., Dietz, M., Blair, K. S., van Beek, M., Rees, G., Vestergaard-Poulsen, P., ... Roepstorff, A. (2012). Cognitive-affective neural plasticity following active-controlled mindfulness intervention. *Journal of Neuroscience, 32*, 15601–15610.

Alterman, A., Koppenhaver, J., Mulholland, E., Ladden, L., & Baime, M. (2004). Pilot trial of effectiveness of mindfulness meditation for substance abuse patients. *Journal of Substance Use, 9*, 259–268.

Anderson, N., Lau, M., Segal, Z., & Bishop, S. (2007). Mindfulness-based stress reduction and attentional control. *Clinical Psychology & Psychotherapy, 14*, 449–463.

Arch, J. J., & Craske, M. G. (2006). Mechanisms of mindfulness: Emotion regulation following a focused breathing induction. *Behaviour Research and Therapy, 44*, 1849–1858.

Baerentsen, K. B. (2001). Onset of meditation explored with fMRI. *Neuroimage, 13*, S297.

Baerentsen, K. B., Stodkilde-Jorgensen, H., Sommerlund, B., Hartmann, T., Damsgaard-Madsen, J., Fosnaes, M., & Green, A. C. (2009). An investigation of brain processes supporting meditation. *Cognitive Processing, 11*, 57–84.

Barnes, V. A., Treiber, F. A., & Davis, H. (2001). Impact of transcendental meditation on cardiovascular function at rest and during acute stress in adolescents with high normal blood pressure. *Journal of Psychosomatic Research, 51*, 597–605.

Baron Short, E., Kose, S., Mu, Q., Borckardt, J., Newberg, A., George, M. S., ., & Kozel, F. A. (2010). Regional brain activation during meditation shows time and practice effects: An exploratory FMRI study. *Evidence-Based Complementary and Alternative Medicine, 7*, 121–127.

Baxter, L. R., Jr., Schwartz, J. M., Phelps, M. E., Mazziotta, J. C., Guze, B. H., Selin, C. E., ... Sumida, R. M. (1989). Reduction of prefrontal cortex glucose metabolism common to three types of depression. *Archives of General Psychiatry, 46*, 243-250.

Bench, C. J., Friston, K. J., Brown, R. G., Frackowiak, R. S., & Dolan, R. J. (1993). Regional cerebral blood flow in depression measured by positron emission tomography: The relationship with clinical dimensions. *Psychological Medicine, 23*, 579–590.

Berg, J., Appelbaum, P., Lidz, C., & Parker, L. (2001). *Informed consent: Legal theory and clinical practice.* New York, NY: Oxford University Press.

Bergomi, C., Tschacher, W., & Kupper, Z. (2013). The assessment of mindfulness with self-report measures: Existing scales and open issues. *Mindfulness, 4*, 191–202.

Berkovich-Ohana, A., Glicksohn, J., & Goldstein, A. (2012). Mindfulness-induced changes in gamma band activity—Implications for the default mode network, self-reference and attention. *Clinical Neurophysiology, 123*, 700–710.

Blumberg, H. P., Kaufman, J., Martin, A., Charney, D. S., Krystal, J. H., & Peterson, B. S. (2004). Significance of adolescent neurodevelopment for the neural circuitry of bipolar disorder. *Annals of the New York Academy of Sciences, 1021*, 376–383.

Bowen, S., Witkiewitz, K., Clifasefi, S. L., Grow, J., Chawla, N., Hsu, S. H., ... Larimer, M. E. (2014). Relative efficacy of mindfulness-based relapse prevention, standard relapse prevention, and treatment as usual for substance use disorders: A randomized clinical trial. *JAMA Psychiatry, 71*, 547–556.

Brefczynski-Lewis, J. A., Lutz, A., Schaefer, H. S., Levinson, D. B., & Davidson, R. J. (2007). Neural correlates of attentional expertise in long-term meditation practitioners. *Proceedings of the National Academy of Sciences USA, 104*, 11483–11488.

Brewer, J. A., Elwafi, H. M., & Davis, J. H. (2013). Craving to quit: Psychological models and neurobiological mechanisms of mindfulness training as treatment for addictions. *Psychology of Addictive Behavior, 27*, 366–379.

Brewer, J. A., Sinha, R., Chen, J. A., Michalsen, R. N., Babuscio, T. A., Nich, C., … Rounsaville, B. J. (2009). Mindfulness training and stress reactivity in substance abuse: Results from a randomized, controlled stage I pilot study. *Substance Abuse, 30*, 306–317.

Brewer, J. A., Worhunsky, P. D., Gray, J. R., Tang, Y. Y., Weber, J., & Kober, H. (2011). Meditation experience is associated with differences in default mode network activity and connectivity. *Proceedings of the National Academy of Sciences USA, 108*, 20254–20259.

Briggs, J., & Killen, J. (2013). Perspectives on complementary and alternative medicine research. *Journal of the American Medical Association, 310*, 691–692.

Britton, W. B., Bootzin, R. R., Cousins, J. C., Hasler, B. P., Peck, T., & Shapiro, S. L. (2010). The contribution of mindfulness practice to a multicomponent behavioral sleep intervention following substance abuse treatment in adolescents: A treatment-development study. *Substance Abuse, 31*, 86–97.

Britton, W. B., Haynes, P. L., Fridel, K. W., & Bootzin, R. R. (2010). Polysomnographic and subjective profiles of sleep continuity before and after mindfulness-based cognitive therapy in partially remitted depression. *Psychosomatic Medicine, 72*, 539–548.

Britton, W. B., Lindahl, J. R., Cahn, B. R., Davis, J. H., & Goldman, R. E. (2014). Awakening is not a metaphor: The effects of Buddhist meditation practices on basic wakefulness. *Annals of the New York Academy of Sciences, 1307*, 64–81.

Britton, W. B., Shahar, B., Szepsenwol, O., & Jacobs, W. J. (2012). Mindfulness-based cognitive therapy improves emotional reactivity to social stress: Results from a randomized controlled trial. *Behaviour Therapy, 43*, 365–380.

Broderick, P. (2005). Mindfulness and coping with dysphoric mood: Contrasts with rumination and distraction. *Cognitive Therapy and Research, 29*, 501–510.

Brown, K., Creswell, J., & Ryan, R. (Eds.). (2015). *Handbook of Mindfulness: Theory, Research, and Practice*. New York, NY: Guilford.

Buckner, R. L., & Vincent, J. L. (2007). Unrest at rest: Default activity and spontaneous network correlations. *Neuroimage, 37*, 1091–1099.

Campbell-Sills, L., Barlow, D., Brown, T., & Hofmann, S. (2006). Effects of suppression and acceptance on emotional responses of individuals with anxiety and mood disorders. *Behaviour Research and Therapy, 44*, 1251–1263.

Carlson, L. E., Speca, M., Faris, P., & Patel, K. D. (2007). One year pre-post intervention follow-up of psychological, immune, endocrine and blood pressure outcomes of mindfulness-based stress reduction (MBSR) in breast and prostate cancer outpatients. *Brain, Behavior and Immunity, 21*, 1038–1049.

Carter, C. S., Perlstein, W., Ganguli, R., Brar, J., Mintun, M., & Cohen, J. D. (1998). Functional hypofrontality and working memory dysfunction in schizophrenia. *American Journal of Psychiatry, 155*, 1285–1287.

Chiesa, A., Calati, R., & Serretti, A. (2011). Does mindfulness training improve cognitive abilities? A systematic review of neuropsychological findings. *Clinical Psychology Review, 31*, 449–464.

Chiesa, A., & Serretti, A. (2011). Mindfulness-based interventions for chronic pain: A systematic review of the evidence. *Journal of Alternative and Complementary Medicine, 17*, 83–93.

Chiesa, A., & Serretti, A. (2014). Are mindfulness-based interventions effective for substance use disorders? A systematic review of the evidence. *Substance Use and Misuse, 49*, 492–512.

Clark, L., Iversen, S. D., & Goodwin, G. M. (2002). Sustained attention deficit in bipolar disorder. *British Journal of Psychiatry, 180*, 313–319.

Creswell, J. D., Pacilio, L. E., Lindsay, E. K., & Brown, K. W. (2014). Brief mindfulness meditation training alters psychological and neuroendocrine responses to social evaluative stress. *Psychoneuroendocrinology, 44*, 1–12.

Cumming, G. (2014). The new statistics: Why and how. *Psychological Science, 25*, 7–29.

Davidson, R. J., Irwin, W., Anderle, M. J., & Kalin, N. H. (2003). The neural substrates of affective processing in depressed patients treated with venlafaxine. *American Journal of Psychiatry, 160*, 64–75.

Davidson, R. J., Jackson, D. C., & Kalin, N. H. (2000). Emotion, plasticity, context and regulation: Perspectives from affective neuroscience. *Psychological Bulletin, 126*, 890–909.

Davidson, R. J., Kabat-Zinn, J., Schumacher, J., Rosenkranz, M., Muller, D., Santorelli, S. F., … Sheridan, J. F. (2003). Alterations in brain and immune function produced by mindfulness meditation. *Psychosomatic Medicine, 65*, 564–570.

Desbordes, G., Negi, L. T., Pace, T. W., Wallace, B. A., Raison, C. L., & Schwartz, E. L. (2012). Effects of mindful-attention and compassion meditation training on amygdala response to emotional stimuli in an ordinary, non-meditative state. *Frontiers in Human Neuroscience, 6*, 292. doi:10.3389/fnhum.2012.00292.

Disner, S. G., Beevers, C. G., Haigh, E. A., & Beck, A. T. (2011). Neural mechanisms of the cognitive model of depression. *Nature Reviews Neuroscience, 12*, 467–477.

Dobkin, P., Irving, J., & Amar, S. (2012). For whom may participation in a mindfulness-based stress reduction program be contraindicated? *Mindfulness, 3*, 44–50.

Draganski, B., Gaser, C., Busch, V., Schuierer, G., Bogdahn, U., & May, A. (2004). Neuroplasticity: Changes in grey matter induced by training. *Nature, 427*, 311–312.

Dryden, W., & Still, A. (2006). Historical aspects of mindfulness and self-acceptance in psychotherapy. *Journal of Rational-Emotive and Cognitive Behavior Therapy, 24*, 3–28.

Eberth, J., & Sedlmeier, P. (2012). The effects of mindfulness meditation: A meta-analysis. *Mindfulness, 3*, 174–189.

Erisman, S. M., & Roemer, L. (2010). A preliminary investigation of the effects of experimentally induced mindfulness on emotional responding to film clips. *Emotion, 10*, 72–82.

Farb, N. A., Anderson, A. K., Mayberg, H., Bean, J., McKeon, D., & Segal, Z. V. (2010). Minding one's emotions: Mindfulness training alters the neural expression of sadness. *Emotion, 10*, 25–33.

Farb, N. A., Segal, Z. V., Mayberg, H., Bean, J., McKeon, D., Fatima, Z., & Anderson, A. K. (2007). Attending to the present: Mindfulness meditation reveals distinct neural modes of self-reference. *Social Cognitive and Affective Neuroscience, 2*, 313–322.

Feil, J., Sheppard, D., Fitzgerald, P. B., Yucel, M., Lubman, D. I., & Bradshaw, J. L. (2010). Addiction, compulsive drug seeking, and the role of frontostriatal mechanisms in regulating inhibitory control. *Neuroscience and Biobehavioral Reviews, 35*, 248–275.

Fox, K. C., Nijeboer, S., Dixon, M. L., Floman, J. L., Ellamil, M., Rumak, S. P., … Christoff, K. (2014). Is meditation associated with altered brain structure? A systematic review and meta-analysis of morphometric neuroimaging in meditation practitioners. *Neuroscience and Biobehavioral Reviews, 43*, 48–3.

Gallagher, S. (2000). Philosophical conceptions of the self: Implications for cognitive science. *Trends in Cognitive Science, 4*, 14–21.

Gard, T., Holzel, B. K., & Lazar, S. W. (2014). The potential effects of meditation on age-related cognitive decline: A systematic review. *Annals of the New York Academy of Sciences, 1307*, 89–103.

Garland, E. L., Froeliger, B. E., Passik, S. D., & Howard, M. O. (2013). Attentional bias for prescription opioid cues among opioid dependent chronic pain patients. *Journal of Behavioral Medicine, 36*, 611–620.

Gentili, C., Ricciardi, E., Gobbini, M. I., Santarelli, M. F., Haxby, J. V., Pietrini, P., & Guazzelli, M. (2009). Beyond amygdala: Default mode network activity differs between patients with social phobia and healthy controls. *Brain Research Bulletin, 79*, 409–413.

Geschwind, N., Peeters, F., Huibers, M., van Os, J., & Wichers, M. (2012). Efficacy of mindfulness-based cognitive therapy in relation to prior history of depression: Randomised controlled trial. *British Journal of Psychiatry, 201*, 320–325.

Goldin, P. R., & Gross, J. J. (2010). Effects of mindfulness-based stress reduction (MBSR) on emotion regulation in social anxiety disorder. *Emotion, 10*, 83–91.

Goldin, P., Ramel, W., & Gross, J. (2009). Mindfulness meditation training and self-referential processing in social anxiety disorder: Behavioral and neural effects. *Journal of Cognitive Psychotherapy, 23*, 242–257.

Goldin, P., Ziv, M., Jazaieri, H., & Gross, J. J. (2012). Randomized controlled trial of mindfulness-based stress reduction versus aerobic exercise: Effects on the self-referential brain network in social anxiety disorder. *Frontiers in Human Neuroscience, 6,* 295.

Goldstein, R. Z., Craig, A. D., Bechara, A., Garavan, H., Childress, A. R., Paulus, M. P., & Volkow, N. D. (2009). The neurocircuitry of impaired insight in drug addiction. *Trends in Cognitive Sciences, 13,* 372–380.

Goldstein, R. Z., & Volkow, N. D. (2011). Dysfunction of the prefrontal cortex in addiction: Neuroimaging findings and clinical implications. *Nature Reviews Neuroscience, 12,* 652–669.

Goleman, D. J. (1984). The Buddha on meditation and states of consciousness. In D. Shapiro & R. Walsh (Eds.), *Meditation: Classic and contemporary perspectives* (pp. 317–362). New York, NY: Aldine.

Goyal, M., Singh, S., Sibinga, E. M., Gould, N. F., Rowland-Seymour, A., Sharma, R., … Haythornthwaite, J. A. (2014). Meditation programs for psychological stress and well-being: A systematic review and meta-analysis. *JAMA Internal Medicine, 174,* 357–368.

Grabovac, A., Lau, M., & Willet, B. (2011). Mechanisms of mindfulness: A Buddhist psychological model. *Mindfulness, 2,* 154–166.

Grant, J. A. (2014). Meditative analgesia: The current state of the field. *Annals of the New York Academy of Sciences, 1307,* 55–63.

Greenberg, M., & Harris, A. (2012). Nurturing mindfulness in children and youth: Current state of research. *Child Development Perspectives, 6,* 161–166.

Hamilton, J. P., Furman, D. J., Chang, C., Thomason, M. E., Dennis, E., & Gotlib, I. H. (2011). Default-mode and task-positive network activity in major depressive disorder: Implications for adaptive and maladaptive rumination. *Biological Psychiatry, 70,* 327–333.

Hargus, E., Crane, C., Barnhofer, T., & Williams, J. M. (2010). Effects of mindfulness on meta-awareness and specificity of describing prodromal symptoms in suicidal depression. *Emotion, 10,* 34–42.

Hasenkamp, W., Wilson-Mendenhall, C. D., Duncan, E., & Barsalou, L. W. (2012). Mind wandering and attention during focused meditation: A fine-grained temporal analysis of fluctuating cognitive states. *Neuroimage, 59,* 750–760.

Hester, R., & Garavan, H. (2004). Executive dysfunction in cocaine addiction: Evidence for discordant frontal, cingulate, and cerebellar activity. *Journal of Neuroscience, 24,* 11017–11022.

Hofmann, S. G., Sawyer, A. T., Witt, A. A., & Oh, D. (2010). The effect of mindfulness-based therapy on anxiety and depression: A meta-analytic review. *Journal of Consulting and Clinical Psychology, 78,* 169–183.

Holmes, D. S. (1984). Meditation and somatic arousal reduction. *American Psychologist, 39,* 1–10.

Holzel, B. K., Carmody, J., Evans, K. C., Hoge, E. A., Dusek, J. A., Morgan, L., … Lazar, S. W. (2010). Stress reduction correlates with structural changes in the amygdala. *Social Cognitive & Affective Neuroscience, 5,* 11–17.

Hölzel, B. K., Carmody, J., Vangel, M., Congleton, C., Yerramsetti, S. M., Gard, T.& Lazar, S. W. (2011). Mindfulness practice leads to increases in regional brain gray matter density. *Psychiatry Research: Neuroimaging, 191,* 36–43.

Holzel, B. K., Lazar, S., Gard, T., Schuman-Olivier, Z., Vago, D. R., & Ott, U. (2011). How does mindfulness meditation work? Proposing mechanisms of action from a conceptual and neural perspective. *Perspectives on Psychological Science, 8,* 537–559.

Holzel, B. K., Ott, U., Gard, T., Hempel, H., Weygandt, M., Morgen, K., & Vaitl, D. (2008). Investigation of mindfulness meditation practitioners with voxel-based morphometry. *Social Cognitive & Affective Neuroscience, 3,* 55–61.

Hoppitt, L., Mathews, A., Yiend, J., & Mackintosh, B. (2010). Cognitive bias modification: The critical role of active training in modifying emotional responses. *Behavior Therapy, 41,* 73–81.

Hugdahl, K., Specht, K., Biringer, E., Weis, S., Elliot, R., Hammar, A., … Lund, A. (2007). Increased parietal and frontal activation after remission from recurrent major depression: A repeated fMRI study. *Cognitive Therapy and Research, 31,* 147–160.

Jadad, A. R., Moore, R. A., Carroll, D., Jenkinson, C., Reynolds, D. J., Gavaghan, D. J., & McQuay, H. J. (1996). Assessing the quality of reports of randomized clinical trials: Is blinding necessary? *Controlled Clinical Trials, 17*, 1–12.

Jain, S., Shapiro, S. L., Swanick, S., Roesch, S. C., Mills, P. J., Bell, I., & Schwartz, G. E. (2007). A randomized controlled trial of mindfulness meditation versus relaxation training: Effects on distress, positive states of mind, rumination, and distraction. *Annals of Behavioral Medicine, 33*, 11–21.

Kabat-Zinn, J. (2011/2016). Foreword. In D. McCown, D. Reibel, & M. Micozzi (Eds.), *Teaching mindfulness: A practical guide for clinicians and educators* (2nd ed.). New York, NY: Springer.

Kabat-Zinn, J. (2011b). Some reflections of the origins of MBSR, skillful means and the trouble with maps. *Contemporary Buddhism, 12*, 281–306.

Kabat-Zinn, J., Santorelli, S., Blacker, M. J., Brantley, J., Meleo-Meyer, F., Grossman, P., ... Stahl, R. (2014). *Training teachers to deliver mindfulness-based stress reduction: Principles and standards*. Center for Mindfulness in Medicine, Health Care, and Society, University of Massachussets Medical School.

Khoury, B., Lecomte, T., Fortin, G., Masse, M., Therien, P., Bouchard, V., ... Hofmann, S. G. (2013). Mindfulness-based therapy: A comprehensive meta-analysis. *Clinical Psychology Review, 33*, 763–771.

Kuehner, C., Huffziger, S., & Liebsch, K. (2009). Rumination, distraction and mindful self-focus: Effects on mood, dysfunctional attitudes and cortisol stress response. *Psychological Medicine, 39*, 219–228.

Kuyken, W., Crane, W., & Williams, J. M. (2012). *Mindfulness-based cognitive therapy (MBCT) implementation resources*. Oxford University, University of Exeter, Bangor University.

Lazar, S. W., Kerr, C. E., Wasserman, R. H., Gray, J. R., Greve, D. N., Treadway, M. T., ... Fischl, B. (2005). Meditation experience is associated with increased cortical thickness. *Neuroreport, 16*, 1893–1897.

Lilienfeld, S. O., Ritschel, L. A., Lynn, S. J., Cautin, R. L., & Latzman, R. D. (2013). Why many clinical psychologists are resistant to evidence-based practice: Root causes and constructive remedies. *Clinical Psychology Review, 33*, 883–900.

Liotti, M., & Mayberg, H. S. (2001). The role of functional neuroimaging in the neuropsychology of depression. *Journal of Clinical and Experimental Neuropsychology, 23*, 121–136.

Liotti, M., Mayberg, H. S., McGinnis, S., Brannan, S. L., & Jerabek, P. (2002). Unmasking disease-specific cerebral blood flow abnormalities: Mood challenge in patients with remitted unipolar depression. *American Journal of Psychiatry, 159*, 1830–1840.

Luders, E., Toga, A., Lepore, N., & Gaser, C. (2009). The underlying anatomical correlates of long-term meditation: Larger frontal and hippocampal volumes of gray matter. *Neuroimage, 45*, 672–678.

Lugo, L. (2012). *Nones' on the rise: One-in-five adults have no religious affiliation*. Pew Research Center's Forum on Religion & Public Life.

Lustyk, M., Chawla, N., Nolan, R., & Marlatt, G. (2009). Mindfulness meditation research: Issues of participant screening, safety procedures, and researcher training. *Advances in Mind-Body Medicine, 24*, 20–30.

MacCoon, D. G., Imel, Z. E., Rosenkranz, M. A., Sheftel, J. G., Weng, H. Y., Sullivan, J. C., ... Lutz, A. (2012). The validation of an active control intervention for Mindfulness Based Stress Reduction (MBSR). *Behaviour Research & Therapy, 50*, 3–12.

MacCoon, D. G., MacLean, K. A., Davidson, R. J., Saron, C. D., & Lutz, A. (2014). No sustained attention differences in a longitudinal randomized trial comparing mindfulness based stress reduction versus active control. *PLoS One, 9*, e97551.

MacDonald, A. W., Carter, C. S., Kerns, J. G., Ursu, S., Barch, D. M., Holmes, A. J., ... Cohen, J. D. (2005). Specificity of prefrontal dysfunction and context processing deficits to schizophrenia in never-medicated patients with first-episode psychosis. *American Journal of Psychiatry, 162*, 475–484.

Maclean, C., Walton, K., Wenneberg, S., Levitsky, D., Mandarino, J., Waziri, R., & Schneider, R. H. (1994). Altered responses of cortisol, GH, TSH and testosterone in acute stress after four months' practice of Transcendental Meditation (TM). *Annals of the New York Academy of Sciences, 746*, 381–384.

Maguire, E. A., Woollett, K., & Spiers, H. J. (2006). London taxi drivers and bus drivers: A structural MRI and neuropsychological analysis. *Hippocampus, 16*, 1091–1101. doi:10.1002/hipo.20233.

Marciniak, R., Sheardova, K., Cermakova, P., Hudecek, D., Sumec, R., & Hort, J. (2014). Effect of meditation on cognitive functions in context of aging and neurodegenerative diseases. *Frontiers in Behavioral Neuroscience, 8*, 17.

Mayberg, H. S., Liotti, M., Brannan, S. K., McGinnis, S., Mahurin, R. K., Jerabek, P. A., ... Fox, P. T. (1999). Reciprocal limbic-cortical function and negative mood: Converging PET findings in depression and normal sadness. *American Journal of Psychiatry, 156*, 675–682.

McCown, D. (2013). *The ethical space of mindfulness in clinical practice*. London, England: Jessica Kingsley.

McCown, D., Reibel, D., & Micozzi, M. (2010). *Teaching mindfulness*. New York, NY: Springer.

Meyer, S. E., Carlson, G. A., Wiggs, E. A., Martinez, P. E., Ronsaville, D. S., Klimes-Dougan, B., ... Radke-Yarrow, M. (2004). A prospective study of the association among impaired executive functioning, childhood attentional problems, and the development of bipolar disorder. *Developmental Psychopathology, 16*, 461–476.

Miller, E. K., & Cohen, J. D. (2001). An integrative theory of prefrontal cortex function. *Annual Reviews of Neuroscience, 24*, 167–202.

Moher, D., Hopewell, S., Schulz, K. F., Montori, V., Gotzsche, P. C., Devereaux, P. J., ... Consolidated Standards of Reporting Trials, G. (2010). CONSORT 2010 explanation and elaboration: Updated guidelines for reporting parallel group randomised trials. *Journal of Clinical Epidemiology, 63*, e1–e37.

Morgane, P. J., Galler, J. R., & Mokler, D. J. (2005). A review of systems and networks of the limbic forebrain/limbic midbrain. *Progress in Neurobiology, 75*, 143–160.

NCCAM/NIH. (2014). *Meditation: Side effects and risks*. National Center for Complementary and Alternative Medicine (NCCAM). National Institutes of Health (NIH). doi:http://nccam.nih.gov/health/meditation/overview.htm#sideeffects.

NICE. (2009). *Depression: Management of depression in primary and secondary care*. London, England: National Institute for Health and Clinical Excellence.

Nutely, S., Walters, I., & Davies, H. (2007). *Using evidence, how research can inform public services*. Bristol, England: Policy Press.

Ochsner, K. N., & Gross, J. J. (2005). The cognitive control of emotion. *Trends in Cognitive Science, 9*, 242–249.

Ortner, C. M. N., Kilner, S., & Zelazo, P. D. (2007). Mindfulness meditation and emotional interference in a simple cognitive task. *Motivation and Emotion, 31*, 271–283.

Papageorgiou, C., & Wells, A. (2000). Treatment of recurrent major depression with attention training. *Cognitive & Behavioral Practice, 7*, 407–413.

Penades, R., Catalan, R., Salamero, M., Boget, T., Puig, O., Guarch, J., & Gasto, C. (2006). Cognitive remediation therapy for outpatients with chronic schizophrenia: A controlled and randomized study. *Schizophrenia Research, 87*, 323–331.

Qin, P., & Northoff, G. (2011). How is our self related to midline regions and the default-mode network? *Neuroimage, 57*, 1221–1233.

Rajguru, P., Kolber, M., Garcia, A., Smith, M., Patel, C., & Hanney, W. (2014). Use of mindfulness meditation in the management of chronic pain: A systematic review of randomized controlled trials. *American Journal of Lifestyle Medicine*. doi:10.1177/1559827614522580.

Reibel, D. K., Greeson, J. M., Brainard, G. C., & Rosenzweig, S. (2001). Mindfulness-based stress reduction and health-related quality of life in a heterogeneous patient population. *General Hospital Psychiatry, 23*, 183–192.

Ritskes, R., Ritskes-Hoitinga, M., Stodkilde-Jorgensen, H., Baerntsen, K., & Hartman, T. (2003). MRI scanning during Zen meditation: The picture of enlightenment? *Constructivism in Human Sciences, 8*, 85–90.

Roberts-Wolfe, D., Sacchet, M. D., Hastings, E., Roth, H., & Britton, W. (2012). Mindfulness training alters emotional memory recall compared to active controls: Support for an emotional information processing model of mindfulness. *Frontiers in Human Neuroscience, 6*, 15.

Rodrigues, A., Loureiro, M., & Paulo Caramelli, P. (2010). Musical training, neuroplasticity and cognition. *Dementia e Neuropsychologia, 4*, 277–286.

Santorelli, S. (2014). *Mindfulness-based stress reduction standards of practice*. Center for Mindfulness in Medicine, Health Care, and Society. University of Massachusetts Medical School.

Santorelli, S., & Kabat-Zinn, J. (2014). *Stress reduction program brochure*. Center for Mindfulness in Medicine, Health Care, and Society. University of Massachusetts Medical School.

Schilbach, L., Eickhoff, S. B., Rotarska-Jagiela, A., Fink, G. R., & Vogeley, K. (2008). Minds at rest? Social cognition as the default mode of cognizing and its putative relationship to the "default system" of the brain. *Consciousness and Cognition, 17*, 457–467.

Sears, S. R., & Stanton, A. L. (2001). Expectancy-value constructs and expectancy violation as predictors of exercise adherence in previously sedentary women. *Health Psychology, 20*, 326–333.

Sedlmeier, P., Eberth, J., Schwarz, M., Zimmermann, D., Haarig, F., Jaeger, S., & Kunze, S. (2012). The psychological effects of meditation: A meta-analysis. *Psychological Bulletin, 138*, 1139–1171.

Segal, Z. V., Williams, J. M., & Teasdale, J. (2011). Handout 6.1: Introduction to mindfulness-based cognitive therapy. *Mindfulness-based cognitive therapy for depression*. New York, NY: Guilford.

Shapiro, D. H., Jr. (1982). Overview: Clinical and physiological comparison of meditation with other self-control strategies. *American Journal of Psychiatry, 139*, 267–274.

Sheline, Y. I., Barch, D. M., Price, J. L., Rundle, M. M., Vaishnavi, S. N., Snyder, A. Z., … Raichle, M. E. (2009). The default mode network and self-referential processes in depression. *Proceedings of the National Academy of Sciences USA, 106*, 1942–1947.

Siegle, G., Ghinassi, F., & Thase, M. E. (2007). Neurobehavioral therapies in the 21st century: Summary of an emerging field and an extended example of cognitive control training for depression. *Cognitive Therapy & Research, 31*, 235–262.

Siegle, G. J., Steinhauer, S. R., Thase, M. E., Stenger, V. A., & Carter, C. S. (2002). Can't shake that feeling: event-related fMRI assessment of sustained amygdala activity in response to emotional information in depressed individuals. *Biological Psychiatry, 51*, 693–707.

Siegle, G. J., Thompson, W., Carter, C. S., Steinhauer, S. R., & Thase, M. E. (2007). Increased amygdala and decreased dorsolateral prefrontal BOLD responses in unipolar depression: Related and independent features. *Biological Psychiatry, 61*, 198–209.

Spring, B. (2007). Evidence-based practice in clinical psychology: What it is, why it matters; what you need to know. *Journal of Clinical Psychology, 63*, 611–631.

Strauss, C., Cavanagh, K., Oliver, A., & Pettman, D. (2014). Mindfulness-based interventions for people diagnosed with a current episode of an anxiety or depressive disorder: A meta-analysis of randomised controlled trials. *PLoS One, 9*, e96110.

Sudsuang, R., Chentanez, V., & Veluvan, K. (1991). The effect of Buddhist meditation on serum cortisol and total protein levels, blood pressure, pulse rate, lung volume and reaction time. *Physiology & Behavior, 50*, 543–548.

Tang, Y. Y., Ma, Y., Wang, J., Fan, Y., Feng, S., Lu, Q., … Posner, M. I. (2007). Short-term meditation training improves attention and self-regulation. *Proceedings of the National Academy of Sciences USA, 104*, 17152–17156.

Tavris, C. (2003). The widening scientist-practitioner gap: A view from the bridge. In S. Lillienfeld, S. J. Lynn, & J. M. Lohr (Eds.), *Science and pseudoscience in clinical psychology*. New York, NY: Guilford.

Taylor, V. A., Grant, J., Daneault, V., Scavone, G., Breton, E., Roffe-Vidal, S., … Beauregard, M. (2011). Impact of mindfulness on the neural responses to emotional pictures in experienced and beginner meditators. *Neuroimage, 57*, 1524–1533.

Travis, F. (2014). Transcendental experiences during meditation practice. *Annals of the New York Academy of Sciences, 1307*, 1–8.

Travis, F., Haaga, D. A., Hagelin, J., Tanner, M., Arenander, A., Nidich, S., ... Schneider, R. H. (2010). A self-referential default brain state: Patterns of coherence, power, and eLORETA sources during eyes-closed rest and transcendental meditation practice. *Cognitive Processes, 11*, 21–30.

Vago, D. R., & Nakamura, Y. (2011). Selective attentional bias towards pain-related threat in fibromyalgia: Preliminary evidence for effects of mindfulness meditation training. *Cognitive Therapy and Research, 35*, 581–594.

van Aalderen, J. R., Donders, A. R., Giommi, F., Spinhoven, P., Barendregt, H. P., & Speckens, A. E. (2012). The efficacy of mindfulness-based cognitive therapy in recurrent depressed patients with and without a current depressive episode: A randomized controlled trial. *Psychological Medicine, 42*, 989–1001.

van den Heuvel, O. A., Veltman, D. J., Groenewegen, H. J., Cath, D. C., van Balkom, A. J., van Hartskamp, J., ... van Dyck, R. (2005). Frontal-striatal dysfunction during planning in obsessive-compulsive disorder. *Archives of General Psychiatry, 62*, 301–309.

Wenk-Sormaz, H. (2005). Meditation can reduce habitual responding. *Advances in Mind-Body Medicine, 21*, 33–49.

Whitfield-Gabrieli, S., Thermenos, H. W., Milanovic, S., Tsuang, M. T., Faraone, S. V., McCarley, R. W., ... Seidman, L. J. (2009). Hyperactivity and hyperconnectivity of the default network in schizophrenia and in first-degree relatives of persons with schizophrenia. *Proceedings of the National Academy of Sciences USA, 106*, 1279–1284.

Williams, J. M., Crane, C., Barnhofer, T., Brennan, K., Duggan, D. S., Fennell, M. J., ... Russell, I. T. (2014). Mindfulness-based cognitive therapy for preventing relapse in recurrent depression: A randomized dismantling trial. *Journal of Consulting and Clinical Psychology, 82*, 275–286.

Williams, J. M., Teasdale, J. D., Segal, Z. V., & Soulsby, J. (2000). Mindfulness-based cognitive therapy reduces overgeneral autobiographical memory in formerly depressed patients. *Journal of Abnormal Psychology, 109*, 150–155.

Wilson, J. F., & Drakeman, D. L. (2003). *Church and state in American history: Key documents, decisions, and commentary from the past three centuries.* Boulder, CO: Westview.

Witkiewitz, K., Bowen, S., Harrop, E. N., Douglas, H., Enkema, M., & Sedgwick, C. (2014). Mindfulness-based treatment to prevent addictive behavior relapse: Theoretical models and hypothesized mechanisms of change. *Substance Use and Misuse, 49*, 513–524.

Wood, A. G., & Smith, E. (2008). Pediatric neuroimaging studies: A window to neurocognitive development of the frontal lobes. In V. Anderson, R. Jacobs, & P. J. Anderson (Eds.), *Executive functions and the frontal lobes: A lifespan perspective* (pp. 203–216). Philadelphia, PA: Taylor & Francis.

Zgierska, A., Rabago, D., Chawla, N., Kushner, K., Koehler, R., & Marlatt, A. (2009). Mindfulness meditation for substance use disorders: A systematic review. *Substance Abuse, 30*, 266–294.

Chapter 6
Training Mindfulness Teachers: Principles, Practices and Challenges

Rebecca S. Crane and Barbara Reid

Introduction

Interest in the development and application of mindfulness-based interventions (MBIs) is expanding around the world; there is an associated increase in demand for good teachers. While a range of different stakeholders are involved in supporting this growth, teacher training materials, programmes and resources are central to the process of teacher development and have not been developed to keep pace with the demand.

The rapid pace of development poses particular requirements for safeguarding the integrity of teacher training. For example, in the UK the impact of the incorporation of mindfulness-based cognitive therapy (MBCT) into the NICE guidelines[1] (NICE, 2004) has been considerable. Ten years later, in 2014, a UK All-Party Parliamentary Group for mindfulness was established, now bringing to the fore widespread interest in the use of mindfulness in education, health care, social policy fields, the workplace and the criminal justice system (The Mindfulness Initiative, 2014). With rapidly increasing recognition of the value of mindfulness-based approaches, there is pressure to train teachers quickly but without risking dilution in standards.

Now when there is strong pressure to expand capacity, long-standing experts are asking how to design and deliver mindfulness-based teacher training programmes and develop a professional context in ways that remain true to the founding principles of mindfulness-based approaches (Kabat-Zinn, 1990; Segal, Williams, & Teasdale, 2002). What should shape our approach to establishing and maintaining the teacher training standards and integrity that undergird our programmes? Good teachers

---

[1] The National Institute for Clinical Excellence (NICE) is responsible for UK government recommendations on what treatments to include within National Health Service treatment protocols.

R.S. Crane, Ph.D. (✉) • B. Reid, Ph.D.
Centre for Mindfulness Research and Practice, School of Psychology, Bangor University,
Brigantia Building, Bangor, Gwynedd LL57 2 AS, UK
e-mail: r.crane@bangor.ac.uk; beereid@googlemail.com

© Springer International Publishing Switzerland 2016   121
D. McCown et al., *Resources for Teaching Mindfulness*,
DOI 10.1007/978-3-319-30100-6_6

become ambassadors for mindfulness-based approaches. They become leaders in the expanding field of mindfulness. In essence, therefore, teacher training must not only be about developing skills and knowledge, but must also be concerned with a wider teacher educational *formation process*. Teacher training organisations thus have a key leadership role and responsibility in defining standards, ethics and codes of conduct (e.g. McCown, JKP Press; McCown, Reibel, & Micozzi, 2010) for the emerging community and profession of teachers of mindfulness-based approaches.

There is a multiplicity of responsibilities associated with educational programme development and delivery. This reality is perhaps one reason why, in the UK, leadership of the teacher training agenda has been centred on the university sector. From this vantage point, it has been possible to ensure that teacher training is grounded in the research evidence base; that the processes of teaching, learning and assessment are systematically examined and researched; and that the needs of individual learners in their different contexts are responded to. The benefits of this evidence-based approach are that teaching and learning can extend outwards beyond technique to enable deep experiential *and* scholarly learning. The trainee teacher thus engages in a formation process, a 'coming into being' as a member of the professional community of mindfulness-based teachers.

In this chapter, we draw on the UK experience of university initiatives in helping lead the development of mindfulness-based teacher training programmes. We explore some of the principles and approaches to teacher training that have both shaped and emerged from this experience. We start by looking at what is being sought in trainee teachers—the defining features of mindfulness-based teaching and teacher presence in a mindfulness context. We then discuss how these sometimes abstract notions can be mapped in such a way that they help us understand what is happening when we see good teaching in progress. Finally, we look at how this mapping is informing an approach to teacher competence assessment, and we consider some of the challenges that lie ahead for educational leadership in this field.

Mindfulness-Based Teacher Training Principles

Given the distinctive features of mindfulness-based teaching, what are the key principles that underpin the design of teacher training programmes, and how do these shape the programmes?

Underpinning Principles

Within the MBI field, in common with many other psychotherapeutic/educational approaches to reducing distress and increasing wellbeing, strong emphasis is placed on the importance of thorough preparation of the teacher/therapist.[2] A distinction

---

[2] Although the term 'therapist' is common in psychotherapy research and practice, we will refer here to 'teacher' as this better conveys the mindfulness learning process.

about the mindfulness context lies in its focus on a particular aspect of the development process, namely, the capacity of the teacher to embody mindfulness as they teach (Crane, Kuyken, Hastings, Rothwell, & Williams, 2010; Santorelli, 1999; Segal, Williams, & Teasdale, 2012).

Dobkin et al. describe embodiment as 'the quality of instantiating into one's being, actions and phenomenological experience the skills that are cultivated through mindfulness practice' (Dobkin, Hickman, & Monshat, 2013, p. 4). The process of developing embodiment—of integrating the qualities of mindfulness practice into one's being—is in its nature an emergent one, rather than being a set of skills which can be systematically taught. This situation, in part, creates a paradox at the heart of the teacher development process with which programmes must fully engage. Mindfulness practice is a process of learning to compassionately listen to and trust one's being. This process is the source of authenticity that enables the teacher to congruently embody the practice. However some of the trainee's learning necessarily involves reaching out for new skills. This combination of evocational and acquisitional learning must be brought together in teacher training—a process of learning to teach and live life from the actuality of the present moment experience.

A central theoretical principle that underpins mindfulness-based teaching is that the human mind can operate in different modes (Williams, 2008). In 'doing' mode the mind is processing in a conceptual way how to resolve 'problems' and has a directional energy away from the present moment experiencing. In 'being' mode the mind is processing in a sensory way what is being experienced in the present moment without trying to 'resolve' it. Both are essential for healthy living. However, an over-reliance on doing mode of mind—particularly when it tips into 'driven doing' (Segal et al., 2012)—is strongly implicated in emotional distress, depression and anxiety.

Accordingly, a key learning aim of MBIs is to enable participants to develop an embodied recognition of doing mode of mind, and the capacity to move into a new relationship with experience. Importantly, being mode is not about eliminating or suppressing doing-mode-reactive patterns of thinking. Rather it enables new perspectives on them. Doing-mode patterns ultimately are driven by adaptive primal survival instincts and are both deeply conditioned and hard wired into the human species. Mindfulness practice therefore becomes an on-going orientation which enables practitioners to inhabit the inherent tensions of being human while also being aware of the tendency to become entangled in trying to resolve the inherently unresolvable. The role of the teacher in creating space for course participants to take on this learning is an important foundational consideration in the design of teacher training.

The pedagogic aim for the MBI teaching space is to create the conditions within which course participants can experiment with residing in and responding from being mode of mind. There is an explicit intention to minimise processes that trigger doing mode. This intention can be illustrated through a typical scenario within a mindfulness-based class, which appears. See scenario in Section IV, Chapter 24, B, which illustrates the often subtle difference between the teacher offering a response to a participant from an orientation of 'doing' and from that of 'being'. How does the teacher training process meet both the acquisitional and evocational learning needs of trainees, including their need for space to discover their own authenticity?

Learning Outcomes and the Pedagogic Process

A well-designed training programme has clear learning outcomes which enables students and tutors to focus their work around developing the required skills, knowledge and attitudes. These are then cultivated within the training programme through a carefully designed pedagogic approach. The dynamic and creative tension at the heart of mindfulness is continually at play within the training environment. Although the learning outcomes for a training process can be clearly articulated, the manner in which they are achieved can be subtle. Of course, trainees want to acquire new skills and knowledge, but a large proportion of the work is an inherently personal journey of connecting with one's own inner authenticity through mindfulness practice and then developing skills in bringing this internal way of relating into the fabric of the classroom.

Particular approaches to teaching and learning are needed to support this emergence. If too much emphasis is placed on a directional push towards gaining particular skills and knowledge, the most important vehicle for the teaching can be lost—that is, the trainees' intimate connection with, and trust in, their own being. Thus a balance needs to be struck within a training programme where trainee teachers align their work towards the particular *form* of mindfulness-based approach, while simultaneously being empowered to personally discover and inhabit the *essence* of the MBI.

The whole teacher training process thus mirrors the teaching and learning process in MBI courses; it is mindfulness *based*. Trainees are supported towards being able to fully draw on their capacities to plan, organise and conceptualise ('doing-mode' skills), while they sustain and widen their mindful connection to all that arises within the teaching space ('being-mode' skills). They learn to integrate their 'doing' and their 'being' modes of mind skills (Crane et al., 2010). Table 6.1 summarises the key skills that trainees are developing during mindfulness-based training in the domains of 'being' and 'doing'.

Table 6.1 Examples of being and doing mode of mind skills developed during mindfulness-based teacher training

Being mode of mind skills	Doing mode of mind skills
– Recognising and describing direct experience	– Understanding and articulating rationales for processes
– Being in touch with direct sensory perception moment by moment	– Connecting direct experience with conceptual understandings
– Approaching internal and external experience non-judgementally	– Knowing the form/structure of the curriculum
– Letting go of agendas and ambitions	– Basing clinical programs and curriculum choices on clear rationale and evidence based underpinnings
– Being open to the emergence of fresh perspectives	– Measuring outcomes routinely to check efficacy

Source: Crane (2010)

Ingredients of a Teacher Training Programme

The pedagogy of the teaching and training of MBIs is thus orientated around the premise that learning is conveyed as much through the essential qualities of the teaching (i.e. the implicit qualities of mindfulness that are embodied and communicated during teaching) as through the actual content form of the programme (i.e. the curricular elements). The explicit and implicit learning processes are thus aligned and equally valued. The journey of developing a mindfulness practice on a personal level, and then developing skills in offering it to others, takes time and requires specific conditions. What are these conditions? What are the tangible ingredients within a training programme which support these particular development processes? Table 6.2 sets out and summarises the core aims, focus and programme elements within a training pathway.

Approaching Assessment

An effective training programme develops learning in line with clearly defined learning outcomes. How in the context of mindfulness-based teaching do we assess how successfully these outcomes are achieved? When training is embedded within a validated academic programme there is a clear imperative to address this issue. Master's programmes[3] are required to demonstrate that progress towards achieving learning outcomes is assessed, using reliable and appropriate methods. Even within nonvalidated continuing professional development programmes, there is an increasing emphasis on assessing outcomes. Assessment is therefore an intrinsic part of course design and of the learning process in general. Though it is a challenging process, for trainee teachers, assessment at particular markers in time during their training journey offers developmental feedback and supports on-going learning. It also has far greater potency and credibility than does a simple certificate of attendance.

Supporting Learning Through Assessment

Given the particular characteristics of mindfulness-based teaching and learning that have been discussed above, creating appropriate approaches to assessment is particularly challenging. Assessment is a necessary feature of formal educational programmes, but it is also the aspect of the learning process that can be most difficult for both teachers and students, whatever the field. Teachers must be clear that

---

[3] In the UK, Bangor, Exeter and Oxford Universities offer some of their teacher training in the context of master's programmes.

Table 6.2 Core ingredients of a mindfulness-based training pathway

Training stage and core aims	Key focus	Training processes within the program
Foundation: Personal exploration and experimentation with mindfulness practice Clarifying intention and motivations for engaging in teacher training	Experiential engagement with the practice with a particular intention to: 1. Cultivate awareness in formal and informal practice 2. Begin a journey of discovering a personal way to embody the attitudinal qualities of mindfulness 3. Develop an embodied (i.e. through direct personal engagement) understanding of human vulnerability	• Experiential participation in an MBSR or MBCT program • Support to development a regular on-going personal mindfulness meditation practice through engagement with teachers, through guided practice opportunities, through attendance on retreats and through personal study
Level 1: Development of early level competencies in offering mindfulness-based teaching	Development of: 1. Knowledge (e.g. of theoretical underpinnings; program form; aims of curriculum elements) 2. Skills (across all domains of the teaching process but with particular emphasis on guiding the core meditation practices and facilitating inquiry) 3. Attitudes (investigating an embodied experiential engagement in mindfulness practice, and the potential for expressing this tangibly within the classroom) Deepening personal engagement with the practice of mindfulness	• Further experiential participation in the program from a participant/observer perspective to develop understanding of aims/intentions/pedagogical approach through the program and within individual curriculum elements • Skills training in guiding the three main meditation practices (body scan, mindful movement and sitting meditation) and leading inquiry • Intentional relational engagement between trainees and trainers/supervisor to support development of key attitudes, personal reflective skills, teaching skills and underpinning understanding • Teaching and personal study focused on development of understanding: – of core theoretical underpinnings to the programs through teaching and personal study, with a particular emphasis on the way the program interfaces and intervenes with the universal and specific vulnerabilities of the participants/populations being taught – of the evidence base for mindfulness-based programs and of the value of evaluating routine delivery of classes • Focused skills training on key aspects of the program (tailored to trainees needs)—particularly holding the group, understanding the development process of groups, and delivery of key pivotal themes • Training processes which enable trainees to understand the core similarities and differences between MBSR and MBCT • Attendance on silent guided mindfulness meditation retreats • Development of understanding of ethical/professional practice related to teaching MB courses • Supervised delivery of first classes—ideally alongside an experienced teacher

(continued)

Table 6.2 (continued)

Training stage and core aims	Key focus	Training processes within the program
Level 2: *(For trainees who have taught a minimum of three MBCT or MBSR courses):* Deepening and developing competencies across all the domains of the teaching process with particular emphasis on embodiment and holding the wider group learning process	• Cultivating the capacity to embody mindfulness while teaching • Developing capacity to engage in an authentic, compassionate relationship with participants • Strengthening teaching skills • Developing awareness and confidence to appropriately support participants to turn towards difficulty • Enhancing group process skills as they relate to mindfulness-based teaching • Developing awareness of and responsiveness to the ethical processes in action during mindfulness-based teaching	• Further integration of silent mindfulness practice in retreat conditions with training processes, with the aim of enabling trainees to practice developing a continuity of awareness between personal meditation practice and teaching practice • Opportunities to reflect and inquire into the personal journey of developing as a teacher • On-going engagement with regular supervision with experienced MB teacher/trainer, including periodic review via video recordings of teaching sessions • Continued engagement with personal practice including regular attendance on silent guided mindfulness meditation retreats • Further development of skills in working skilfully with the organisational context for implementing MB courses • Further development of skills in evaluating classes • Formal assessment of teaching competency by submission of video recordings of a full 8-week course and accompanying written review
On-going	• Deepening and developing competencies • Supporting on-going connection to the practice and to personal learning and development • Inspiring a reflective inquiring approach to life and teaching	• Engagement with regular supervision including receiving periodic review of teaching via DVD • Attendance on silent guided mindfulness meditation retreats • Attendance on workshops/trainings to refresh practice and network with colleagues • A commitment to on-going development as a teacher through further training, keeping up to date with the evidence base, recording and reflecting on teaching sessions, participation in webs forums, etc. • As appropriate development of skills as a mentor/supervisor/trainer of less experienced trainees

assessment methods actually assess the knowledge, skills and attitudes they are seeking to evoke through their teaching and learning strategy. A reductionist or mechanical approach to assessment risks interrupting the very learning that it is intended to support. Integrating assessment within the teaching and learning strategy is therefore critical—but also delicate—requiring careful attunement to the student learning process.

Learners are at the heart of the process of creating learning, and the learner sits at the crossroads of a complex system. Trainee teachers of MBIs are part of a class of student teachers; they are simultaneously beginning teachers and students; they are in relationship with other teacher trainers, teachers and students; they may move between different teaching and learning settings and may also move between different institutional settings in their working lives. These social and contextual relations define their learning experiences. And these circumstances offer a further challenge to the assessment process: how can the assessment tools that are used evoke the student's full experience of understanding (coming both from within and beyond the classroom), thereby encourage learning to take place across the whole of this wider terrain? Here assessment approaches that encourage integration and 'meaning making' have a wider role to play: they help establish a wider culture of reflective practice and self-assessment that extends well beyond individual assessment 'events' or the requirements of defined learning programmes.

Designing the Approach

Effective course design thus rests on creating an approach to assessing student achievement that coheres with both the intended programme objectives and curriculum and with the ways that the student is making meaning out of their whole learning experience. Biggs (1996) expressed how the degree of connection between these two areas directly influences the likelihood of 'deep learning' being evoked in the student and described this connection as 'constructive alignment'. Deep learning is the opposite of accepting new facts without critical appraisal or discernment, or relying on 'rote' learning or cataloguing of information. In mindfulness terms, it is the sum of acquisitional plus evocational learning: the interweaving of 'doing' and 'being' modes of learning. It requires curiosity, engagement and appropriate contextual knowledge. Further it is about taking on new information and ideas, evaluating these critically and with discernment, applying and relating them appropriately and making connections and links with real-life settings (Biggs, 1999; Entwistle, 1988; Ramsden, 1992).

There are two main approaches to assessment design that can be used in education and training programmes: competence-based and standards-based.

Competence-based assessments articulate what behaviours at a range of benchmark levels are required to demonstrate the relevant skill, which are then used by assessors to assess trainees. Trainees undertake assessment activities, the purpose of which is to determine their level of competence. More generally, skills (e.g. teaching to a specific level of proficiency), knowledge and attitudes may form the basis of competence assessment (though competenc-based tools cannot access the more qualitative and experiential dimensions of attitudes). Competence is achieved when a skill (such as teaching) is assessed as taking place at defined benchmark levels. So, for example, in a mindfulness-based teaching context, a trainee may submit a video of their teaching for feedback on their progress towards developing competence in teaching.

Standards-based approaches are based on more general descriptions of required learning which provide an overarching rationale for teaching and learning. Assessment is carried out against the standards, using evidence gathered from trainees and generated from participation in a range of activities where trainees may, for example, be creating, designing, performing, researching or otherwise participating. In mindfulness-based teaching, for example, this kind of activity could involve leading practices, reflecting on the experience and then setting that experience in the context of relevant literature. An assessor infers capability by examining the evidence. Because it actively engages with the trainee's meaning-making world, the standards-based approach is considered to be meaningful to the individuals being assessed. It also gives assessors a degree of discretion in their assessment of the evidence submitted, for example, in terms of the type of evidence that is considered acceptable, with the onus on the trainee to demonstrate relevance. The process accordingly requires horizontal accountability among assessors.

Robust teaching and learning programmes draw from both approaches, often underpinning competence-based tools with standard-setting activity. Standards-based methods are used to create balance, to respond to teaching and learning priorities and to draw on evidence-based research to guide the rationale for the overall approach. In this way, the assessment strategy reflects the pedagogy (the teaching and learning strategy) of the training programme.

Practical Considerations

There were a number of additional 'beyond-the-classroom' educational factors to bear in mind when assessment tools and approaches have been developed within UK university mindfulness centres. Reliable methods to assess skills development and growing competence are needed in research trials as well as within the master's programmes. There is also a wider educational and professional priority around protecting the integrity of MBIs by devising a framework capable of both supporting reflective practice and the personal development of the teacher beyond the training program.

Accordingly, three additional practical considerations are important in shaping assessment strategy within MBI teacher training:

1. *What is the purpose of the assessment?*

Assessment may often serve different purposes. Newton (2007), for example, cites as many as 18 differentiated purposes for educational assessment. Many of these echo the priorities of MBI teacher training curriculum development, such as student monitoring and attainment, qualification, guidance, programme evaluation, formative identification of learning needs, providing a measure of student achievement, discovering more about the results and wider impacts of the training programme, safeguarding the integrity of the approach and encouraging compliance with emerging teaching standards.

2. *What is being assessed?*

The main focus within MBI teacher training is on the developing mindfulness-based teaching skills and the underpinning knowledge and attitudes required. Here, we have established that acquisitional as well as evocational learning both need assessing. There are also wider potentials for using assessment to gather evaluation information about the effectiveness of the teacher training programme as a whole.

3. *How is the assessment designed and organised?*

A key challenge is integrating core principles of MBIs into assessment design. How can assessment methods capture moment-to-moment insights, and experiential learning, and achieve a balance of 'doing' and 'being' modes. Inevitably the assessors' judgements and decisions are a highly significant influence in this process. Their own teaching and training contexts, their relationship to the assessment process and the manner in which they frame student feedback are all important aspects of the relational activity which enlivens the assessment process.

In responding to this wider context when framing an approach to assessment that meets the needs of MBI teacher training, what combination of methods enables reliable assessment of the range of skills that trainee mindfulness-based teachers are developing? It would be impossible to capture or distil down the complexity of mindfulness-based teaching to any single method of assessment (Crane, Kuyken, et al., 2012). A combined 'whole strategy' approach enables progressive and developmental assessment to happen within the framework of a developed teaching and learning strategy. Where competence-based tools are used, they are underpinned by a standards-based approach to on-going reflective learning. Likewise, where standards-based tools are used, they are underpinned by competence-referenced reflection as students come to learn through more reflective styles of assignment what is expected of them concretely 'in the classroom' when they teach.

A key ingredient within the range assessment methods used in UK training programmes is the Mindfulness-Based Interventions: Teaching Assessment Criteria (MBI-TAC) (Crane, Soulsby, Kuyken, Williams, & Eames, 2012). This assessment is a competence-based tool developed to directly assess teaching skills and is described further in the next section. Table 6.3 summarises the various assessment methods used in UK training programmes.

The Mindfulness-Based Interventions: Teaching Assessment Criteria

Mindfulness is intimate and interior work and it can sometimes seem countercultural to set it within an assessment context. But the issue of maintaining standards and integrity in the delivery of MBIs is an important concern and invites a response that is as clear as possible. This requirement in turn demands clarity about the nature of the teaching skills needed and how they are formed and developed.

The MBI-TAC was developed in this combined context of educational accountability, scholarly accountability and accountability to the beneficiaries of MBA teaching (the wider public). There were several motivations for its development:

Table 6.3 Methods for assessing mindfulness-based teaching skills, knowledge and attitudes

Tool	Description	Primary assessment tool	Type of learning
Teaching portfolios	Accumulated experience gathered in the form of a portfolio or dossier which can include detailed narrative of session by session teaching processes including personal reflections on the experience, publicity materials, participant feedback forms, and outcomes of evaluation/audit of the class. Teaching portfolios do not provide direct evidence of competencies but are useful accompaniments to other methods	Standards-based (underpinned by competence-based approach as students come to learn what is expected of them)	Acquisitional (with reflective practice leading to evocational)
Reflective assignments	Given that the teaching process strongly relies on the teacher having a sophisticated capacity to attune to internal experience in the form of sensations, thoughts, and emotions, training programs include assessment of the particular style of reflective capacity required for mindfulness-based teaching	Standards-based (underpinned by competence-based approach as students come to learn what is required of them)	Evocational (with reflective practice leading to acquisitional, in that teaching practice takes place in a real setting and requires skills and knowledge to be practiced)
Academic assignments	Training programs require trainees to produce written assignments on the theory and background underpinning MBSR and/or MBCT teaching. Commonly, these require students to synthesise their own experience with the literature on mindfulness-based teaching	Standards-based (which may engender competence-based reflection)	Acquisitional (leading to evocational, in that reflection occurs as the result of engagement in the assignment)
Self assessment	Explicitly inviting trainees to assess their competencies after teaching can be a way of actively engaging them in an exploration of strengths and areas for development from a different perspective than receiving feedback from others. If trainees develop the capacity to engage in honest reflection of their own teaching this will serve their ongoing development beyond their engagement in formal training processes. The MBI-TAC can be usefully used as a framework for this	Competence-based (underpinned by a standards-based approach to ongoing reflection)	Acquisitional (leading to evocational through engagement in reflection)

(continued)

Table 6.3 (continued)

Tool	Description	Primary assessment tool	Type of learning
Peer assessment	The usual context for practising skills in a training group context is with peers. Peer feedback therefore becomes a key training tool and in itself is a skill which needs training so that the feedback is both honestly and sensitively offered. The process is mutual—in offering feedback trainees are honing their understanding of the competencies required through a direct experience of what works well and less well. Again the MBI-TAC is a useful framework for this process	Competence-based (underpinned by a standards-based approach to ongoing reflection)	Acquisitional (leading to evocational through engagement in reflection)
Review of teaching by an expert panel via video-recording or live observation	This offers a marker that the teacher has made their teaching practice available for external scrutiny and has participated in a robust series of training processes. All such reviews in the UK context employ the MBI-TAC for this process. In Master's programs this element of assessment is progressively developed. In the early stages of training, students are assessed on their skill in teaching elements of the curriculum, whereas at the end they are required to submit DVDs of an entire 8-week MBCT or MBSR course for review	Competence-based (underpinned by a standards-based approach to ongoing reflective practice)	Acquisitional (leading to evocational through reflective practice)

Source: Adapted from Crane et al. (2012)

first was responding to the absence at the time of a systematic approach to directly assessing MBSR/MBCT teaching competency and bringing rigour and substance to understanding the constituent elements of 'good teaching' in the context of training and research programmes. Additional motivations were to enable coordination among teams of programme assessors, to offer transparency to students, to establish national benchmarking between training centres, and to provide a tool for reflective practice.

The MBI-TAC Development Process

In 2009, Bangor, Oxford and Exeter Universities, all of whom were interested in assessing teaching as part of their respective master's and research programmes, came together to collaborate by pooling expertise and experience. The development of the MBI-TAC was effectively a piece of grounded theory generation: the work was the expression of an on-going process of learning from experience. Theory building—in this case, the creation of the categories and themes—was grounded in actual observations of MBSR and MBCT teaching practices. Trainers from the three university centres gradually refined the MBI-TAC through a series of developmental stages in which the face and content validity of the tool were tested by practical application of the tool in the mindfulness-based classroom (Crane et al., 2013).

The Structure of the MBI-TAC

The MBI-TAC (Crane, Soulsby, et al., 2012) contains six general 'domains' or themes of teaching in practice, as follows:

1. Coverage, pacing and organisation of session curriculum
2. Relational skills
3. Embodiment of mindfulness
4. Guiding mindfulness practices
5. Conveying course themes through interactive inquiry and didactic teaching
6. Holding of the group learning environment

Within each domain a number of features are articulated which unpack the various aspects of this element of the teaching process. For example, domain 2 includes 'curiosity and respect', while domain 3 includes 'present moment responsiveness'. A scale for assessing competence based on the work of Dreyfus and Dreyfus (1986) enables indicative differentiation of competence based on six bands ranging from 'advanced' to 'incompetent', in turn providing a means of giving detailed and context-specific feedback to trainees on their development. Table 6.4 shows how the domain and competence levels interact using domain 3 (embodiment) as an example.

Cautions and Limitations to the MBI-TAC

There are important caveats and limitations to the use of the MBI-TAC. Teaching skills do not develop in isolation nor as the simple direct result of having participated in a training course. There is a 'hidden curriculum' for every student: what the individual brings to the training, how they relate to the personal development process and how they integrate the new learning into their lives are all influencing

Table 6.4 Sample page of the MBI-TAC illustrating how the domains and competence levels interact

Domain 3: Embodiment of mindfulness	
	Examples
Incompetent	Embodiment of mindfulness is not conveyed
	Examples include: absence of present moment focus/responsiveness. Attitudinal qualities of mindfulness are not in evidence and those that are conveyed have the potential for harm
Beginner	At least one of the five key features is present at a level that would be desirable for adequate MBI teaching, but significant levels of inconsistency exist across all key features
	Examples include: lack of consistent present moment focus/responsiveness; teacher not calm, at ease and alert; attitudinal qualities often not clearly in evidence; teacher manner conveys restlessness and unease; teacher does not seem 'at home' in themselves or in the space
Advanced Beginner	At least two of the five key features are present at a competent level, but difficulty and/or inconsistency is clearly evident in others; participants' safety is not compromised; no aspects of the embodied process is destructive to participants
	Examples include: teacher evidences embodiment of several principles of mindfulness practice within the teaching process, but there is a lack of consistency (i.e. teacher demonstrates some skilful present moment internal and external connectedness, but this is not sustained throughout); the teacher might seem 'steady', but there is a lack of vitality in the space or vice versa; teacher's bodily expression at times conveys qualities that are different from mindfulness (e.g. a sense of hurry, agitation and/or striving)
Competent	All key features present to a good level of skill with some minor inconsistencies
	Examples include: teacher generally demonstrates an ability to communicate the attitudinal qualities of mindfulness practice through his/her bodily presence and is mostly present moment focused/responsive; teacher mostly seems natural and at ease
Proficient	All key features consistently present with a good level of skill
	Examples include: sustained levels of present moment focus through the teaching and demonstration of the range of attitudinal qualities of mindfulness throughout with very minor inconsistencies; the bodily expression of the teacher implicitly conveys the qualities of mindfulness; teacher is natural and at ease; teacher is authentic both to themselves and to the qualities of mindfulness
Advanced	All key features present to a high-skill level
	Examples include: teacher demonstrates exceptionally high levels of awareness of and responsiveness to the present moment throughout the teaching process; teacher has high levels of internal and external connectedness; teacher has attitudinal qualities of mindfulness present in a particularly inspiring way; teacher is highly authentic both to him/herself and to the qualities of mindfulness. Difficult for reviewer to find further 'learning needs' to feedback

factors of teacher development. What might be observed in students teaching in their classrooms may not always be the result of what has been formally taught to them, but more the reflection of their manner of appropriating, internalising and integrating their learning. Then while there are visible aspects of the teachers' skills or their classroom presence that can be observed and described, there are also less-visible processes which cannot be assessed by observation. It is important to acknowledge that any one teaching assessment represents one moment in time in the context of a long journey of development. An observer assessor cannot gain an entire picture of the trainee's learning from a single observation. It is a 'soil sample' only. The importance of using the MBI-TAC as only part of a framework of teaching, learning and assessment should therefore be strongly emphasised.

Looking to the Future: Supporting the Emerging Professional Context for MBI Teaching and Teachers

Training processes that have integrity need to take account of the context within which trainees will practise and implement new skills. What does appropriate governance and professional practice in this context look like? What frameworks are needed within which practitioners can optimally operate? What standards are needed to support appropriate conduct and competence levels? How can the field maintain public confidence and ensure that professionals working with integrity are not undermined by those who are not?

Mindfulness as a part of mainstream life is a new phenomenon. It is increasingly being integrated into a range of contexts including political life, education, health care and the justice system. There are tensions between the urgency to respond to the demand for greater teaching capacity and the urge to ensure that developments are sustainable and have integrity. If skilful forms of governance are not developed from within the profession, there is a risk that integrity is weakened, which in turn could lead to compromised public confidence.

The Implementation Challenge

It is critical that any new approach is implemented in ways which are consistent and congruent with the developers' intentions and with the evidence base. Implementing new evidence is always challenging. It requires deliberate and active effort and relies on having the right people working in a supportive context to enable the change to happen. Any action is contextually situated, and so the evidence is frequently interpreted in different ways as it is implemented, which can dilute or change the intervention (Rogers, 2002). In addition to the generic challenge of implementing new approaches, there are some particular aspects to the mindfulness implementation process which render it liable to being offered in ways which do not have integrity. There are three features of mindfulness-based teaching that potentially create this vulnerability—the deceptive simplicity of the practice, the way in which ethics are held within mindfulness-based teaching and the way in which integrity rests on the teacher's inner work:

1. *The deceptive simplicity of the practice*

Anyone who has engaged with mindfulness practice in a sustained way will realise that the process is tremendously subtle, multidimensional, multilayered and inherent with paradox. It is an easy step for mindfulness practice to be taken up as another way to address problems within oneself or within an organisation—a way to 'fix' what is 'broken' (Kabat-Zinn, 2011). It is an easy step for mindfulness practice to be taken up as a way to step back, and gain some relief, from the pressures of life. In fact, the practice is a radical paradigm shift that challenges the status quo within ourselves and within the cultural context in which we live. The term 'mindfulness' can easily become a catch-all phrase for a spectrum of practices, many of which are just a small aspect of the original intentions of the practice.

2. *An implicit—rather than explicit—ethical underpinning*

Within the Buddhist context for mindfulness practice, there is a surrounding explicit ethical framework. It is completely appropriate that the ethical framework for delivering mindfulness in contemporary secular contexts is implicit within the process. Within MBSR and MBCT, the emphasis is on enabling an ethical orientation towards oneself and then others to emerge through the personal learning process. At its best this practice naturally grows into an ethical shift towards our human ecology—the interconnected system that surrounds the individual.

The integrity of teacher training programmes however is deeply reliant on the teacher evoking within the personal and collective learning process a clear ethical framework. This integrity in turn relies on the teacher having a high degree of personal clarity regarding their own ethical orientation and the intentions for the practice. If the approach is being taught as a 'management tool' in a workplace context without a deeper understanding of the potential of the approach, it is possible that it could be used, for example, to enhance performance or increase an individual's competitive edge. These outcomes could come at the expense of personal and collective wellbeing which is counter to the core intention of mindfulness. A basic underpinning ethic of mindfulness is that it is offered in the spirit of reducing suffering experienced by the individual and in the interconnected system around that individual. Purser and Loy frame it thus: 'Mindfulness is a *distinct quality of attention* that is dependent upon and influenced by many other factors: the nature of our thoughts, speech and actions; our way of making a living; and our efforts to avoid unwholesome and unskilful behaviours, while developing those that are conducive to wise action, social harmony, and compassion' (Purser & Loy, 2013).

3. *Integrity relies on inner work*

As discussed earlier, the integrity of the approach relies on and emerges from the teacher's personal internal engagement with practice. This quality is not possible to quantify and is difficult to operationalise within a governance process. As discussed above, the process of assessing competence largely relies on assessing the visible ways in which the practice becomes tangible within the classroom. This appearance is deeply personal and culturally specific. It is entirely appropriate therefore that there are diverse ways in which embodiment is expressed. The assessment of competence is thus complex and prone to subjective bias.

Furthermore, there are a range of pathways along which teachers journey as they gather personal experience with the practice before and as they engage with teacher training. Many do not come through the doorway of professional practice, and many come from a wide range of different professional settings. Accordingly, the 'teaching work' of teachers cannot be assumed to be situated within the scope of any specific professional body which provides oversight in terms of integrity and ethical approaches.

In sum, the scope that exists for confusion is manifest. How can a member of the general public wanting to take a mindfulness-based class be sure that what is being offered is not just a caricature of mindfulness? Safeguarding integrity therefore is in the service of enabling the receivers of mindfulness services—i.e. participants in classes—to have clarity. Clear, accurate communication is needed, both of the approach being offered and of the training which the teacher has engaged in. The general public needs to know that the teacher adheres to recognised standards, has engaged in appropriate levels of training and has reached a recognised level of competence.

The Building Blocks for Good Governance

How is the field ensuring that robust foundational building blocks to support integrity are being put in place? How are we stepping up to the challenge of protecting the integrity of mindfulness when it is offered in secular contexts, at a time of unprecedented interest and demand?

The process of safeguarding integrity is requiring the generation of new knowledge and the development of fresh insights. It is requiring collaboration on national and international levels to develop consistent and coherent approaches to integrity. It is a reflexive process of dialogue between the contemplative context for mindfulness practice and the emerging professional contexts of MBIs in the mainstream. There is a parallel emphasis on developing integrity both from the 'inside out' (training teachers so that there are expectations regarding on-going attention to self-integrity) and from the 'outside in' (developing anchor points in the form of governance and standards to which people from both within and without the professions can relate).

The process requires that everyone working within the field takes on a measure of responsibility for upholding and developing clarity around integrity. Much rests upon the teachers themselves. They are the main vehicle and conduit for their work in the world. As Kabat-Zinn said: 'It has always felt to me that MBSR is at its healthiest and best when the responsibility to ensure its integrity, quality, and standards of practice is being carried by each MBSR instructor him or herself' (Kabat-Zinn, 2011, p. 295).

However, teacher training organisations also have a special role in leading the development of supportive professional contexts for their teaching practice communities. It is not enough to simply focus on good training. Trainers need to care about the implementation context for trainees' on-going practice and teaching work.

Training organisations are in a particularly strategic position in this regard. They interrelate with trainees, with the mainstream contexts where implementation is taking place and with each other. They are uniquely placed to facilitate developments and lead dialogue which support the development of good governance. They have a responsibility to communicate the cornerstones of ethical and professional practice to all stakeholders in the process and to cultivate a culture of ethical self-regulation and self-responsibility within their trainees.

There are of course other stakeholders. Teachers and trainers need to be aware of this contextual landscape of organisations and institutions where MBAs are being implemented. This context can include pressures for swift or low-cost implementation. In these cases it is vital that a lone teacher is able to draw on the collective voices of leaders within the field to communicate consensual views on what governance needs to ensure integrity during implementation (Rycroft-Malone et al., 2014).

Moving now to the specific building blocks to support integrity: what processes and governance are in place to which people from both within and without the profession can relate and what is needed to take these forward?

- *Good practice standards for teachers and trainers* (e.g. Santorelli, Goddard, Kabat-Zinn, Kesper-Grossman, & Reibel, 2011; UK Network for Mindfulness-Based Teacher Training Organisations, 2012): Further work is now needed to lift these standards up to an international level so that there is overarching leadership on good practice standards to which each country can relate.
- *National and international networks of teacher training organisations which are institutionally independent* (e.g. EAMBA, 2014; UK Network for Mindfulness-Based Teacher Training Organisations, 2012): These networks are crucial in enabling training organisations to come into alignment on common areas of interest and to give collective attention to the wider vision for the work. Networks are needed at both a national level to support collaborative working within the local context, and at an international level to support the development of a coherent international voice on integrity issues.
- *Conceptualisation of the nature of teaching competence and the development of a system to assess it* (Crane et al., 2013; Crane, Soulsby, et al., 2012): Further work is needed to refine the tool, to develop other methods for assessing skills which can sit alongside, and to adapt the tool to the range of MBIs.
- *Development of a framework for the particular form of supervision needed by mindfulness teachers and standards for supervisors* (Evans et al., 2014): Considerable attention is being given to this requirement in the UK context. Attention is now needed on the development of international standards for supervision, as supervision is a key way in which the strengths of individual teachers are cultivated and supported.
- *Conceptualising how training models and pedagogy align with intended learning outcomes* (Crane et al., 2010): Research on the range of training models which are being employed internationally is needed to support the development of empirically underpinned understanding of best practice.

- *Governance in the settings where MBAs are being implemented:* Successful implementation relies on tailoring national and international guidance on good practice to the specifics of the local context for implementation. Reflexive practice, continually responsive to dialogue between grassroots practice and the wider context for implementation, is needed so that best practice informs the whole (Rycroft-Malone et al., 2014).

Conclusion: The Work Ahead

In the midst of this live and emerging process, it is hard to predict the ways in which our community of mindfulness-based teachers and trainers will develop, and the specific forms that the professions' governance structures will take. It is clear that much groundwork is taking place to support good practice. At its best, regulation can empower by giving impetus to learning, can facilitate best practices and promote public confidence. The key challenge is to navigate a line between participatory, inclusive approaches which bring the field towards consensus on good practice, while also ensuring clarity in relation to what constitutes a divergence from agreed integrity standards.

To accomplish this goal successfully, all stakeholders need to collaboratively contribute to dialogue on training, integrity and governance developments. Training organisations have a particular responsibility and are well placed to provide leadership on these issues. Ultimately, it should be borne in mind that the purpose of this work is to serve our wider community—the general public who are the recipients of the services that mindfulness teachers offer. Our collective hopes for the potential of mindfulness practice to serve in this way are best supported by rich and on-going dialogue and collaboration.

References

Biggs, J. (1996). Enhancing teaching through constructive alignment. *Higher Education, 32*, 346–364.

Biggs, J. (1999). *Teaching for quality learning at university*. Berkshire, UK: SHRE and Open University Press.

Crane, R. S., Eames, C., Kuyken, W., Hastings, R. P., Williams, J. M. G., Bartley, T., … Surawy, C. (2013). Development and validation of the Mindfulness-Based Interventions—Teaching Assessment Criteria (MBI:TAC). *Assessment, 20*, 681–688. doi:10.1177/1073191113490790.

Crane, R. S., Kuyken, W., Hastings, R., Rothwell, N., & Williams, J. M. G. (2010). Training teachers to deliver mindfulness-based interventions: Learning from the UK experience. *Mindfulness, 1*, 74–86.

Crane, R. S., Kuyken, W., Williams, J. M. G., Hastings, R., Cooper, L., & Fennell, M. J. V. (2012). Competence in teaching mindfulness-based courses: Concepts, development, and assessment. *Mindfulness, 3*(1), 76–84. doi:10.1007/s12671-011-0073-2.

Crane, R. S., Soulsby, J. G., Kuyken, W., Williams, J. M. G., & Eames, C. (2012). *The Bangor, Exeter & Oxford mindfulness-based interventions teaching assessment criteria (MBI-TAC) for assessing the competence and adherence of mindfulness-based class-based teaching.* Retrieved from http://www.bangor.ac.uk/mindfulness/documents/MBI-TACJune2012.pdf

Dobkin, P. L., Hickman, S., & Monshat, K. (2014). Holding the heart of mindfulness-based stress reduction: Balancing fidelity and imagination when adapting MBSR. mindfulness. *Mindfulness, 5,* 710–718.

Dreyfus, H. L., & Dreyfus, S. E. (1986). *Mind over machine: The power of human intuition and experience in the age of computers.* New York: Free Press.

Entwistle, N. (1988). *Styles of learning and teaching.* Abingdon, UK: David Fulton.

European Associations of Mindfulness based Approaches (EAMBA). (2014). Retrieved from http://eamba.net/

Evans, A., Crane, R. S., Cooper, L., Mardula, J., Wilks, J., Surawy, C., … Kuyken, W. (2015). A framework for supervision for mindfulness-based teachers: A space for embodied mutual inquiry. *Mindfulness, 6*(3), 572–581. doi:10.1007/s12671-014-0292-4.

Kabat-Zinn, J. (1990). *Full catastrophe living, revised edition: How to cope with stress, pain and illness using mindfulness meditation.* London, UK: Piatkus.

Kabat-Zinn, J. (2011). Some reflections on the origins of MBSR, skillful means, and the trouble with maps. *Contemporary Buddhism, 11*(1).

McCown, D., Reibel, D., & Micozzi, M. S. (2010). *Teaching mindfulness.* New York: Springer.

Mindfulness All Party Parliamentary Group, 2015-last update, Mindful Nation UK. Retrieved from http://www.themindfulnessinitiative.org.uk/images/reports/Mindfulness-APPGReport_Mindful-Nation-UK_Oct2015.pdf.

National Institute for Clinical Excellence (NICE). (2004). *Depression: Management in primary and secondary care.* (Guideline 23 p.76. ed.)

Newton, P. E. (2007). Clarifying the purposes of educational assessment. *Assessment in Education, 14*(2), 149–170.

Purser, R., & Loy, D. (2013, July 1). Beyond McMindfulness. Retrieved from http://www.huffingtonpost.com/ron-purser/beyond-mcmindfulness_b_3519289.html

Ramsden, P. (1992). *Learning to teach in higher education.* New York: Routledge.

Rogers, E. M. (2002). The nature of technology transfer. *Science Communication, 23,* 323–341.

Rycroft-Malone, J., Anderson, R., Crane, R. S., Gibson, A., Gradinger, F., Owen-Griffiths, H., … Kuyken, W. (2014). Accessibility and implementation in UK services of an effective depression relapse prevention program—Mindfulness-based cognitive therapy (MBCT): ASPIRE study protocol. *Implementation Science, 9,* 62.

Santorelli, S. (1999). *Heal thy self.* New York, NY: Bell Tower.

Santorelli, S., Goddard, T., Kabat-Zinn, J., Kesper-Grossman, U., & Reibel, D. (2011). Standards for the formation of MBSR teacher trainers: Experience, qualifications, competency and ongoing development. In *Investigating and Integrating Mindfulness in Medicine, Health Care, and Society. 9th Annual International Scientific Conference for Clinicians, Researchers and Educators,* Boston, USA.

Segal, Z. V., Williams, J. M. G., & Teasdale, J. D. (2002). *Mindfulness-based cognitive therapy for depression.* New York, NY: Guilford Press.

Segal, Z. V., Williams, J. M. G., & Teasdale, J. D. (2012). *Mindfulness-based cognitive therapy for depression.* New York, NY: Guilford Press.

UK Network for Mindfulness-Based Teacher Training Organisations. (2012). *Good practice guidance for teaching mindfulness-based courses.* Retrieved from http://mindfulnessteachersuk.org.uk/

Williams, J. M. G. (2008). Mindfulness, depression and modes of mind. *Cognitive Therapy Research, 32,* 721–733. doi:10.1007/s10608-008-9204-z.

Part II
Teaching MBI Curricula Everywhere: Global Cultural Situations

Chapter 7
Teaching MBSR in Korea with a Special Reference to Cultural Differences

Heyoung Ahn

Introduction

The purpose of this chapter is to share my personal experience of teaching MBSR in Korea for the past 10 years or so. I address cultural differences in teaching MBSR in Korea, paying particular attention to what I have added to the template MBSR curriculum in my class and how and why I have chosen to do so. I will proceed with Hall's poignant remark in mind: "Culture hides much more than it reveals, and strangely enough what it hides, it hides most effectively from its own participants" (1959, p. 29).

I do know from my own experience that the template MBSR program as taught at the Center for Mindfulness in UMASS works well in Korea, regardless of the cultural differences between the two countries, in light of the following factors:

1. The template MBSR program has evolved through a combination of (a) Jon Kabat-Zinn's long-term mindfulness practice and creativity, (b) collaborative work by Saki Santorelli and his colleagues, and (c) continuous research experimentation. It is a powerful program based on a confluence of two distinctive epistemologies of contemplative wisdom and scientific research.
2. The template MBSR program is about "M," mindfulness, which refers to the universal quality of mind. Stripping away the various layers of culture and language, we humans are left with an essential core or "the common pathway" as members of *Homo sapiens*. MBSR intrinsically orients all toward this dimension of "deep down" within us, transcending linguistic and cultural trappings.

My first intention in teaching is to maintain the integraty of MBSR and help my participants optimize their potential when taught in a culture enormously different

H. Ahn, Ph.D. Ed.D. (✉)
Korea Center for MBSR; Seoul University of Buddhism,
1038-2, Doksan-Dong, Geumcheon-Gu, Seoul 153-831, South Korea
e-mail: mbsr1@hanmail.net

© Springer International Publishing Switzerland 2016   143
D. McCown et al., *Resources for Teaching Mindfulness*,
DOI 10.1007/978-3-319-30100-6_7

Table 7.1 Individualistic and collectivistic cultures (adapted from Gudykunst & Kim, 1997)

Individualistic	Collectivistic
Emphasis on individual goals	Emphasis on group goals
Self-realization	Fitting into the group
Little difference between in-group and out-group communication	Large difference between in-group and out-group communication
Independent self-construction	Interdependent self-construction
"I" identity	"We" identity
Saying what you are thinking	Avoiding confrontations in group
Low-context communication: direct, precise, and absolute	High-context communication: indirect, imprecise, and probabilistic

from its place of origin. This experience resonates well with the McCown, Reibel, and Micozzi (2010) observation that "…the metastructure [of MBSR] has remained unchanged for decades simply because it has an extremely powerful intuitive logic… [and] has an undeniable integrity (p. 139)."

Cultural Differences Between the United States and Korea

I now highlight the cultural accommodations that I employ in my class which may be specific to my country and possibly to other East Asian countries as well. Considering there are different ways to discuss the cultural differences, certain kinds of operational concepts or framework are in order. Above all, I find it very useful to selectively borrow Hofstede's dimensions of cultural variability—(1) individualism–collectivism, (2) uncertainty avoidance, and (3) power distance. A sketch of these dimensions helps pave the way for the discussion that follows.

Among the three concepts, the dichotomy of individualism–collectivism can be the most salient feature illustrating cultural differences between these two populations. Table 7.1 shows the main characteristics differing between individualistic and collectivistic cultures.

Examples of more individualistic cultures include, but are not limited to, Canada, France, Germany, Great Britain, South Africa, Sweden, and the United States. Examples of more collectivistic cultures include Brazil, China, India, Japan, Korea, Saudi Arabia, and Venezuela (Gudykunst & Kim, 1997). These contrasting cultures are said to represent their own characteristic communication styles respectively, that is, low-context communication and high-context communication. Low-context communication is predominantly used by members of individualistic cultures, while high-context communication is predominantly used by members of collectivistic cultures (Gudykunst & Kim). As shown in Table 7.1, a low-context communication or message is said to be more direct, precise, and absolute, compared to its counterpart, which is indirect, imprecise, and probabilistic.

I find my participants differ from one person to another, demonstrating the important role of individual personality, as well as culture. Although many appear

Table 7.2 Low and high uncertainty avoidance cultures (adapted from Gudykunst & Kim, 1997)

Low uncertainty avoidance	High uncertainty avoidance
A weak desire for consensus; deviant behavior is acceptable	A strong desire for consensus; deviant behavior is not acceptable
Less display of emotions	More display of emotions
Lower stress levels and weaker superegos	Higher stress levels and stronger superegos
Acceptance of dissent and more risk-taking	Less acceptance of dissent and less risk-taking
Less resistance against change	More resistance against change
Lower levels of anxiety	Higher levels of anxiety
More tolerance for ambiguous instructions, less conflict avoidance, approval of competition	Preference for clear instructions, conflict avoidance, and disapproval of competition
Higher motivation for achievement	Lower motivation for achievement

to be under the influence of collectivistic characteristics, some show those of the individualistic culture shown in Table 7.1. As indicated above, my participants have a general tendency to be "group oriented": more sensitive to the class atmosphere (i.e., relationships or opinions of others) and more hesitant to stand out or express their opinions clearly when it is likely to clash with those of others.

Another useful concept or framework for categorizing cultural similarities and differences is uncertainty avoidance proposed by Hofstede. It accounts for "the degree to which the members of a culture feel threatened by uncertain or unknown situations (Hofstede, 1997, p. 113). Table 7.2 was designed to show the difference between a low uncertainty avoidance culture and a high uncertainty avoidance culture.

High uncertainty avoidance cultures include France, Greece, Japan, Korea, and Spain, while low uncertainty avoidance cultures include Canada, England, India, Sweden, and the United States (Gudykunst & Kim, 1997). My participants have a relatively strong tendency that matches well with those in a high power distance culture. They tend to show a high level of anxiety and less risk-taking in confronting others. They appear to be afraid of other people's opinions or disrupting the class atmosphere. For example, when someone is late for the class, he or she often mentions during the dialogue and inquiry session that they felt really sorry or guilty simply because they were late. In their minds, being tardy is associated with disrupting others. Some people even have a hard time attempting to suppress their coughs or sneeze because they worry about causing any inconvenience to others.

Another useful dimension is power distance. It means "the extent to which the less powerful members of institutions and organizations within a country expect and accept that power is distributed unequally (Hofstede, 1997, p. 28).). The following table was made, drawing on Hofstede's and Gudykunst & Kim's description.

Egypt, India, Malaysia, Saudi Arabia, and Venezuela are cultures where high power distance predominates, while low power distance is predominant in Austria, Canada, Germany, Sweden, and the United States (Gudykunst & Kim, p. 73). Korea belongs to a slightly high power distance culture.

In general, my participants demonstrate those characteristics described in Table 7.3. It is very rare that any participant challenges the teacher's authority by

Table 7.3 Low and high power distance cultures (adapted from Gudykunst & Kim, 1997)

Low power distance	High power distance
Less acceptance of power as part of society	Acceptance power as part of society
Limited dependence of subordinates on boss; interdependence between boss and subordinates	Considerable dependence of subordinates on boss
Emotional distance between boss and subordinate is relatively small	Emotional distance between boss and subordinate is relatively large
Students value self-direction and display egalitarian attitudes	Students value conformity and display authoritarian attitudes
Open supervision, less fear of disagreement with a supervisor	Close supervision, fear of disagreement with a supervisor

inappropriate behavior or asking challenging questions. They appear to accept the teacher's power as an authority without any resistance. Some do not stretch out their legs or lie down during the class, even though I tell them that they can do anything as long as it does "no harm" to others.

Most people attending my MBSR class come from the collectivistic cultural background. This fact does not necessarily mean that each and every individual operates from these characteristics. Although each participant is different, the class as a whole tends to display this collectivistic dynamic.

There are two guiding questions that I believe are very useful in conducting class in this typical collectivistic culture.

1. How can I create a safe holding environment for participants living in a high uncertainty and power distance distance country?
2. How can I help each participant cultivate and maintain commitment to mindfulness practice throughout the course?

These two considerations lead me to employ the following methods: (a) class activities, such as the rubber band throw game and mindful dancing for the holding environment, (b) emphasis on the right attitudes, and (c) the building buddy system and using Kakaotalk to enhance ongoing commitment to mindfulness practice.

Korean Society

Collectivism runs deep in Korean society as a whole, despite the fact that South Korea's market economy ranks 12th in the world by GDP. The society appears to be more vertical than horizontal, compared to its American or European counterparts. Nisbett (2003) points out that "there is good evidence that for East Asians the world is seen much more in terms of relationships than it is for Westerners, who are more inclined to see the world in terms of… categories" (p. 162). It is not uncommon that an individual sense of Korean identity is buried behind the collectivist pronoun *we*. For example, foreigners are surprised to hear their Korean friend says "our wife" instead of "my wife."

In a collectivistic culture, people tend to be more conscious of other peoples' opinions of themselves. They generally are afraid of making social blunders in their interpersonal relationships. Losing *chemyon* (or face), traditionally is one of the strongest sources of fear for Confucian-influenced countries like Korea where people have developed and maintained very strict rules and social etiquettes over long periods of time. In this hierarchical society, what is called "in-group" pressure is relatively strong. For example, if a son or a daughter of a family fails a college entrance exam, it could become not only the child's problem but also the problem for the whole family. If a member of the family or organization behaves badly, the whole group to which he or she belongs could be stigmatized as such. Disrupting the harmony of the group could be considered a great source of shame to those in a collectivistic culture. So it is important to read another person's *kibun* (or feeling or mood). Accurately sounding out the general *bunuiki* (or atmosphere) of the situation has long been considered one of the most important social skills in Korea.

The tendency for Koreans to be overly considerate of others' opinions is bolstered by Park's (1994) argument that a traditional Korean communication style is characterized by an affective or situation-oriented approach where nonlinguistic elements such as feelings and attitudes play an important role. Since the harmony of the whole group is more important than the well-being of an individual, people learn from their childhood how to read others' feelings (or *kibun*) and the whole atmosphere (or *bunuiki*). In this kind of society, expressing one's feeling or opinion publically or saying "no" to others is not easy.

The world is shrinking due to unprecedented advances in science and technology. Although global society is becoming more diversified and complex in some ways, there are also some strong tendencies to move toward a universal culture. The advent of a universal culture influences people, whether they come from an individualistic or collectivistic culture, to become more akin to each other in appearance, communication, and lifestyle.

In summary, while members of a society are all different from one another, each society has a general tendency or preference for certain communication styles. In that sense, the Korean culture shows stronger collectivistic or group-oriented characteristics that make people more susceptible to others' opinions. Effective interpersonal communication is dependent upon how individuals manage the anxiety and uncertainty they experience when communicating with others (Gudykunst & Kim, 1997, p. 309). It can be surmised that if the level of anxiety and uncertainty in my class communication situation is reduced, the nature of the communication will change accordingly.

Approaches That Did Not Work Well

My first 2 years of MBSR teaching were done mainly with outpatients in a local psychiatric clinic. In my first few months of teaching MBSR in Korea, I began to use PowerPoint in every class in order to deliver the themes of each weekly lesson at the repeated request of concerned psychiatrists with whom I had to work. Although I had learned otherwise and knew that using PowerPoint can increase the possibility of misleading my participants into endless analysis and judgment, the demands from the doctors and patient participants were such that I decided to experiment with it any way. Before long, I came to see for myself that the use of PowerPoint is both misleading and even counterproductive, contributing to participants' more thinking. So I dropped the whole idea of using it in my class. Since then, I minimize the use of PowerPoint in my MBSR class (except for a few examples when I felt it appropriate to for effective delivery).

Another approach I took in my initial teaching of MBSR, but discarded later, is the use of different physical exercises and activities in my class. For example, to engage more people and make the class more fun and engaged, I invested some of my class time in relaxation mood-enhancing activities. Though helpful in some ways, I came to realize before long that these activities ultimately reduce precious class time and steer participants away from the core curriculum. Relaxation and fun can simply substitute for awareness.

The important lesson for me was to return to the original intention and purpose of the program, without sacrificing precious class time for unessential elements. MBSR is meant to be a very skillful means for optimizing the mind-body connection for individual and social transformation. I returned to the template MBSR curriculum by cutting down on many exercises and activities I had added. This does not necessarily mean following the CFM curriculum in a "cookie-cutter" manner. Now, I feel more comfortable following the template curriculum without feeling stuck in the curriculum. I am much more familiar with what is called "live" curriculum which constantly arises in each moment as I grow in my teaching years.

MBSR teachers are granted the license to teach class in a creative way as long as we do not "decontextualize," *dharma*, or "distort" the authenticity of MBSR. MBSR has to be based on the deep cultivation of mindfulness and thus grounded in the universal dharma. As Jon Kabat-Zinn says, since its quality is only as good as each and every MBSR teacher, anyone who desires to become an authentic MBSR teacher should receive adequate training in mindfulness meditation and MBSR teaching. In this sense, teaching MBSR requires both embodied presence of the teacher through ongoing mindfulness practice and pedagogical skillful means for teaching MBSR. My own research (Ahn, 2006) also indicates that teaching MBSR is embedded in teaching from presence, multifold methods, facilitating inquiry, and weaving actual experience from the class.

In what follows, I focus on the *how* of the pedagogy which deals with underlying cultural factors as I teach in Korea. Even when the template MBSR curriculum is implemented skillfully, if cultural differences remain unnoticed by the teacher, they can influence the whole class dynamics in subtle and sometimes serious ways.

Approaches That Work Well

Over the past several years, my MBSR teaching has evolved to implement the following three activities in order to nurture a better holding environment for my participants: (A) reducing anxiety and tension ((1) Ice-breaking game in Class 1 or 2 and (2) pair and group mindful dancing in Classes 3 or 4 (B) establishing the right attitudes for mindfulness practice, and (C) helping participants maintain commitment through pair and group work. I believe these skillful means for creating a holding environment in Korea are congruent with the template MBSR curriculum.

Reducing Anxiety and Tension

Ice-Breaking Game in Class 1 or 2

About 15–20 people sit in a circle, and usually, there is a slight sense of "tension" in the room. Before class, people are invited to have tea, coffee, or snacks. Not much talking is heard except for a few people conversing with each other. At the beginning of Class 1, I welcome participants and give a short summary introduction of MBSR. A short opening meditation and sharing of that experience follow. Class guidelines are explained. And there is a go-round when people introduce themselves in terms of their names, jobs, motivations, and expectations from the program. The atmosphere is different from one class to another. Usually, people introduce themselves in the order they are seated. Some classes look more active, lively, and relaxed. Others somewhat look more shy and tense.

When I find the class atmosphere is low and tense I suggest to the class that we play some game together. I explain what we are supposed to do; class divides into two teams. I provide one target for each team. To make the game more fun, participants are asked to decide what will be the reward for the winning team. Usually, they end up choosing to receive a massage from the losing team. Each person starts throwing a rubber band toward their assigned target. At the end of the game, the team having more bands located closer to the center of their target is the winner.

A number of things happen during the game, depending on the personality of the participants. Some class cycles are full of laughter and fun, while others appear more reserved. At the end of the game, I ask participants to go back to their seats and do a guided reflection on what has happened to them during the game. My questions include:

What happened to your mind and body when you first heard that we are going to play the game?
What happened when you were assigned to a team?
How did you feel when it was your turn to throw?
What happened to you when you threw it "right" or "wrong"?
How did you feel when your team or the other team member did a good/bad job?
How did you like it when it was time to do massage?
What was your overall experience of this game?
Was it fun or boring?
Where did you feel it in your body?
Did it remind you of any past experience?

After that reflection, all participants are asked to share their experience in dyad.

When they return to a big circle I encourage them to voluntarily share their experience. Usually by this time, people tend to develop some rapport and they feel more at home and ready to engage in a larger group activity in a more relaxed way. Usual responses include: "I was very glad when I heard the word 'game.' It reminds me of my childhood days." "I felt like running away from the class because I hate the game, I always lost game." "My mind was busy figuring out what was the best way I can do it well." "I was disappointed/guilty/shame when my shot was worse than I had expected." "I was excited/proud when my shot was a great success." "I didn't want to play games, because I didn't like to stand out, I could not help but follow the instructions." At that point, I switch gears to bring attention to what is happening in that moment to their bodies, emotions, and thoughts. I encourage them to redirect their attention to within, without analyzing or assessing the experience.

My intention to introduce the game is twofold: one is to relax the class atmosphere, which is often filled with some degree of anxiety and tension. These uncomfortable feelings, if ignored, can erect a big wall between the teacher and the class and among members of the class, thus blocking effective class communication. The other intention, which is more subtle, is to let the participants know from the outset of the program that there are so many things we forget/miss in each passing moment, and that being aware of what is happening while we experience the moment is of crucial importance in life.

The tension level in the room usually drops noticeably. Each and every individual who has come to the class as a total stranger with some uneasy feelings about what's waiting for them in this first session now looks more lively, more energized, and more connected to one another and thus "psyching" themselves for the next thing to be taught in the class, whatever that is.

Pair and Group Mindful Dancing

Mindful movement is introduced in Class 3 or 4 and is often liked by a majority of my participants. I introduce it along with mindful Yoga when class energy is low or participants become tired of sitting.

All participants stand up and clear the classroom of any object on the floor including pens and pencils and cushions. Everyone pairs up. One person becomes a leader, and the other is assigned the role of follower. The leader puts an arm out toward the face of the follower, with the palm about 30 centimeter away from the follower's face. The leader leads the follower with a stretched-out palm, while the follower does his or her best maintaining distance between the face and the leader's palm. This activity requires a lot of attention on both parts. This exercise is usually done with lively music playing. The leader is asked to move around the room, so everyone is constantly on the move. Everyone is encouraged to pay full attention to what's happening in each movement.

Many participants say mindful dancing is really fun and relaxing. There is music, interaction among different partners, physical movement—and a sudden stop when participants are instructed to a complete standstill. There are also different postures (standing, slow and fast moving, leading and being led, sitting and lying, etc.) and paying attention to different objects, inside and outside. The lively dancing element associated with exercise helps increase the likelihood of easing anxiety and tension, possibly helping participants move from the head to the heart. This exercise could be useful in creating a safe place where participants feel more relaxed, less defensive, more concentrated, and more connected. The real value of this exercise lies in helping participants turn attention from the outside world full of changing movements, music, and sounds to exploration of the interior world with curiosity and openness. The overall purpose is not just to have fun but to be aware of our ability to react or respond to moment-to-moment experience.

From the traditional perspective of Vipassana meditation, playing music for practice is not regarded as a norm. People just practice seeing things as they are. Given that the present moment is constantly changing, there are endless objects of which to be aware. So there is no need to create an artificial environment, and using music is not an essential element in practicing mindfulness. The main reason for using music for this kind of exercise in my MBSR class is that people get more engaged in learning. Traditionally, Korean people are known to enjoy dance and music to the extent that even the ancient neighboring Chinese people knew about this propensity.

In recent years, it is evidenced by the spread of K-pop to other regions of the world. It is known for a diversity of audiovisual of content, systematic training of singers, and synchronized dance formations and key movements into choreography (Wikipedia). Psy, a Korean singer, became an overnight global star, whose music video, *Gangnam Style*, has recently become the first to reach more than 2.1 billion YouTube views. According to Wikipedia, Time magazine recognized the K-pop music market as "South Korea's Greatest Export." Even in ordinary gatherings such as a private party or company field trip, singing and dancing are considered the norm in Korean daily life. Whatever the reason for the Korean people's propensity for singing and dancing, I find it conducive to building a holding environment in my class. With music and dance, the class becomes more energized and lively. When skillfully employed, they help people become more engaged in learning to be.

Establishing the Right Attitudes for Mindfulness Practice

In essence, learning to practice mindfulness is a long journey toward the "being" mode of mind from the "doing" mode of mind. The being mode of mind is often compared to the "lost world," since most people have lost touch with the inner core. This journey requires different attitudes from ordinary activities associated with the doing mode of mind. The attitudinal foundation of mindfulness practice described by Jon Kabat-Zinn (1990) is crucial to meditation in general and mindfulness meditation in particular. It is also crucial in my MBSR class. In this soil of the attitudinal foundation, participants can cultivate their ability for loving hearts and clear seeing. I emphasize the importance of attitude in learning mindfulness practice, right from the beginning to the end of each class. The seven attitudinal factors of mindfulness ascertained by Kabat-Zinn can provide participants with the *what* and *how* of mindfulness practice.

From the perspective of the attitudinal foundation, I would like to touch on some learning difficulties facing my participants. Most of the difficulties that participants experience in their mindfulness practice tend to result from their misunderstanding, or ignorance, of these attitudinal foundations. Accordingly, these difficulties can be transformed into powerful learning tools when they develop a better understanding of these obstacles and begin to have the right attitudes.

Nonjudging

There are some participants who think of nonjudging as "living a daily life without any judgment at all." It is no wonder that they often develop a certain level of resistance in learning mindfulness, because they doubtlessly see the value of having good judgment in their lives. This kind of uneasy feeling or resistance can be easily found especially among those who hold logic and judgment in high esteem. It is important to note that nonjudging does not mean that we deny the positive side of good judgment. They need to understand that what is meant by nonjudging means becoming an impartial witness to whatever happens in each moment. It just means that meditators need to assume the stance of an impartial witness to their own experiences, because if we keep ourselves stuck in our thinking/judging mind, we cannot enter the realm of nonconceptual awareness. I remind these participants that they just learn to practice the impartial stance, which when deepened, can help them think and judge more clearly. After all, this nonjudging will help them step out of their automatic tendency to be boxed into thinking/judging and eventually see more widely, and clearly, all things as they are. Learning that the nonjudging attitude is not meant to be anti-intellectual, or emptying of the mind, but eventually promotes good judgment, can be a powerful motivator.

Patience

It is not unusual to find participants who expect quick results or ready solutions for their problems. Since they have heard of the fame and popularity that MBSR enjoys worldwide, some participants expect to gain a lot from the program within a short period of time, without realizing it requires a great effort to attain their goals, whatever they might be. It is common for them to assume that a program of the magnitude of MBSR should have a powerful "magic" formula that will miraculously work for all participants. To their disappointment, however, they find themselves faced with a situation like "nothing has happened yet," despite their efforts for the past week or so. They should learn that everything has its own time line; flowers bloom, water boils, and a caterpillar becomes a butterfly, only in their own good times. Depending on an individual's "readiness," the length of the time needed can widely vary to realize the effects of meditation.

Beginner's mind

According to Jon Kabat-Zinn, beginner's mind means willing to see everything as if for the first time. However, many participants come to class with some unrealistic expectations or beliefs that often prevent them from seeing what is required to cultivate mindfulness. For example, Korea is traditionally rich in various kinds of life-nurturing healing arts: Zen meditation, breath training methods, martial arts and dietary regimens, etc. Many have experience with some of these practices before they join the MBSR program. Their previous exposure to these practices often gets in the way of their proper learning of MBSR. Despite repeated instruction, some readily mistake the awareness of breathing for "breath training," while others mistake mindfulness meditation for intensive concentration training. To some, meditation is a synonym for "enlightenment." Others just regard all meditation as sheer religious practices. Some people have a tendency to regard meditation as something "undesirable," or even taboo. Learning to be free of expectations, mistakes, and prejudices and seeing without the veil of thoughts and opinions are pillars of mindfulness practice. It is often this type of non-beginner or pseudo-beginner who has unusual ideas about meditation. They often believe that meditation is tantamount to gaining some supernatural power, or psychic energy, or even physical levitation. Helping them disengage from their fixed misunderstanding regarding meditation is sometimes very challenging.

Trust in Self

Trusting in oneself and one's feeling is integral to all kinds of meditation including mindfulness practice. However, many participants tend to seek outside of themselves for guidance and problem-solving. They constantly ignore their inner voice and look for outside authority. This seems to be more common in Asian society where people are taught to respect authority and social hierarchy. Habitually believing that "teachers know everything" or "teachers are better than me" can seriously undermine mindfulness practice grounded in the learners' innate goodness and authority. Learning to honor one's own feelings and inner wisdom can prevent learners from constantly going on "wild goose chases" through meditation, never arriving at home, however hard one tries.

As Jon Kabat-Zinn (2005) said, mindfulness practice is a radical act of love. In order for meditation to be real, compassion and self-compassion are essential. It is actually not uncommon to meet long-term meditators who still lack this inner capacity for boundless trust in themselves. The ability to trust oneself is an essential part of mindfulness practice. It should be taught through the attitudinal foundations of mindfulness practice from the beginning to the end. Without taking this approach, mindfulness meditation can be "a cold attention training without heart."

Non-striving

Non-striving is another area with which many participants have problems. Lopsidedly believing that meditation is always "something extraordinary," some participants put in too much effort and energy in order to achieve their own unrealistic goals or get to where they want to be. One famous Burmese meditation teacher is known to have made a joke to a group of Korean meditators about their serious efforts at meditation, saying "I love you guys, but your efforts scares me sometimes." This rigorous effort at meditation may partly stem from a general tendancy among Korean people who often see meditation as enlightment. For example, Zen meditation stress a complete commitment to study *Kongan* or *Koan* (a story, dialogue, question, or statement used in Zen practice to provoke the "great doubt" in Zen practice (Wikipedia)). In this tradition, a serious meditator needs to die before dying in order to get enlightenment. To solve the *Koan*, totally giving yourself up to engage in "*yongmangjungjn*" (meaning fearless efforts) is considered a norm rather than an exception.

Another reason for this "endlessly strenuous" effort could be that the term meditation has been identified as "a concentration practice" by many practitioners. Concentration on any object entails an exclusion of other objects. This practice is focused attention. To be mindful, we need to open our attention. I often hear participants say,

> "I have long practiced meditation in terms of concentration. Now my meditation becomes more relaxed and open, thanks to my MBSR class. It is very helpful to learn that mindfulness means 'paying an open and compassionate attention' to my experience. This is amazing."

I encourage my participants to assume an attitude of non-striving, which is non-doing and "trying less and being more." For those who have learned meditation in a very serious way, a touch of this non-striving attitude can open new possibility.

Acceptance

In the context of MBSR, acceptance accounts for coming to terms with things as they are. We know that acceptance comes first and then change follows. However, many of my participants want things to be different from what they are now, thus wasting energy while denying, suppressing, and forcing, etc. Whenever I notice a participant getting stuck in these habitual resistant patterns, I encourage them to understand that our mind state is like the weather outside; if it is raining, it is raining. If it shines, it shines. Nothing else. Most of them do not have any problem with that. However, a majority of people do not know how to notice or observe their mind-body states just as they are. I point to the fact that both the outside weather and the interior mind-body states are just part of the natural phenomenon. Many things around us happen without our consent. It is about the whole universe, not about something as personal as I/my/me/mine.

Letting Go (Nonattachment)

Letting go (meaning nonattachment) involves letting things be and accepting things as they are. It is the antonym of holding on, clinging or grasping. From the perspective of awareness or the spaciousness of the mind, nothing remains the same. In each moment, everything arises and passes away, comes and goes. It is Nature's Way. In Way (*Tao*), when we are hungry, we eat. When we feel sleepy, we go to sleep. However, in civilized society, the doing mode of the mind presides over, and the rules of the game become completely different. People want everything to be different, but only to their benefit. However, it is also true that we humans constantly experience letting go in everyday life. Without this natural process of letting go, life simply cannot go on. If we stick to thinking too much, we cannot easily go to sleep. If we are seriously stuck in one state of mind, our minds will not flow naturally.

Although nature unfolds in its own natural rhythms, repeating the process of letting go and holding on, people tend to attach to something they desire without knowing that they cannot have it forever. To the degree they cling, they suffer. It is no wonder that letting go constitutes an ultimate pillar of mindfulness meditation. Many participants often say that they understand what letting go means in their head, but it is still difficult to actually let things go. Through repeated mindfulness practice, they manage to learn that they have been practicing in the doing mode of mind, rather than in the being mode. For example, they struggle to create the state of letting go by constantly changing or pushing objects (thoughts, emotions, sensations, outside stimuli) away. It is not easy for them to differentiate the being mode of mind from the doing mode of mind, not to mention dwelling in the being mode in their daily lives. Some participants even mistakenly believe that letting go means that they should give up everything they hold dear in their lives and live like a monastic.

Table 7.4 presents a summary of the attitudinal foundation of mindfulness practice by Kabat-Zinn, typical learning difficulty questions of my participants and my teaching suggestions.

From beginning to end, I place emphasis on assuming the right attitude and understanding what mindfulness practice is. The right attitude is both foundation for good meditation practice and direction to the final destination. I deliver its importance to my participants throughout the program, formally and informally, through whatever means available (lecturing, meditation practice, dialogue and inquiry, etc.). Oftentimes, participants become better prepared for class and home practice, as they come to understand these attitudes and learn how they should approach mindfulness meditation

Table 7.4 Seven attitudinal foundations and learning difficulties

Attitude	Learning difficulty	Teaching suggestion
Nonjudging	"How can we live without judgment?"	We are not trying to discard thinking or judgment but cultivate impartial witness
Patience	"Nothing happens even if I practice meditation"	It takes time. Meditation effects requires "critical mass"
Beginner's mind	"I've done this kind of practice many times"; a "big or strange" idea about meditation	Every experience is different; every meditation is different
Trust in self	"My teachers are better than me"	As far as my experience is concerned, I am the best authority. There is genius in everyone
Non-striving	"Always pushing myself to the limits is the best way to practice mindfulness"; "too big expectation"	Less trying, more being
Acceptance	"Acceptance means giving up, or failure"	Like outside weather, accepting whatever unfolds opens new possibility
Letting go	"I need to 'control' every situation to live better"	No need to "control" everything. Just watch things come and go

Helping Participants Maintain Commitment Through Pairs and Group Building

Building Buddy System for Homework

MBSR throughout the course requires lifestyle modification on the part of each participant. They need time out of their fixed busy schedule to do formal meditation. Until participants progress to a certain point in learning, when they find the program interesting and rewarding, they easily forget to do homework or find themselves not in a mood to practice when they are alone.

In this situation, making a class friend can be very helpful. I ask the class to find a partner and exchange mobile phone numbers in Class 2 or 3. For every day of the week, they are encouraged to send a simple text message two or three times a day to their assigned partner, just asking, "Are you being mindful at this moment?" This sounds simple, but many of my participants report that it is very helpful to be reminded of the practice through cell phone contacts. Eventually, they come to the class, becoming more eager to voluntarily share their experiences, including the common problems they faced during the week. It is likely that participants in a collectivistic culture become more expressive when they work in small groups or teams, rather than working on their own.

Using Kakaotalk Service for the Whole-Class Networking

Kakaotalk is like a Facebook-style social networking service. In class, participants and I sometimes create our own Kakao Space where we can simultaneously exchange opinions and pictures. Since many of us these days tend to be living in a virtual reality, contantly connected to computers, cell phones and wireless palm devices etc, I make it a rule to keep this exercise to the minimum.

Participants can ask questions regarding their daily practice in the Kakao Service. The use of this service continues until the class ends. In the end, a decision is made as to whether the class will keep or disband this service.

Another thing for which Kakao Service is useful in group activity is the Class 2 theme: Perception and creative responding. How we see things, or don't see them, will determine how you will respond to them. I ask all participants to take pictures of the class room and send two pictures of their choice to the Kakao Space we have created together. I also send pictures of my own choosing. While we look at the pictures, we talk about many things regarding the pictures that were taken (who, what, why, how, etc.). Many of the participants are pleasantly surprised to know that there are a variety of ways they can perceive and interpret the classroom they are in. Some say that they never imagined that the classroom could be seen so differently. Using Kakao Space in this way can be fun and conducive to helping learners further expand their perspectives.

Inquiry and Dialogue

Pedagogically speaking, there has been strong emphasis on exploration of the participants' first-hand experience of their mindfulness practices. MBSR teachers are supposed to create a safe holding space conducive to classroom dialogue "arising out of the freshness of the present moment." To achieve this goal, it is essential for the teacher to "suspend judgment, to attempt to understand as much as possible the experience of the participants, to refrain from using formulaic responses when confronted with difficult or uncomfortable classroom experiences, and to listen keenly as well as redirect participants as required within the class discourse."

According to the MBSR curriculum, the dialogue and inquiry require the teacher to listen closely, allow space, refrain from the impulse to give advice, and instead, to inquire directly into the actuality of the participant's experience. This requirement can be interpreted as the most challenging aspect of teaching MBSR. A teacher's ability to do so in the spontaneity of each arising moment, without reacting, can be a litmus test for a skillful MBSR teacher. It is clear that this teaching ability is grounded in mindfulness practice.

Even if the MBSR teacher is skillful at facilitating the dialogue and inquiry, the other end of the communication line is important as well. The term *communication appreciation* can be a very useful concept for my MBSR teaching. It means "a person's level of fear or anxiety associated with either real or anticipated talk with one of more persons" (Park, 1994). Those who have a high degree of apprehension

"prefer large lecture classes over those small classes" and prove to be "low produc-
ers of original ideas in group discussions" (p. 153). For this reason, I often invite
participants to work in pairs, in fours, and then return to the large group. The tend
to talk more in smaller groups. When an individual more speaks up when he or she
is assiged the role of "the representative" of the small group. It is after the small
group activity that it looks easier for them to talk in the whole class.

Skillfully engaging participants in dialogue and inquiry is both challenging and
exciting for me. This process is challenging for two reasons. One is the participant's
assumption about the teacher–student relationship. Traditionally, this relationship is
inherently hierarchical, especially in East Asia. Students expect their teacher to give
them the right answers, because they assume that their teacher knows "everything"
about the subject they study or at least "knows better than themselves." The teacher
has the authority, and the student adapts a passive role in learning. Even though the
influence of this tradition has been on the wane in twenty-first-century Korean society (as Korea is increasingly more exposed to globalization), it is more common for
an active discussion and sharing to predominate in Korea. I surmise that Nisbett's
(2003) claim is losing ground or is only partially true as far as my MBSR class is
concerned that "debate is almost as uncommon in modern Asia as in ancient China."

In order to engage participants more actively in the dialogue and inquiry process,
I emphasize two things: First I emphasize that the MBSR program is not a unidirec-
tional, ready-made class but a special journey that participants and the teacher
embark upon together. Those who are eager to actively express what they experience in, and outside, class can learn better and also contribute more to the learning
of the whole class. There is "no lecturing," "no advice," and "no teaching," in this
class. But we can still learn from each other in the spirit of mutual respect, non-
harming, direct experiment, and openness to the possibility.

Second I also emphasize that we are each our own best authority in our experience and inner feeling. Every one of us has genius, so that it is crucial for us to trust
our own, whatever situation we are in. We are intrinsically whole regardless of our
current mind-body condition and surrounding situation. Each participant is the best
authority, as far as their own experience is concerned. It is clear that the template
MBSR curriculum contains all of these principles.

Conclusion

This chaper has been based on my assumption that the template MBSR curriculum
developed by Kabat-Zinn works well in Korea, despite the striking cultural differences between Korea and the US. MBSR is about mindful awareness which is universal. It is my belief that the MBSR curriculum allows experienced teacher to be
creative enough to meet their learners as they are coming from their own specific
culture and provide a holding environment conducive to learning and growth. This
is why I have decided to utilize some class activities descrived above which I believe
help my participants in the high collectivist, high uncertainty avoidance and

relatively high power distance culture. The pedagogy of *what* and *when* to teach in MBSR is well provided by the template curriculum of the Center for Mindfulness. The pedagogy of *how* to teach the curriculum can be varied from one teacher to another and from one culture to another. All the things I have added to the template curriculum are just about this *how*, rather than what, and when.

Looking back over the past 10 years of my MBSR teaching, I have come to realize that there is some paradox involved. It seems that the distance between me and "the hidden dimension of MBSR" has not shrunk, contrary to my initial expectation. I would like to summarize my MBSR teaching in Korea by paraphrasing Hall's remark cited in the introduction, as follows:

MBSR hides much more than it revels, and strangely enough what it hides, it hides most effectively from me as my MBSR teaching goes on.

References

Ahn, H. Y. (2006). *A phenomenological case study of the practicum in Mindfulness-Based Stress Reduction: Insights into mindfulness and its connection to adult learning.* Unpublished doctoral dissertation, Teachers College, Columbia University, New York, NY.

Gudykunst, W. B., & Kim, Y. Y. (1997). *Communicating with strangers: An approach to intercultural communication* (3rd ed.). New York, NY: McGraw-Hill.

Hall, E. T. (1959). *The silent language.* New York, NY: Anchor Books Doubleday.

Hofstede, G. (1997). *Cultures and organizations: Software of the mind.* New York: McGraw-Hill.

Kabat-Zinn, J. (2005). *Coming to our senses: Healing ourselves and the world through mindfulness.* New York, NY: Hyperion.

Kabat-Zinn, J. (1990). *Full catastrophe living. Using the wisdom of your body and mind to face stress, pain, and illness.* New York: Delta Trade Paperbacks.

McCown, D., Reibel, D. K., & Micozzi, M. S. (2010). *Teaching mindfulness: A practical guide for clinicians and educators.* New York, NY: Springer.

Nisbett, R. E. (2003). *The geography of thought: How Asians and Westerners think differently... and why.* New York, NY: Free Press.

Park, M. S. (1994). *Communication styles in two different cultures: Korean and American* (2nd ed.). Seoul: Han Shin.

Chapter 8
Teaching in Italy

Antonella Commellato and Fabio Giommi

In the limited space of this chapter, we highlight a few themes and cultural traits that we have experienced in our work as especially relevant for teaching Italians.

We have been teaching MBSR, MBCT and Interpersonal Mindfulness classes since 2003 and have designed and serve as the guiding teachers of a year-long Mindfulness Professional Training program since 2009.

Our classes have been offered in Milano, where our center is located, and in other cities in Northern Italy, Torino, Padova, Piacenza, and Parma as well as in the Italian speaking region of Switzerland. We have also offered mindfulness workshops in the Netherlands, Poland, and Sweden.

XXVIII

knowing now
that the life
at which I aim
is a circumference
continually expanding
through sympathy and
understanding
rather than an exclusive centre
of pure self-feeling
the whole I seek
is centre plus circumference
and now the struggle at the centre is over
the circumference
beckons from everywhere.

Kenneth White

A. Commellato, M.A. • F. Giommi, Ph.D. (✉)
Associazione Italiana per la Mindfulness, Via Piranesi 14, Milano 20137, Italy
e-mail: antonella.commellato@gmail.com; fabiomario.giommi@gmail.com

© Springer International Publishing Switzerland 2016
D. McCown et al., *Resources for Teaching Mindfulness*,
DOI 10.1007/978-3-319-30100-6_8

Our participants come from different social backgrounds, though mainly urban: upper-, middle-, working-class. Before starting the course we ask them by letter to not disclose their professional status to others.

In this chapter, when speaking of the original contemplative and Buddhist context of mindfulness, we use expressions like "Mindfulness Meditation" or "Insight Meditation." When we refer to the vast and multifaceted context of its applications as MBSR, MBCT, MBIs, and to the spreading of mindfulness into society, we use expressions like "mindfulness-world" or "mindfulness subculture."

To speak about the overall cultural traits of a country can be challenging. On the one side, anything that can be said always somehow appears schematic, simplistic, overgeneralized, superficial, approximative, if not stereotyped and preconceived. In handbooks of cultural anthropology, sociology, and social psychology, there are hundreds of different definitions of what constitutes a culture. We find them neither remotely exhaustive nor useful to effectively define or describe one specific culture. Of course, anthropologists have also long recognized that there are variations within cultures based upon different personalities.

On the other side, when we are native to a culture, or know it well from within, we immediately *feel* how it is perceiving and experiencing reality *through* its own lenses, and we are clearly able to recognize its most typical aspects when they manifest.

In describing the Italian cultural context, it is unavoidable to speak by generalizations. However, we are convinced that the most prominent characteristics and traits in a culture are not unilateral and "stand-alone" aspects. Instead they may manifest as part of a process of *polarization*: when a cultural trait/quality appears at an intensified level, it is often the case that its complementary, reciprocal quality also appears enhanced.

For example, a centuries-old feature of Italian culture is a strong propensity to the so-called *familism* or *amoral familism*[1] a form of selfish family-centered behavior and indifference to others outside the inner circles.

At the same time—perhaps *just because* of such widespread and pervasive diffusion of familism—Italy is perhaps the European country with the highest number of people volunteering their time for nonprofit works: the latest 2014 figure from ISTAT, the national statistical agency, show that 12.6 % of population, millions of people, is actively involved in some kind of nonprofit activities for the benefit of the community.[2]

---

[1] Social action persistently oriented to the economic interests of the nuclear family. In a controversial account of poverty in a village in southern Italy (*The Moral Basis of a Backward Society*, 1958), Edward C. Banfield argued that the backwardness of the community was to be explained "largely but not entirely" by "the inability of the villagers to act together for their common good or, indeed, for any end transcending the immediate, material interest of the nuclear family." This was attributed to the ethos of "amoral familism."

[2] ISTAT—Unpaid activities to benefit others, July 2014 [http://www.istat.it/en/archive/129122]

The Role and Expression of Emotions

One of the most popular stereotypes about Italians is that they are "emotional" in the sense that they communicate emotions more freely and with more expressivity, through verbal and nonverbal behaviors, than other Western European cultures. As with most stereotypes, this one is partially true.

Another stereotype about Italians, also well known, and connected to the previous one is that they are theatrical (or operatic) and their style of communication appears to foreign eyes somehow as a spectacle, or a performance. This observation is also partially true. Taken together these stereotypes suggest something important that has to be understood about the relationship of Italians with their emotions. The adjective *theatrical* indicates the art of acting. While acting, an actor makes use of his emotions to give life to a character but it is not fully identified with them, he elicits and employs them to accomplish a task, as those emotions are not his real, personal sentiments.

The shadow side of the Italian theatrical expression of emotions (the complementary polarity of their "freedom" in emotional expressivity) is a disposition and ability to *use* emotions as an effective social communication tool. This skill can easily become a manipulatory relational talent, a tacit competence in how to strategically manage their emotions and their expression. Not by chance the construct of "Machiavellian intelligence" is named after the famous Italian Renaissance philosopher. This cultural background has a strong implication for the way Italians relate to their inner, intimate lives. Precisely because often in the social life there is a display of fake and manipulative emotions, the real, intimate feelings and sentiments are carefully protected and shielded.

Italians are actually quite reserved and reluctant in showing their real vulnerability and suffering.

Given such a context, the themes of vulnerability and authenticity become of extraordinary relevance during a mindfulness class. The teacher has to take particular care and effort to embody authenticity. This cultural trait has therefore a profound impact on the mindfulness group process and a number of consequences, which we now describe.

1. Familiarity with the "handling" of emotions makes Italians highly sensitive and impervious to inauthentic, emphatic, or sentimental expressions of emotional contents. The usage of affected, artificial or emotionally overcharged interactions might be accepted or even promoted in the "mundane" social dimension, but it becomes suspect, doubtful, or ambiguous within a more intimate dimension. When intimacy is involved, the communicative style of Italians is much more discreet and self-restrained than appears at first glance.

Therefore, for a mindfulness teacher it is crucial to be "real" and to embody mindfulness as honestly as possible, not pretending any wisdom, or meditative knowledge or compassion that he or she has not actually realized and is unable to bring into the room.

A teaching style that is not fully and deeply honest in its intention and genuine in its manifestations is quickly felt and spotted by an Italian audience. Italians, in general, do not believe so easily in what is only uttered or merely asserted. Even if combined with a display of sincerity and disclosure of emotional feelings. They do observe and scan the consistency and the actual behaviors of the teacher over time, within and outside the class.

During a mindfulness protocol, participants are invited to come closer to their intimate experience. With an Italian group, this implies that we also come closer to a place of caution and high sensitivity to the hints and signs of sincerity from the teacher. When the teacher appears affected or insincere, the participant's reaction, though covered and masked, can be intense and irreparable. And, even worse, this effect can shift the entire group process into the "mundane" social dimension, mentioned above, triggering the automatized schema of inauthentic emotional interactions and eventually spoiling the whole endeavor of mindfulness.

In short, the intention of the instructor to be "real" that is certainly so crucial for mindfulness in any cultural context— is particularly important in Italy.

While teaching we dedicate as much awareness and energy we can to guard and be mindful of our own motivations and dispositions. We also insist on this aspect during our mindfulness professional training and our supervision with the instructors-in-training. In this respect, strong support comes from the fact that we often co-teach our classes: the mutual and honest feedback is precious and challenging, and helps us to regain each time more sincerity. We recommend co-teaching to our instructors when possible.

The authenticity of the instructor and of what he/she brings to the class, of course, raises a big issue: that of the instructor's depth of training and meditation practice. Nowadays, in Italy (and in Europe and the USA as well...) we see a trend of "mass production" of MBIs instructors, not only by local self-appointed mindfulness "experts," but also by well-known important international mindfulness institutions which train cohorts of 80–90 or more trainees at a time during periods of less than 10 days. This trend fosters pretended expertise in teachers and results in superficial and shallow experiences in MBI's participants, wasting precious opportunities to invite people into the liberative power of awareness.

2. In our cultural context a wariness about intimacy implies that some time is needed in order to develop trust in the authenticity of the teacher. Sometimes a slower pace is also needed for the group process to mature and to allow personal contents to emerge in the class. Rarely is this threshold passed before the mid-path, the fourth session, and it requires from the instructor a capacity for patience, internal stability, and deep confidence in the process.

3. Even so, a characteristic of Italian groups is that many participants will not share anyway their most personal troubles and intimate stories in front of the whole group during the inquiry. In our experience, it is much less common to hear from participants narratives of intense personal pain (e.g., a trauma or their daughter's psychological illness) in Italy than, for example, in the USA. In our groups, it is more usual to have people sharing difficulties related to the meditation practice or the homework. During the inquiry, it may well happen that participants share very

challenging emotional events as they occur in their experience. However, these events are often emerging in a somehow episodic way from their current life, but seldom are they framed as part of some personal and painful narrative, which totality, the background reasons of suffering, are not shared in public. One example, is the case of a participant suffering from panic attacks who never named them aloud during the 8 weeks, although working actively and effectively on them all the time. He mentioned the attacks only at the follow-up meeting one month after the end of the MBSR program.

This cultural trait has to be met with specific care and attention in the way inquiry is conducted. The point here for the instructor is to be particularly ready to make use of the relatively intense challenges usually brought in by participants, in order to teach them a way, a "method," to deal also with the really difficult ones, even if these are not openly alluded to in the class. Focusing on this is really essential for the teacher and often quite subtle. It can be described as a sort of "playing off the cushion" in pool, using what is present in a participant's experience here and now to deal indirectly, by "rebound," with what is not openly present.

4. Given this context, it would be an error to try pushing the group process towards a more explicit sharing of painful personal contents, or a more emotional style of interaction. The group process becomes a free territory where each one feels at ease in offering and taking what is felt moment by moment as commensurate to one's true need.

An aspect of our mindfulness pedagogy might be described as taking a "less is more" teaching style: guiding the inquiry with a sort of light touch, offering hints and exploring a method that participants will be able to deepen when by themselves; trying to avoid a didactic approach; and being careful not to, even implicitly, elicit or suggest any expectation of "emotional stuff" and "moving stories".

A clear sample of this Italian cultural trait is evident in the following episode which neatly challenges some well-known stereotypes about the British versus the Italian way of dealing with emotions. During our 2013 Mindfulness Professional Training, Rebecca Crane,[3] who is member of the Faculty, was teaching a workshop on inquiry in Milano. The audience was a group of 30-plus instructors-in-training, with an average age of about 40 years, the majority of which were psychotherapists, psychologists, psychiatrists, … : . Therefore, they were not a youthful or naive group. Rebecca showed a video of a British instructor inquiring with participants after a mindfulness practice. The video had been selected by Rebecca as a good example of embodiment of mindfulness, care, loving kindness, and of an inviting and accepting attitude from the instructor…and it actually was, but only according to British tacit cultural parameters.

At the end of the video there was a rather long silence and then an eruption of comments expressing annoyance or perplexity: "if I had been there, after all those mushy smiles and sham tones of voice I would have rushed out of the room…," "I felt the instructor as too much inviting, she exaggerates in showing gentleness,… she looks fake…too much mirroring."

---

[3] Director of the Centre for Mindfulness Research and Practice at Bangor University in Wales, UK.

Rebecca was surprised, since, in the English context, the video had never been received in this way. We learned something about how even the slightest "suspicion" of inauthenticity is potentially able to trigger rejection. Of course, these reactions are only visible when people feel free to express openly their opinions; otherwise, they just say (…and apparently with a lot of Italian emotionality…) what is perceived as "socially" appropriate and implicitly desirable in the class context.

An Eloquent Silence

In the context of the "mindfulness subculture," it is not uncommon for Europeans attending a workshop, a seminar, even a retreat in the USA, to find themselves a bit bewildered and embarrassed at the end of the event, having witnessed the amount of time devoted to what is perceived by them—as it is apparent from their reciprocal eye gazing or is openly confessed afterwards—as a sort of strange mandatory social ritual.

The majority of participants usually declare their satisfaction using linguistic expressions and tones which to European ears might often sound overly emotional or rhetorical. Each time there is a final outpouring of: "I offer deep gratitude," "This was tremendously transformative," "Deep bow," and "A life changing experience," together with intense emotional activation and lots of tears.

The point, however, is that this seems to happen almost every time. Therefore, one starts to suspect that these are a set of culturally shaped behaviors, tacitly assumed as expected in such circumstances, a sort of "social desirability bias" required as a mutual confirmation that things went well. In other words, it seems that the American cultural norms in this context contemplate what would be called a *crescendo ending*.

It might be surprising to know that in Italy, when an MBSR class or a mindfulness workshop goes well and reaches depth, it is often the case that there is a *decrescendo* ending. The more the experience is touching, the more people become silent and private.

In the traditional Italian popular culture when one comes to the most sensitive and delicate issues (although it might seem paradoxical) silence may become an important vehicle for communication. Silence is not meant here in the sense of something the person is not aware of, or unconscious, or repressed and inhibited, and the like; but is related to a content that is too sensitive, private, and delicate to be expressed in words. A possibly extreme but very fitting example of this attitude is a typical communicative usage of traditional culture in Sicily and in Southern Italy to underline—to point out—*by the means* of silence what is most important, the sensitive issue in a conversation. What is kept tacit by the speaker (or nonspeaker, in this case) is inferred as the most relevant thing by the listener. This probably used to be more true in the past, as the contemporary industrial and consumer mass culture have changed this refined and subtle skill. Yet this example is representative of the value attributed to the power of silence in Italian culture, which still emerges in contemporary Italian culture.

Sometimes, there are participants who never speak a word to the instructors throughout the whole program. When someone is quiet all the time, we are always a bit concerned, and sometimes rightly so. However, we have learned to trust silence much more than we used to. Sometimes silence is just the expression of lack of motivation and interest, or lack of diligence in doing the homework, and therefore coming to the class with no significant experience to share. Even less is silence, in our experience, a sign of difficulties and problems with the practice. In the latter case, people sooner or later show up—possibly not in front of the group during the class but in the corridor before or after the session or by mail—asking for clarification and help or complaining that mindfulness does not work for them. However, we have been surprised several times in discovering only afterwards how intensely a silent participant was actually committed, involved in the practice and how deep his/her experiences and insights were. One way we use to communicate at a deeper level with each participant (especially with those who have been less exposed) is to ask them in the eighth session to write about their experience.

This exercise is not meant as feedback in the usual sense, and we are not asking for an evaluation of any sort.

We ask them to write following specific instructions, and introduce it as just another mindfulness exercise. The exercise starts with sitting meditation. In the silence, a few questions are repeated. Then, the instruction is to write anything that emerges, without stopping. The aim is to contact and give voice to a deeper stratum of participants' experiences during the course; in a way that is much more open and free from preoccupation about evaluation and feedback, as well as from the "social desirability" effect implicit during communication with teachers, and from the pressure of group conformity implicit during communication in front of the class. They do not know in advance that we are going to collect the papers.

These papers provide us with the possibility to touch the richness and the discoveries of our participants vividly. We have often been surprised by the reports of persons who kept consistently silent during the frequent moments of open exchanges during the 8 weeks. One example is a medical doctor in an MBSR class we taught in the town of Bellinzona, in Italian Switzerland. He was completely silent during the course, though always present and attentive. Finally, we were persuaded that he was diligent but had simply not appreciated the course.

A few months later, we were sent an article he had written for a local newspaper in which he described his experience with deep and rich details and lively insights, saying it was life-saving for him.

Another time, we were a bit concerned about a psychiatrist who never ever spoke in front of his MBSR class in Milano. After the end of the course, he came to us expressing the intention to become a mindfulness instructor, as he had been deeply touched by the practice and the potential of mindfulness.

Over time we have realized that the "rule" that MBI participants are totally free to choose whether or not to share their experience with the instructor, is really a profound principle. The practice is guarded by silence and does not need words or explicit expression to mature. Allowing the possibility to explore mindfulness with privacy is for some participants an important and necessary support offered by the instructor.

Self-Discipline and Commitment: The Daily Homework

Meditation practice at home is probably the most important and at the same time the most challenging aspect of the MBSR curricula. It is the most important for a number of reasons. First, the experience of mindful mental states can only be realized by continuity and graduality of practice. Second, the self-observation exercises which orient towards a closer intimacy with actual daily life (like the pleasant and unpleasant event calendars) are perhaps the richest and most meaningful sources of insight for participants. These exercises represent one of the truly distinctive features of MBSR, in comparison with other more traditional ways to learn meditation. At the same time, it is the most challenging because home practice requires a quite high level of personal commitment, as well as energy and self-discipline. However, attitudes towards engagement and discipline are not related only to individual personality traits but they also involve the cultural background.

The Italians' attitude towards the role of teacher, and towards homework, is influenced by the more general disposition towards authority roles and hierarchy.

Two well-known features of Italian culture are creativity and a strong tendency to individualism. These are usually portrayed as positive qualities, and rightly so. Yet, as any aspect of a culture, they can show a flip side. Individualism can take the shape of a tendency to anarchism and aversion against any form of authority. We attempt to clarify by a comparison. In the American culture, individualism is balanced by a strong sense of community, as well as by a strong sense of being part of one Nation. A centuries-old trait belonging to the dark side of Italian culture is a tendency to *familism*, that is to identify with and to feel genuine commitment only to members of the closest social circle, the family or very small inner circles and networks. Over centuries of foreign invasions alternating with localistic governments, individuals turned to tight-knit family networks. A few years ago, a poll was published in the most important Italian newspaper, *La Repubblica*: "What's your best employment agency?" The more common answer: "Your family, friends, and their connections." This can entail widespread indifference for the larger communities, a sense of caution and suspicion against the State and public institutions.

This trait explains also why, generally speaking, Italians do not trust and do not like hierarchy. They dislike receiving external direction, which is often perceived as "rigid," "bureaucratic," and "obtuse." They are not prone to recognize the authority of a certain role only because it is set by a hierarchic structure. They have first to acknowledge the significance *for them* of that structure, and only then it is possible to respect and accept the person holding that role.

A related aspect is the Italian cultural attitude towards rules, their usage and enforcement. The perception of rules and how to implement them is quite peculiar.

From an Anglo-Saxon or German perspective, for example, a rule is a rule and it has to be applied in a straight and simple way with no exception (precisely because it is a rule).

From an Italian perspective a "rule" is almost never 100 % mandatory. All rules have to be contextualized and adapted to the actual conditions. Most rules are perceived with "fuzzy borders" and they are usually considered 60 % as mandatory and 40 % as contextual, i.e., they have to be interpreted to fit each occasion within the specific circumstances. The positive side is that this attitude grants a high degree of mental flexibility and ability to recognize what is called for in the moment. The negative side is a sort of resistance to accept a rule simply as it is, and a tendency to reshape, and to reformulate it. Of course, this practice is especially true in "normal" conditions, and much less within particular contexts like rigidly organized companies or the military.

Such cultural attitudes can be seen also in the way a task assignment is received from a teacher, particularly if the students are adults and paying clients, as in the case of MBIs.

A homework task may be perceived strange to the point of being puzzling and meaningless, or difficult to the point of not being doable, or boring to the point of lacking any possible interest. This perception means, within the Italian context, that as MBSR teacher you cannot rely and leverage on a deeply and culturally rooted "automatic pilot" behavior based on "I must accomplish my task assignment" (as Jon Kabat-Zinn said "like it or dislike it, just do it!"). Italians can simply choose not to comply with a "command" and, moreover, they do not feel either guilty or wrong in doing so. They can even feel "right" in adapting the rule to their personal needs or in simply dropping what seems to them strange or absurd.

This cultural trait implies that during the preparatory phase of the mindfulness class, extra effort and attention is needed in setting the expectations and the "contract" with the participants. It is important to fully persuade the participants of the crucial importance of keeping a continuity of practice, both formal and informal, at home between the weekly sessions. The trivial yet inescapable matter of fact is that commitment and self-discipline can only be brought to the learning process by the participant. It is a responsibility that is exclusively in his/her own hands.

In addition, there is another important cultural trait. Giuseppe De Rita, one of our most famous and influential sociologists, says "Italians tend to give their best when they are in trouble,"[4] meaning that they perform better under difficult conditions than under favorable or easy conditions. In our experience with mindfulness groups, we have checked this statement several times. It is much more helpful and fruitful for the participants' motivation and commitment to "raise the bar" high at the beginning, insisting on the difficulties they will meet during the protocol.

We explain the fundamental aims of mindfulness in terms of more intimacy with our own experience, more freedom from automatic pilot reactions, more awareness,

---

[4] Giuseppe De Rita *48th Annual Report on the Social Condition of the Country*—CENSIS [http://www.censis.it/10?shadow_ricerca=121016]

and more presence. We do not put much emphasis on lists of expected practical benefits like symptoms reduction, well-being, or happiness.

We have translated this extra attention in setting the right expectations into a number of actions. They can be summarized as being clear and demanding with participants about what is needed in terms of effort and persistence, while at the same time stimulating curiosity and motivation, and remaining gentle and inviting. Yet, one of the main messages we try to convey before the journey starts is that mindfulness doesn't have to be pleasant and that we are not pursuing psychological or physical comfort per se.

First, we always send a preparatory letter to the participant before the start, based on the "classical" MBCT "green book" (Segal, Teasdale, & Williams, 2012) model letter which has been then expanded with several more passages explaining the need for patience and tolerance even when the results are not immediately visible. And the need to be willing to accept that mindfulness as a deep, against-the-stream and counterintuitive deconditioning process, which takes time. One should not expect "to get" it before the third or even the fourth week of practice.

Second, these warnings are gently yet carefully repeated in the introductory phase at the opening of the first class.

Third, during the first 2–3 weeks we are prepared to take advantage of any opportunity occurring during the classes to reassert that the process requires patience and persistence.

The Energy Issue

During the last 20 years, the working habits of large layers of the Italian population (with a few exceptions like the public sector, retail banks, and certain industries) have been modified by the pressure of competitive markets in the direction of longer working hours (up to 6.30–7.30 pm).

In Italy most of the MBIs classes are offered in a private practice context, after work. In addition, in the case of big cities and metropolitan areas (where at the moment most MBIs in Italy are offered) there is also the time needed to travel to the class location.

In Milano, we have to start our class at 8.00 pm (which in Italy is the usual dinner time); otherwise, several participants cannot manage to be on time.

This scheduling requires us to deal with participants who are tired, often overdriven and exhausted, have had no time to eat dinner (apart perhaps a snack), and rush into the room just in time for the beginning of the session.

The energy issue is therefore a huge one in conducting our groups. It must be addressed, first of all, in our own minds as teachers.

A way we have developed to meet this difficulty is to name it and make it explicit as much as possible. We always start with 2–3 minutes of silence inviting people to notice the transition. Then, just before the beginning of the first practice, we ask about the level of energy present in the room that evening, doing a sort of quick and semi-serious poll of how each one feels.

We carefully attend to signs of tiredness in the group throughout the session, and we try to directly manage fatigue inducing activities that increase activation, like speaking in triads or body movements.

In addition, we have also made use of technology to help our participants to sustain their energy level. In the meditation room of our center, we invested in the installation of a special lighting system—*Dynamic Lighting*[5] from Philips—that mimics the natural rhythm of daylight to deliver different specific lighting effects. The system is able to influence in participants the physiological levels of activation corresponding to different states of concentration, alertness, and performance.

The Power of Clichès: The Role of Yoga

A difficulty we have been experiencing with yoga (and was probably not existing in the 1980s when it was introduced in the MBSR curricula) is related to the cultural background of our participants. For contemporary Italian urban population, yoga is a well-known "construct", popular and, more important, often already experienced in one form or another. Proposing "yoga" immediately implies that more than half of the group starts projecting its previous experience and knowledge. This is a rather serious obstacle to mindful yoga, or to the possibility of using simple asanas as a way to feel the body from within without any particular agenda. People start doing yoga following their own habits or are misled by their preconceptions.

Moreover, those who have already attended yoga courses are accustomed to practicing with the idea of looking at the yoga teacher showing the asanas, and they are quite reluctant to do it alone at home. At the same time, those who had never done yoga before find it too uneasy and confusing having to repeat and learn the sequence of movements relying only on the audios and on the drawings distributed by the instructors. These tools are often reported as poor and inadequate, in comparison to the actual presence of the teacher, to make it possible to "get it." The result is that people show a tendency to discouragement and to skip the yoga homework, and they often prefer to turn to other practices.

Therefore, although we do propose yoga extensively in the group sessions, we introduce it only after class three, so that people already have a clear idea what could a mindful movement be. We offer also the possibility to substitute yoga homework with mindful walking (the original mindful movement practice of mindfulness meditation) instead of skipping it altogether.

---

[5] http://www.lighting.philips.com/main/applications/office-and-industry/dynamic-lighting

Finding a Language

The "language of mindfulness" is of extraordinary importance for MBIs.

The language we use (or, may be better, the language that uses us) shapes in depth and often with irreversible effects our mental settings, projections and ways of seeing. This fundamental truth is particularly evident with mindfulness, as we use language not only to describe but also as a means to transform our minds.

In the case of the propagation of MBIs in Italy, there is a double issue.

There is the issue of the translation of the original Dhamma vocabulary in English, its transference into the mindfulness world, and the meaning resulting from its circulation and actual use. There is also the issue of the retranslation of many of those English words into Italian.

Is it evident that the risk of such a sequence of steps would be in a lexicon that has lost most of its original meanings and had become a vehicle of misunderstanding and confusion.

Luckily in Italy, we are supported by the work of Corrado Pensa. He is a scholar in Indian Philosophies and Religious Studies who was a student of Giuseppe Tucci, one of the world's top scholars in Eastern Religious Study. He has spent part of his academic career translating text from pali and sanskrit. At the same time, he was trained as a Jungian psychoanalyst and, most important, he became a Vipassana teacher. He is a faculty member of the Insight Meditation Society of Barre as senior teacher. Therefore, he integrates several precious skills with a firsthand and in depth knowledge of the original Buddhist literature and of its English and Italian translations. He knows the language of contemporary psychology, and above all, he has a long and extensive personal meditation practice. These talents have made him able to forge a precise, lucid, faithful, and vibrant Italian vocabulary to translate the most important Mindfulness Meditation and Theravada terms and concepts. We are now in the fortunate condition to use Pensa's heritage not only for Insight Meditation but in the context of the "mindfulness world".

In addition, we have a beautiful single word *consapevolezza* that translates *sati* and mindfulness quite well.

However, in Italy the predominant English vocabulary of "mindfulness" words is generating extensive misunderstandings.

We select here only a couple of examples among the many possible ones.

One of the words probably eliciting the highest rate of misapprehension is "compassion." The main problem being (in Italian as well as in English) that its original meaning in the context of the Buddhist meditation traditions refers to a state of mind—not to a sentiment or to an emotion per se. But this cannot be understood without the actual experience, coming from personal meditation practice, of how it is to be in the mental state named "compassion." Without this first-person, embodied meaning, the word "compassion" (again, in Italian as well as in English) can only be misunderstood as something emotional, sentimental.

Or, even worse, in a moralistic, prescriptive sense, something that one *ought* to feel in order to be a "good" mindful person. A "should" that often becomes an attitude, a pose.

However, in Italy the situation is even more complicated because in Italian the word *compassione* has also a negative nuance. To say to someone "*mi fai compassione*" (literally: "you make me feel compassion") is insulting. It means "I disdain you, I feel contempt towards you."

The range of reactions induced by the word *compassion* may be differentiated. Yet, the point is that it almost always does produce a reaction among participants.

Also to be considered is the influence of the deep strata of clerical culture still buried in our Italians minds. Because of consumeristic contemporary culture, only 30 % or less of Italians remain practicing Catholics, but the influence of the old culture is still resonating and producing effects that can be described as producing a polarization.

One pole is a sort of "allergic" reaction to anything that might taste as clerical, and *compassione* has definitely such taste. In our classes, we have experienced several times that participants who were curious and confident in following us along the path of mindfulness practice become suddenly cautious and perplexed at the moment we introduced the word *compassione*. Some were explicit during the inquiry in showing his/her dismay ("I thought, here we are: eventually the religious background of mindfulness had to came out, and I felt repulsion" or "I am here to explore and I dislike feeling pushed in taking a moral attitude"). This kind of reaction is not infrequent in people with an urban middle class profile who think they had struggled to free themselves from their religious education.

The other pole is appreciation because "at last this MBSR protocol is showing some spiritual content"… This reaction happened particularly when we offered metta (loving kindness) meditation during the full day. The appreciation came mainly from participants who attended the course with previous interests in meditation or in "spiritual" themes and came with "spiritual" expectations who may find the style of MBIs somehow too dry.

A second example of misunderstanding is the now popular expression "non-judgmental" (*non giudicante* in Italian).

Stripped away from its original meditation context, "non-judgmental" has been diverted from naming the intention to become more and more aware of the deeply rooted habits of the mind to meet experience through any sort of preconceived concepts. It has been somehow reduced and narrowed to refer only to value judgments. As a consequence, in the mindfulness subculture (in the USA as well as in Italy) the cultivation of a non-judgmental mind, a mind aware of its own judgments, has been misunderstood as the blame for any occurrence of judgment towards others or ourselves. This misunderstanding suggests the idea that judging has to be banned if you are cultivating mindfulness. Paradoxically, this quite restricted view has become itself a moralistic judgmental attitude, a posture. It happens to hear people blaming others for being judgmental…. Whereas contemplative traditions differentiate between blind, automatic judgment, and discernment, which according to the Buddhist tradition is an essential aspect of wisdom.

A third example is the spreading of the use of the adjective "mindful" with a strong positive valence applied to everything. From mindful therapist to mindful eating, from mindful person to mindful leadership. It has taken the function of a marker of identity and membership to a trendy subculture. In Italian, the phenomenon is even more annoying because the word "mindful" is circulating *not* translated, so that we have the English adjective with an Italian noun: *un approccio* mindful, *mangiare* mindful, and so on.

In our classes, we make an effort to avoid as much as possible the use of words too charged by the "mindfulness subculture" such as compassion, acceptance, and loving-kindness.

We are especially careful in the first half of the eight sessions. We aim to minimize the risk of an implicit prescription of a moralistic attitude, or the tacit induction of a "right," expected way to think or feel.

We try to use a language that is at the same time simple, precise, warm, and yet able to resonate and to convey, at least in part, the meanings rooted in the mindfulness meditation contemplative tradition.

Only later during the protocol, when participants have developed some degree of personal, direct experience of what those traditional words like acceptance or compassion are pointing to, we introduce them with great wariness.

Mindfulness and Kitsch

We believe that today, in the western world in general, as well as Italy, one of the most dangerous and deceitful risks generated by the popularity of mindfulness is its spreading into the world in diluted, simplistic versions. These distorted versions are fostering misrepresented views about the nature of mindfulness practice, and can be summarized as an attitude suggesting a form of edifying moralism, or an attitude suggesting a reassuring promise and a guarantee of individual well-being and improved performance. These two attitudes are often blended together.

The edifying view prompts a "mindful life style" of pretended "mindful" thoughts, sentiments, attitudes, and behaviors, and invites people to cultivate a pose to "be good" according to the values of the mindfulness subculture, that is, non-judgmental, compassionate, and accepting. But by inducing the idea of "being good" rather than being aware and real, this moralistic posture becomes a parody and the turning upside down of the original intention of mindfulness to "see things as they are." On the other hand the hedonistic, pleasure-seeking view implicitly assures the removal of stress and an easily gained and sustained state of well-being, physical and mental, often joined with improved performance; thus becoming, again, the reversal and the betrayal of the fundamental intention of mindfulness to open to the unpleasant, to "turn towards" suffering.

Both views share the same background motive: looking at mindfulness practice as a means of psychological comfort and solace. Therefore, neglecting that mindfulness is above all a practice of truth aiming at freedom from a fabricated, self-indulgent relation with our experience, and that the power of mindfulness is therapeutic because it is liberative, and it is liberative because it generates insights penetrating "things as they are."

When these views and attitudes prevail and obscure its original intention, its Dhamma root, the mindfulness subculture becomes a supreme expression of *kitsch*. "Kitsch" is a philosophical, psychological, and sociological as well as an aesthetical category, which seems to us very useful to understand and describe the current phenomena of the trivialization and commodification of mindfulness. It has been elaborated during the twentieth century by several important European philosophers, writers, and artists.

Milan Kundera (1986), the Czech-French novelist, writes *"There is a kitsch attitude. A Kitsch behavior. It is the need to gaze into the mirror of the beautifying lie and to be moved to tears of gratification at one's own reflection."* He notes (Kundera, 1984) that *"kitsch is an integral part of the human condition"* and calls the key quality of kitsch the "second tear": *"Kitsch causes two tears to flow in quick succession. The first tear says: How nice to see the children running in the grass! The second tear says: How nice to be moved, together with all mankind, by children running in the grass! It is the second tear which makes kitsch kitsch."* The appeal of kitsch resides in its formula, its familiarity, and its validation of shared sensibilities.

Hermann Broch (1933), the great Czech novelist and thinker, describes its essence, *"the spirit of kitsch can be seen as a deception: by providing comfort, kitsch performs a denial. It glosses over harsh truths and anesthetizes genuine pain."*

Kitsch is not only an individual attitude, it is also a cultural phenomenon, Clement Greenberg (1939) emphasizes the *"pre-condition for kitsch, a condition without which kitsch would be impossible, is the availability close at hand of a fully formed cultural tradition, whose discoveries, acquisitions, and perfected self-consciousness* Kitsch *can take advantage of for its own ends…. Kitsch does not analyze culture but repackages and stylizes it. Kitsch reinforces established conventions, appealing to mass tastes and gratifying communal experiences. As a result, kitsch is easy to market and effortless to consume."*

These quotations show how well the trivialized versions of mindfulness can fit into the category of Kitsch. It is happening everywhere in the Western world. However, in Italy, we are perhaps more sensitive and more inclined to such risk because our national culture has been deeply impacted by 35 years of the hyper-kitsch TV, media, and political discourse led by the well-known media tycoon and former Prime Minister, Silvio Berlusconi.

All that aside, we are convinced that ultimately the essence of mindfulness meditation practice as an expression of the Dhamma cannot be touched by such superficial trends and phenomena. We are teaching MBIs with this reference point—the Dhamma—always present in our minds. Sadly the present-day mindfulness subculture risks to waste the liberative potential of awareness and to lose any vital connection with its origin, becoming just another lifeless commodity. This is why we put so much intention and effort into trying to be real in our classes, to suit the Italian character, and to honor the spirit and practice of mindfulness.

References

Broch, H. (1933). In G. Gillo Dorfle (ed.). *Kitsch: The world of bad taste* (1968), New York: Universe Books.

Greenberg, C. (1939). *Avant-Garde and Kitsch*, Partisan Review 6.

Milan, Kundera (1984). *The Unbearable Lightness of Being: A Novel*. New York: Harper.

Milan Kundera (1986). *The Art of the Novel*. New York: Harper.

Segal, Z., Teasdale, J., & Williams, J. (2012). *Mindfulness-Based Cognitive Therapy for Depression* Guilford, 2nd Edition.

Chapter 9
Teaching in Israel

Diane (Dina) Wyshogrod

If missiles are fired at Jerusalem and the air-raid sirens go off during class today, is there enough space in the shelter for my MBSR group? Can we get there in time before the rockets hit?

This was no drill. This was reality here in Israel during the summer of 2014. For 50 days, war raged between Israel and Hamas in Gaza, bringing suffering and destruction to people on both sides of the conflict. This was indeed the full catastrophe, as promised: Life. Death. And everything in between. A true test of Mindfulness-Based Stress Reduction (MBSR).

Years back, I saw a cartoon spoofing Rudyard Kipling's famous poem "If." The caption read: "If you can keep your head when everyone around you is losing theirs... Maybe you just don't understand the situation."

Or maybe, you know something that's helping you handle it better.

MBSR is exactly what I, a clinical and medical psychologist, had been looking for years ago, namely, techniques to add to my existing "toolbox" for managing anxiety and stress and enhancing health, job performance, creativity, and resilience. I wanted an evidence-based, grounded, sensible approach that was not faddish or "New Age-y," was robust enough to withstand skepticism yet provide a gentle balm for physical and emotional pain, and did not conflict with religious or spiritual practice. It had to be simple to learn (which, as most of us quickly discover, does not guarantee easy!) and powerful enough to withstand everything that life dishes out.

My search was also personal: in 1991, I moved from my hometown of New York City to Jerusalem, Israel, with my husband and three young sons, and I was excited and apprehensive about the challenges ahead. Any approach I adopted had to help

D. Wyshogrod, Ph.D. (✉)
MBSR-ISRAEL, the Israeli Center for Mindfulness Based Stress Reduction,
Dan 12, Jerusalem 9350912, Israel
e-mail: dr.dina@breathedeep.net

© Springer International Publishing Switzerland 2016
D. McCown et al., *Resources for Teaching Mindfulness*,
DOI 10.1007/978-3-319-30100-6_9

me handle the stresses of everyday life compounded by the adjustment to a new country and culture plus, unfortunately, terrorism and war.

A tall order, to be sure. MBSR, with its research backing, universality of practice, accessibility, clarity, and graceful simplicity, fit the bill. As I began to integrate MBSR into my own life and to experience its relevance and power, I dreamed of bringing MBSR to Israel as a way of bringing a measure of peace to my adoptive country.

The Israeli Scene

Israel is fertile ground for new ideas and approaches. Notwithstanding Israel's tiny population (only eight million people) and size (barely larger than the state of New Jersey), whatever you seek can be found here. Skepticism about fads and intense dislike of being "suckered" are counterbalanced by curiosity, openness and, above all, a hunger for practical, innovative solutions promising effective relief from the considerable challenges we face.

Israel is on the cutting edge of expertise in trauma treatment, both physical (with world-ranked orthopedic facilities) and emotional. Rubbing shoulders are some of the world's oldest "alternative" or "complementary" approaches including acupuncture and reflexology (which have long been reimbursed by Israeli socialized medicine) and Ayurveda, plus revolutionary new approaches such as energy medicine and psychology.

Meditation has long been part of the Israeli scene: Goenka, approaches inspired by Thich Nhat Hanh and the Dalai Lama (both of whom have visited Israel), Transcendental Meditation (TM), Jewish mindfulness, and Kabbalistic meditation. So although the specific form of MBSR was new, meditation was not.

Since establishing MBSR-ISRAEL in 2002, I have taught MBSR to thousands of people, lay people and health care professionals, businesspeople, and academics, in classic eight-week courses, seminars, workshops, and retreats. My students, although predominantly Jewish, also have included Christians and Muslims as well as foreign diplomats, journalists, and workers for nongovernmental organizations (NGOs) crisscrossing between Israel, the Palestinian territories, and Jordan. They've been men and women, from 16 through 91 years, mostly middle-class though not exclusively so, native-born Israelis and immigrants, the vast majority English-speaking.

I have participated in research on reducing burnout among pediatric oncology workers, and have been part of a new initiative training teachers in mindfulness and MBSR for integration into the nation's education system. MBSR-ISRAEL offers Teacher Training and annual Mindful India trips that integrate mindfulness into itineraries featuring India's fabulous highlights. It's gratifying to see the recent proliferation of MBIs—MBSR, Mindfulness-Based Cognitive Therapy (MBCT), and even Mindfulness-Based Childbirth and Parenting (MBCP) programs around the country, after having been the only MBSR teacher here for over a decade.

Bringing MBSR to Israel

Bringing MBSR to Israel has been a mindfulness practice in its own right, necessitating everything from making the appropriate cultural and linguistic translations, to straddling religious divides and accommodating cultural sensitivities, to teaching a practice of peace in a region at war. Describing this process skillfully in these pages is itself a mindfulness practice. I am a child of Holocaust survivors, immigrants to the United States. I am now myself an immigrant, a status I share with many of my students. As we often discuss, that experience of marginality, that ever-shifting edge between belonging/not belonging graces us at times with some degree of "beginner's mind" with regard to what insiders take for granted, and at other times, renders us blind and ignorant. I'm mindful of the joyous and sober responsibility to do justice to the work that I love in the country I love.

The mindfulness teaching of Right Speech is mirrored in Judaism's concern about *lashon hara* (literally: evil tongue, i.e., slanderous talk). One teaching tale likens *lashon hara* to releasing feathers from a sack: easily scattered and impossible to recapture as they waft from place to place, spreading pain. One of my father's favorite Yiddish aphorisms neatly sums up this metaphor: *Ah patch fargeit, un a vort bashteit.* A slap is forgotten but a word lingers forever. So I will avoid generalizations to the extent possible knowing how hurtful and dangerous, let alone misleading, they can be. As I urge my students, I will seek to "state my truth," sharing my experiences as student, teacher, and trainer of MBSR over the years. May what I write be for the greater good of all.

Practicing in Israel as a clinical psychologist and teacher/trainer of MBSR has proved very different from my work in New York. In New York, it was easier to maintain the separation between practitioner and patient. Israeli society is smaller and more intimate, and whereas conventional wisdom holds there are six degrees of separation between people, here it's more like two or three. The people you treat or teach may live next door, sit near you at prayer services at your congregation (especially if you lead monthly meditation sessions prior to Sabbath morning services, as I do), or be lathering up in the shower stall next to yours at the local gym locker room (true stories!). In addition, I've found the culture to be informal, almost familial, which may account for the lack of self-consciousness in requesting that courses be scheduled around a prospective participant's schedule, or invitations to lead mindfulness practices at engagement parties, weddings, and new baby celebrations. More seriously, these people will be huddling with you in your air-raid shelter or crying next to you at a young soldier's funeral. Most gratifying is that some of my MBSR students have become close friends.

Translating MBSR

Translating MBSR to Israel began with literally translating the word "mindfulness." Hebrew has no word for "mind" but "awareness," "consciousness," "introspection," "self-observation," and "attention" have all been suggested in trying to convey the essence of mindfulness, along with using the word "mindfulness" itself, transliterated into Hebrew as מיינדפולנס and delivered with an Israeli accent. Consultations with the Academy of the Hebrew Language soon after I began teaching yielded the term *ke-shi-vut* (קשיבות) from the root *keshev*, attention. I liked the fact that it was relatively unknown, with few associations. Beginner's mind in three syllables. That newness has its drawbacks; people look askance at me as they test it gingerly on their lips. It is slowly and steadily gaining acceptance, its usage depending to some extent on the speaker's background. Those with prior meditation experience tend to use "mindfulness"; people I've taught or those new to the practices easily adopt *ke-shi-vut*. I myself often use both when introducing the subject, to cover all bases and reach all audiences while making this small linguistic contribution to my adoptive language.

All handouts, home practice assignment sheets, and audio materials used in the course are available in both Hebrew (prepared in consultation with professional translators) and English, and each student gets material in the language of his/her choice. Both Hebrew- and English-speaking classes are offered, though people do "crossover" with Hebrew-speakers in the English-speaking classes and vice versa. In whichever class, students are welcome to speak in their preferred language and someone will translate if necessary. Even in the Hebrew-speaking classes some English creeps in: scientific and mindfulness terms, relevant idioms, and even jokes, though these are immediately translated. Many Israelis know some English, and numerous English phrases have slipped almost unconsciously into everyday parlance society-wide.

The "all-day" class brings together current course participants, course graduates, and often others with suitable backgrounds. The choice of language of instruction depends on participants' proficiency. If everyone is fluent (or fluent enough) in either Hebrew or English (ascertained in advance), that will be the language of the day. The presence of foreign nationals, for example, mandates English. However, if enough participants also require Hebrew, the teaching is done in both by translating back and forth as smoothly as possible throughout the day. Leading fewer (or shorter) language-intensive practices (e.g., the body scan and yoga) in favor of more self-guided practices (e.g., walking and basic sitting practices) reduces the amount of speaking in any language in favor of deepening the silence.

I am fluent in Hebrew, but it is not my native language, as is true for many course participants whose mother tongue is neither Hebrew nor English, but Arabic, French, Hungarian, Russian, or Spanish, among others. As immigrants, we have to adapt for the "loss" of our primary language. When discussing stress reactivity during the course, non-natives often mention language as a stressor, such as when they struggle to express themselves adequately and powerfully especially when angry, or are immediately pegged as "outsider" the minute someone hears their accent. I can relate. I often feel the difference in my face and body when teaching in English versus Hebrew. It has become part of my practice to notice and accept these reactions and I invite students to do the same. Grammatical mistakes or "word fumblings" can become opportunities to practice empathy, acceptance, humility, and a sense of humor.

Hebrew has no neutral "it"; everything is either masculine or feminine. In early versions of the participants' workbook, trying to use neutral language, I alternated between male and female verb forms from section to section. Many participants found this practice artificial, preferring the standard male form, so I have shifted my materials accordingly, although when speaking I still often integrate both (e.g., "each of us noticing *his or her* reactions...").

There is also no gerund in Hebrew, so the "—ing" form (e.g., "raising the leg") is not an option. When guiding meditations, I sometimes speak in the first person plural ("...let's raise the leg") although some complained that this instruction reminded them unpleasantly of the exhortations of their kindergarten teachers. I've alternated between the imperative ("Raise the leg"), the more impersonal, almost disembodied form used by many yoga teachers ("... the leg rises toward the ceiling..."), and more "invitational" language (e.g., "please notice..." or "you are invited to notice...."). In sum, I mix and match, hoping to pique students' curiosity about this most human behavior of speech, because what we say has far-reaching consequences. God "spoke" the world into being, according to the Book of Genesis. What worlds are we creating or destroying, what realities are we highlighting or obscuring, with our words?

In the "raisin" and "Nine Dot" exercises, we explore how our lives are affected by the words and labels we use and the way we box ourselves in and out. Our work in class focuses on the personal ramifications, but if one is paying attention, the geopolitical and sociological implications are ever present. Certainly, the cross section of students in my classes attests to the intersection of labels and "boxes": Jew/Christian/Muslim, outside/inside Jerusalem, outside/inside "the territories," Israel/Palestinian territories/Jordan, religious/secular, observant/nonobservant, and native/immigrant/temporary resident. The task of ensuring that this intersection will be smooth and soothing, warm and welcoming, falls first and foremost to the MBSR teacher.

Religious Sensitivities

The ceremonial Passover meal, the Seder, opens with the following beautiful invitation: "May all who are hungry come and partake; may all who are needy, be welcome here." Making sure each participant feels safe and nurtured at the MBSR "table" necessitates awareness and respect for each one's background and concerns, maneuvering gently yet firmly within a multitude of delicate, sometimes contradictory, needs. One way to do so is by being transparent and honest when presenting the MBSR course, its content, background, and underpinnings, so that nobody feels misled or that anything was misrepresented.

Though it would be easy to call this a "relaxation course" as people often do when inquiring about it, I explain forthrightly this is a course in "mindfulness" and "meditation." *Because* of people's wariness about religious and foreign influences, I specifically and deliberately credit the 2500 year Buddhist contribution to our understanding of the workings of the mind. I also note respectfully that every religious and spiritual tradition teaches its own ways of quieting down and going within in order to connect with the self and/or with some Higher Power or to achieve some other aim. But none of the above is the purview of the course. MBSR is not a course in Buddhist meditation, Jewish meditation, or spirituality. Nor is it "secular" meditation because, especially here, that adjective is hardly neutral.

This course is in mindfulness, paying attention, being aware, being present— innate and *universal* human abilities that people can learn to apply more often, more consistently, and with greater self-understanding and compassion in order to improve their lives and serve their particular needs. I also mention the growing body of research that substantiates it.

Rarely do people balk when the course is presented in this way.

The same candor works for "yoga," a term that's gone mainstream but can still evoke suspicion and distrust. Some, from very traditional religious backgrounds, worry that it derives from "idol worship" and is therefore potentially subversive. The explanation that we are simply moving mindfully in ways that may be familiar from Pilates or physiotherapy usually assuages this concern. I also can produce a ruling from a well-known rabbinic authority stating that yoga and mindfulness are not idol worship, which reassures some Orthodox Jews. These straightforward explanations defuse much reactivity and anything that's left can become grist for the mill during the course.

In general when teaching, using familiar, everyday language enhances safety and the sense of belonging, and reduces the chances of triggering someone unnecessarily. We speak of "group" or "community" rather than *sangha,* and "compassion" or "loving-kindness" rather than *metta* (although I do teach those terms so students will recognize them in other meditation settings).

Loving-kindness itself is a core Judaic value. The Hebrew expression for paying attention is *la-sim-lev*, to place the heart. In a famous story, a cynic challenged one of Israel's ancient sages, Hillel, to boil down the Torah to its essence, something that could be conveyed while standing on one foot. Hillel didn't bat an eye. "Love thy neighbor as thyself," he replied.

Easier said than done, of course, just as translating "loving-kindness" into Hebrew touched on sensitivities requiring tender handling. I ran several options past translators and students. *Rahamim*, from the root *rehem* (womb), denotes mercy, but is too often confused with self-pity and feeling sorry for oneself, cultural "no-nos." *Hesed* means kindness and benevolence, but its association with "doing good works" came too close to religious injunctions for some. I ultimately chose *hemla*, another synonym for compassion tinged with feeling for the suffering of another.

In my experience, the relative nuances of each word can easily touch off an impassioned, almost Talmudic debate—a time-honored tradition in Judaism. For our purposes, I teach that it's fine to notice one's reactions, honor the discussion, appreciate the passion, *and* practice detaching from it all. Students can also always substitute words or phrases that suit them better.

To enhance the sense of comfort and belonging in class, I bring in a selection of quotes, poems, and readings that's balanced between English and Hebrew, Israeli and international sources, and Zen and rabbinic stories; the parallels between some of the latter are often striking (see Chapter 23 for "Rabbi Akiva Taught: This Too is For the Best" and "Good News, Bad News, Who Knows?")

Holding Fast to Curriculum and Yet...

Another way to make the MBSR classroom safe and nurturing for all is to hold fast to the curriculum with its clear, universalist approach. Nobody has yet argued with "breathing in, breathing out."

Hold fast, yes, but gently, embracing needs arising from the different religions, cultures, and backgrounds of the students. My classes in Jerusalem, for example, often include very observant Jews, making me particularly sensitive to certain issues of personal modesty, contact between the sexes, food and eating, and scheduling. Other populations pose other considerations.

Modesty and proximity between men and women: For reasons of modesty, many observant Jewish men and women do not usually interact together the way they do in an MBSR class. Lying down or sitting (whether on mats or in chairs) near each other, raising their legs in the air or undulating or twisting their bodies in front of one another or in the presence of a teacher of the opposite gender, or even listening to one another discuss personal experiences in class, are all a stretch for many — pun intended.

Therefore, some Orthodox Jewish men would never take a course taught by a woman, no matter how Orthodox she is. But keep in mind that no group is monolithic, no matter how its members look or dress. Many very Orthodox men and women do participate in regular mixed-gender, heterogeneous MBSR courses where we all sit together.

Before accepting someone into the course, I always conduct an individual pre-course consultation which takes place in the actual classroom with the mats right there, so prospective participants can assess the space and conditions. I describe the body scan and mindful movement and explain that they will be practicing these near to, *but not touching,* members of the opposite sex; physical contact between students is never required. They're welcome to raise any issues, and I take these into account as much as possible. In class, if necessary, I place those who are more sensitive on different sides of the room for the body scan and yoga. I have also on occasion taught the yoga to men and women separately by having one group in my office and the other in an adjacent room, with me moving back and forth between them. The all-day class is taught in a larger hall where one section can be set off with a divider (a *meḥitza*) affording privacy to those who prefer to practice separately for reasons of modesty.

With mixed-gender groups, engaging in physical contact such as holding hands to form a circle would be unacceptable to very observant Jews *even if they themselves are not directly touching a person of the opposite sex.* It also would be unacceptable to set up a circle of men inside a circle of women.

Modesty of dress: Both sexes may feel uncomfortable seeing or being seen by members of the opposite sex, including the teacher, in poses and positions that are considered revealing. Feeling exposed is a form of feeling immodest.

Many Orthodox women don't wear pants, and certainly not in mixed company. Some women handle this by wearing sweatpants or leggings under their skirts for yoga and sometimes even for the body scan. It's wise to notify them in advance that these practices will be on the agenda so they can prepare accordingly. Being able to cover up with blankets (which I provide) during the body scan for reasons of personal modesty is also often appreciated.

Communication: Pairing men and women for post-meditation check-ins, communication exercises, or as "meditation buddies" can be problematic. At issue might be the close physical proximity or simply having a personal discussion that supersedes acceptable bounds of intimacy with someone of the opposite gender.

Food and eating are central to most cultures. Every tradition has its ways of sanctifying food and the act of eating beyond simply stoking our engines and keeping us alive.

Long before modern science affirmed that pausing and breathing consciously before eating are healthful practices, aiding digestion and metabolism, many cultures taught us to say a blessing before ingesting something. But when doing the "raisin exercise," we slow down the process deliberately and examine each component carefully, so much so that participants sometimes wonder out loud whether they will ever actually eat the object they've been eyeing, sniffing, and handling, and if so, at what point should they say the blessing?

Because this issue arises so frequently, I often incorporate it into the exercise. After we've examined the raisin with our other senses, I inform them that we'll now begin to explore tasting and eating, inviting them to include in their practice the timing of the blessing. For everyone, it can be fascinating to consider what constitutes "eating" and when it begins and ends. Where does this raisin begin and end? (And, for that matter, where do "I"?)

Different religions observe particular dietary laws and restrictions. This chapter by no means provides a comprehensive or definitive guide to them. It just offers "food for thought." Observant Muslims eat *halal* (acceptable according to Islam) food, refraining from certain meats (e.g., pork), alcohol, and gelatin. Observant Jews observe *kashrut*, which applies to all food, including raisins, and drinks. Appropriate certification (on package labels) makes it possible to check that food derivatives and processing did not render something unkosher, or *haram* (forbidden according to Islam). Organic foods are not necessarily kosher.

Kashrut demands strict separation between meat and dairy or their derivatives, between kosher and nonkosher products, and with regard to the utensils, plates, and cookware used to prepare and serve food. Disposable dishes, cups, and utensils offer a simple solution.

Observant Jews also wait a certain length of time between consuming dairy and meat products. So, for example, when planning an eating meditation using chocolate, consider serving one that's labeled "*pareve*" (i.e., neutral, neither meat nor milk, and can be eaten with either) or inform students in advance so they won't come having just eaten a meat meal and be unable to eat anything dairy until several hours later.

Additional considerations include being aware of major and minor fast days and the observance of Lent and Ramadan. MBSR-ISRAEL courses, programs, and retreats are held only at venues which have appropriate *kashrut* supervision and are scheduled only on weekdays, avoiding the Sabbath (which begins Friday at sundown) and any relevant holy days.

Does one really have to take all these factors into consideration? After all, some students opt out of eating the raisin because they don't eat sugar or "hate raisins."

Can't we just suggest that they *imagine* doing the exercise, notice their reactions, and fold that into the experience and subsequent inquiry? Maybe, but *choosing* to sit out an exercise is very different from being *precluded* from participating.

You don't need to have a degree in comparative religion, nor be an expert in kosher raisins. The internet can be an excellent source of information, even pointing you to what questions to ask, and it might be wise to query your students about their needs. Notwithstanding, we'll probably still make mistakes, serve the "wrong" raisins, say the wrong things. Being "right" isn't necessarily the issue. In fact, as Yehuda Amichai, one of Israel's foremost poets, writes (used with permission):

> From the place where we are right
> Flowers will never grow
> In the spring.
> The place where we are right
> Is trampled and hard
> As a yard.
> But doubts and loves
> Dig up the world
> Like a mole, a plow.
> And a whisper will be heard in the place
> Where the ruined
> House once stood.

If we own our doubts and mistakes with grace and humility, these moments of clumsiness might teach us all—teachers and students—to replace hubris with humility, condemnation with curiosity, and criticism with compassion towards ourselves and others.

Working with populations we don't know, and sometimes even more challengingly, with those we *think* we do know, dares us to notice the "place[s] where we are right" and to dig deeper under what's become rote and "trampled and hard as a yard" to hear the whispers of more profound meanings.

It must be emphasized that despite the lengthy discussion above, *none of these religious considerations take up much actual time or space in the classroom.* This limitation is deliberate.

MBSR-ISRAEL classes also include many participants who are secular or even antireligious and who might be uncomfortable or outright fearful of anything smacking of religious influence.

Additionally, by design and intent, MBSR is emphatically not a course in spirituality and is not taught as such.

Notwithstanding, people sometimes do make their own surprising connections. One nonreligious participant realized that the traditional blessings he had dismissed as "fanatical" were actually experiences of mindfulness, a reframing that allowed him to soften considerably and reevaluate his relationship to his Jewish roots and coreligionists.

Another participant was delighted to notice the link between the breath, *neshima,* and the soul, *neshama.*

Many ultra-Orthodox men and women have credited mindfulness for teaching them not only to reduce stress and pain, but to pray and perform rituals with greater focus and intention. I'll never forget the wonder on one woman's face as she realized that this single raisin between her fingertips "contained" within it the sun, rain, earth, human labor, the whole interconnected world. In a word: God. Although she had been blessing her food her entire life, she said, she'd never experienced that connection before.

Finding Our Ways "Home"

Adjustment to immigration, including the adjustment to a new language as discussed above, is yet another significant experience and potential stressor.

Many of us have had the experience of taking a seat upon entering a brand-new classroom and "locking onto" that spot so that, from that moment, woe betide anyone who usurps it. I often challenge this attitude at some point in the course, asking people to observe their reactions as they change places, face into and away from the center of the room, choose whether or not they want to go back to their original seats. This simple yet surprisingly powerful exercise often stimulates a very meaningful exploration of what it means to be *at home* in one's body, in one's "homeland," and in the world. What does it mean to have a place, or to be "displaced"?

This discussion has intense personal relevance in classes which are heavily populated by immigrants like me, and where even the native-born Israelis are often only one generation away from the immigrant experience. Whether here by choice or out of duress, each has left behind everything that was familiar, much that was taken for granted, and is now engaged in putting down new roots, forging a new identity, and merging, not always comfortably, with a still-emerging culture.

With so many groups, identities, and elements jockeying for position, Israel is not so much a "melting pot" as a mosaic, comprised of often jagged and sharp pieces with each seeking to claim its place in this seething, dynamic whole. By being mindful, and without making a big deal of it, all these respective needs, identities, and sensitivities can be accommodated smoothly and unobtrusively, creating a seamless whole where everyone feels safe and welcome.

It's very moving to look out over an audience—say, at an "all-day" or refresher class or MBSR retreat—and see people from many backgrounds, nationalities, ages, religious affiliations and styles of dress, meditating together and engaging mindfully with each other, learning that no matter how different they might seem from one another, they have much in common with each other and with people all over the world. After all, they come to MBSR for many of the same reasons: They're in pain, physical and emotional. There's "too much noise" in their heads. They're afraid of the future—and the present. They come because life is beautiful and taxing and dangerous and sometimes just too much, and they seek peace and quiet and strength. And they discover that some of that strength derives from seeing beneath the stereotypes that separate us into the essence of heart and soul we sometimes share.

... There Are Differences

And yet... there *are* differences, and these blew up in our faces during the summer of 2014. The summer opened explosively with the kidnapping and murder of three Israeli Jewish teenagers by Hamas terrorists. Several days later, three Israeli Jews intent on revenge beat and burned to death a Palestinian teenager from East Jerusalem. The border between Israel and Gaza exploded and we were again at war.

I've taught in the midst of the Second Intifada and various combat operations through the years, but it was my first time teaching during a war like this, where the civilian population country-wide was under direct attack. I had actually not expected Jerusalem to be fired on; surely Hamas wouldn't risk hitting the holy Muslim sites of the Dome of the Rock and the Al-Aqsa Mosque? But they did fire rockets at Jerusalem several times during those subsequent weeks, and we did indeed have to go into the air-raid shelter, while the threat never abated.

I clocked the walk from my office to the shelter to ensure we could get there safely within the 90-second warning time, and then notified my classes that we could meet as scheduled. It was strange to be meditating and conducting an inquiry with an ear cocked for the telltale whining crescendo of the air-raid siren—thankfully, it never went off during class—but otherwise, the war was only one of the stressors we discussed in class, and even that, only minimally. The rest of the time we dealt with the usual: coping with cranky kids, demanding bosses, and sick relatives, balancing work and family, and staying awake during a body scan. In fact, throughout all my years of teaching MBSR and counseling clients one-on-one, people have displayed tremendous resilience, handling "the situation" (the "*matzav*" as we call it), with grace, humor, and fatalism offset by the ubiquitous statement "*yi-yeh b'seder*," everything will be all right. As I often say at the beginning of a course, stress may be serious, but it shouldn't be grim, and even in times of war, classes are usually full of warmth, ease, and laughter.

Body awareness, enhanced by weeks of the body scan (whose relevance so many question initially!), proved an important basis for coping. People monitored how the media barrage affected them physically and emotionally and used that awareness to strike a suitable balance between being informed and "going crazy." I also urged them to observe the body revving up in the face of danger—real and perceived—and to consciously release that tension (e.g., by breathing, jumping, laughing, crying, shaking) when appropriate to reduce the possibility of trauma being stored in the nervous system, particularly when the immediate danger had passed.

The suggestion to "stay in the moment" became a lifeline for many. My advice was to "Keep asking yourself: *at this very moment, to the best of my knowledge, is everything all right?* If you've got someone in active service at the frontlines (which, given Israeli society's two or three degrees of separation, is basically everyone), it's small consolation but true: if they're hurt or worse, you'll know. Fast. Otherwise, it's a safe bet that *at this moment*, that person is fine. Don't let your mind hijack you. Keep coming back to *this* moment. Ground yourself: feel your feet on the floor. Be aware of sounds around you. Focus on *this* in-breath, *this* out-breath. Repeat. Repeat. Repeat."

The students in my classes at the time represented points all along the political, ideological, and religious spectrums, and none of that became the issue as we paused to breathe and take stock, listened and spoke to each other mindfully, shared our thoughts and feelings, and kept our hearts open. When the home of a Christian American NGO worker in the group was caught in the cross fire during the riots following the murder of the Palestinian teenager, other group members (including those living outside Jerusalem in "the territories," i.e., the West Bank) immediately offered sanctuary in their homes until the situation in town calmed down. Notwithstanding the shelter under the building, we built a safe space in that room, with each other, for each other.

The course also teaches us how to create and reinforce our *inner* safe spaces. This knowledge is vital: the constant threat under which we live, with the shadow of the Holocaust ever-looming in the background, means that fight/flight/freeze reactions are easily reactivated and reinforced. Months after the cease-fire, sounds eerily reminiscent of the air-raid sirens, such as a baby beginning to whine or someone gunning an engine, are enough to raise hackles and rev up the nervous system: *what's happening?*

Loving-Kindness in the Face of Threat and War

Mindfulness practices, according to research, can enhance emotion regulation, as can loving-kindness and compassion. These qualities are already embedded in the practices, but given the situation here, for years now, I've been integrating loving-kindness practice even more systematically into the course. I bring each practice to a close with the suggestion that participants thank themselves for having nurtured themselves in this unique way. Then, as early as Class 4 or 5, and certainly before the "all-day" class, I teach the formal loving-kindness practice as another form of concentration practice and include it on the list of home practices.

These practices initially make many people squirm. They're used to being self-critical. But self-compassion or appreciation? That's "kitschy." Over the weeks, many students' attitudes soften toward themselves and they come to appreciate the effects of this practice, particularly in the wake of Classes 4 and 5, during which we cover, in depth, stress reactivity and trauma and the relevant physiology and neuroscience. I intersperse these discussions with frequent pauses using the STOP technique (Stop/Take a breath/Observe sensations, feelings, and thoughts without changing them/Proceed) because the discussion itself often triggers people. I invite participants to notice when they are becoming triggered and to flag me so we can pause in the discussion and "recalibrate." I keep a close eye on how people are reacting in judging when to call for these pauses myself. The loving-kindness practices are then seen as a natural next step, an easily accessible antidote to the feelings of vulnerability and powerlessness that underlie the fight/flight/freeze reactions.

One way to particularly underscore that message is by always beginning the loving-kindness practice with the intention to be safe and protected. When I began teaching MBSR in 2002, the Second Intifada was raging. Bombs were exploding everywhere. Nobody was safe. I vividly remember how moving it was when my teachers at the Center for Mindfulness, Melissa Blacker, Pam Erdmann, and Florence Meleo-Meyer, guiding me through various stages of my training during those years, began their loving-kindness practices with "May you be safe." As they told me later, they were conscious of what I, my family, and my students, were facing back home. I've never forgotten that.

I often introduce the formal loving-kindness practice by having students first send wishes of well-being (e.g., safety/happiness/health/freedom from suffering/peacefulness) to "someone dear or special to you" before focusing on themselves, thus skirting that initial skittishness about self-compassion. In subsequent practices, we follow the traditional order of (1) self; (2) beloved other; (3) neutral other; (4) difficult other; (5) all beings, with some modifications.

I inform my classes that in some meditation circles they might hear the more traditional term "the enemy" for stage 4, but that I deliberately don't use the word because it might prove too loaded for some. I want the practice to comfort and soothe, not agitate, especially when the practice is still new and challenging enough. (This is my rationale for using the term "rest pose" rather than "corpse pose" when guiding mindful movement, while clarifying that they may hear the latter in some yoga classes).

Still, even without being explicit, this issue still crops up when focusing on "the difficult other" or "all beings." Some students regularly send wishes of well-being to the Palestinians—even Hamas—in the hope that we might all someday be peaceful and free from suffering. But others have a harder time. On an MBSR retreat during a period of relative quiet in the country, one man spoke candidly and painfully about his unwillingness to send positive intentions to everyone if this meant including the Arabs. His son was serving in the army; if he wished the other side well, might this not rebound in some way to hurt his child?

The group sat together in respectful silence, holding him as he held the multitude of feelings arising: anguish and fear, self-criticism and defiance, the wish for things to be different, and the acceptance that this was the reality right now. His honesty and candor were a powerful lesson for all present that what shows up when we are mindful is not necessarily pretty, or calm, or politically correct, but authentic and human, and our challenge is to embrace it with awareness, acceptance, and compassion.

As I prepare to lead a loving-kindness practice, tracking my own truth from moment to moment personally and as teacher guides me in choosing whether, and how, to proceed. I want to do more than make sure nobody is harmed. I want to enhance self-regulation and self-efficacy, so people will come away knowing they've now got a powerful resource that can counter helplessness and promote healing, that's accessible to all, for the good of all. Awareness of potentially sensitive issues doesn't mean shirking from them. Should something arise that demands attention, I will deal with it.

I preface any modifications I might make to the loving-kindness practice by stating that what I'm about to lead feels right *to me* at this moment, and invite participants to monitor their reactions and accept/reject/adjust my words as they will. This preface underscores the importance of stepping out of autopilot into conscious choice according to their consciences, not mine.

So during one early-morning practice, when *four* families—three Jewish, one Muslim—sat in mourning over their murdered sons, when the number of casualties was rising on both sides of the border, when many of us felt increasingly helpless and angry and scared and frustrated, we sent intentions of safety, protection, healing, ease, and peace to the four bereaved families and to all victims of terror and violence in both Israel and Gaza. Those practices afforded us a sense of inner refuge, a means of enhancing the sense of self-efficacy and control.

On another occasion, leading a community-wide emergency stress reduction program at my synagogue, I was aware that in the audience were friends and neighbors whose children—kids we all knew since they were babies—were in the fighting. My primary intentions that evening were to soothe and comfort, to reduce the parents' worry and feelings of helplessness. I began the loving-kindness practice by directing our intentions first to our soldiers, our sons and daughters, beginning with safety and protection and moving through comfort, resilience, and well-being. We then extended our scope to include everyone present, gradually widening the circle to include anyone and everyone who needed it, and ending with the whole world. That gave everyone, no matter where they were from, who they were, or their stance on any issue, maximum latitude to use this practice as they wished. We closed with the fervent "May we all be blessed with peace."

Dreaming, Hoping, and Not-Knowing

I learned mindfulness hoping that it could make me and those around me stronger and more resilient in the face of fear. Many of us have indeed learned to find a measure of safety and refuge in *this* moment.

I had also dreamed that MBSR would bring a measure of peace to this beleaguered region of the world. I'm less optimistic about that now. Mindfulness is about seeing clearly. What I see is that the minds of men and women are still too deluded; the labels dividing us still too entrenched; the lines too firmly etched; the boxes still too solid; and brute force still seems like the best, the only solution.

And yet, I still want to believe, along with Anne Frank, that people are basically good at heart; that we have more in common than not; and that we shall overcome.

Both Judaism and Islam teach that whoever saves one person, saves a world (Tractate Sanhedrin 37a; Qur'an 5:32).

The Talmud also teaches that you may not be able to complete a task, but you have to at least start (Mishnah Avot, 2:17).

Perhaps, one person at a time, one breath at a time, we can begin to shift the balance from rage to reconciliation, from fear to forgiveness, from cruelty to compassion, and from war to *salaam*, to *shalom,* to peace.

Chapter 10
Teaching in Australia

Timothea Goddard and Maura A. Kenny

Setting the Scene in Australia

In the highlands of New South Wales where we hold our mindfulness teacher trainings, the early mornings are cold, and warm blankets and colorful shawls envelop the group sitting quietly after the dawn yoga practice. The sun has come up and the wide opalescent sky is now clear and blue and echoing with bird song. The beauty and silence of the Australian bush supports and nurtures us in this endeavor although later the flies will be an invitation into non-judgmental acceptance. But for now, in this moment, the still purity of the morning brings a sense of wonder at the miracle of simply being alive. Is this what being mindful is all about? Or just part of it?

G'day.

We have been asked to write about Mindfulness-based Interventions within the Australian context—a broad remit indeed. We are aware of the responsibility of representing accurately all the ways in which MBIs have unfolded in Australia, and all the views that abound on mindfulness and its teaching in our multicultural society. We have had to reflect carefully about what we could usefully say from an "Australian perspective", especially as one of us originally hails from Scotland, and as our broader teaching and supervisory team and collegial network is a diverse mix of cultures, races, and nationalities.

But this reality is a quintessentially Australian scenario as we are a melting pot of cultures, sensibilities, and views on how we should be governed and our place in the wider world. The national character (if there is such a thing) could be described as

T. Goddard, B.A., Dip. Psychotherapy (A.N.Z.A.P.) Clin Mem P.A.C.F.A. (✉)
Mindfulness Training Institute of Australasia,
Suite 807/251 Oxford St, Bondi Junction, NSW 2022, Australia
e-mail: tim@openground.com.au

M.A. Kenny, M.B.Ch.B., M.R.C.Psych., F.R.A.N.Z.C.P.
Mindfulness Training Institute Australasia, Centre for the Treatment of Anxiety
and Depression, SA Health, 30 Anderson Street, Thebarton, SA 5031, Australia
e-mail: maura@mtia.org.au; maura.kenny@sa.gov.au

having a broad streak of egalitarianism, optimism, and irreverence. There are refreshing qualities of mateship, directness, high energy, good humor, good-naturedness, and nonhierarchical interactions; a kind of deep democracy which resonates well with the nonhierarchical collaboration between teacher and participants in mindfulness classes. The Aussie spirit is summed up in such colloquialisms as "she'll be right" (all manner of things will be well), "no worries, mate" (happy to help/all will be well, my friend), and " this mindfulness lark is ridgey-didge" (the genuine article, trustworthy).

Geographically, Australia is a vast country with a disproportionately small population of 23.6 million despite it having the sixth largest landmass in the world. A two-day drive separates these two teachers (authors) who nevertheless work closely together. We are in the same country yet live in different climates, and there is rugged and sometimes dangerous landscape in between.

Yet we are also an English-speaking, "postmodern" society that participates in developments in the MBI culture in much the same way that Americans, Europeans, the British, New Zealanders, and now many parts of Asia, might (see Chap. 7). And the political landscape is changing too, with some of the Australian-defining characteristics described above arguably being less reflected in our foreign and domestic policies these days. Why is that relevant to a chapter on mindfulness? Our conditions are changing rapidly in this fast-paced world and mindfulness is needed more than ever to facilitate skillful and respectful ways of living.

So, for this book, the best we can offer a view from Australia is to simply and honestly offer the view that is emerging in the authors. Our paths converged in 2009 and a mutually respectful working relationship began due to shared views on teaching. This view focused on what matters in teaching participants in MBI courses, and what matters in training and supporting the next generation of mindfulness teachers here. In essence, this is an overview of Australian causes and conditions, particularly in relation to the topic of pedagogy in the MBIs.

In this way, we might capture something of the three Cs described by McCown (2013). The **Corporeality**—what is immediate, and embodied in us; the **Contingency**—responding to what is arising here, now, in this Aussie scene, while recognizing that some of it will have little to do with being in Australia; and the **Cosmopolitanism**—naming many of the ideas and processes that are arising here and globally, but not presuming to capture the whole (McCown, 2013).

Availability of MBIs for the General Population

In many Australian towns and cities now, there is MBSR and MBCT in health and community settings, mindfulness interventions in education (primary, secondary and tertiary), and mindfulness programs in corporate settings and organizations.

There are other approaches that use mindfulness, too, e.g., Mindfulness Integrated Cognitive Behaviour Therapy (Cayoun, 2011), Dialectical Behaviour Therapy (Linehan, 2014), and Acceptance and Commitment Therapy (Hayes et al., 2011), which are provided both individually and in groups. And there are therapists and counselors who combine elements of all of these models in their work with people. In this way, we are like any other country where mindfulness has proliferated rapidly.

We often have the work springing up in various settings, not because of any policy, but usually because there are individuals trained in MBIs being in the right place at the right time—an unplanned, vibrant and sometimes chaotic unfolding of its development which can make it challenging for potential participants and referrers to find and access. Unlike some places in the UK and in Europe, the MBIs have not been taken up strongly in the public health system. When offered in institutions, courses are often organized around a research focus on a grant by grant basis, with little stability for teachers or participants. In private settings, teachers can struggle to find an economically viable way to generate numbers for their courses.

In rural areas, the provision of any service (including health, education, and mindfulness courses) is yet more challenging, as is supporting the providers of those services in remote places. There is no doubt that technology has helped, but even so, there are limits in what it can overcome.

It is clear that demand is high and the uptake across all walks of life is surprising. What started as an "intervention" for the kinds of suffering arising out of a hospital population in the USA has spread rapidly, and sometimes well ahead of its evidence base. Now there are courses for ambitious corporates, stressed professionals, tired and anxious students, the physically disabled, the socially isolated, and the old and the young, with a variety of physical and mental health issues. People with a range of issues and from a variety of ethnic and socioeconomic backgrounds may find themselves in a mindfulness class meditating together. In those precious moments, all barriers dissolve and the spirit of Aussie mateship and deep democracy arrives.

Training in the MBIs

In the early days of MBIs in Australia, many of the emerging MBI teachers had some background in Buddhist practice (Tibetan Mahayana, Theravdin and Zen traditions), had attended silent meditation retreats in those traditions, had read some of the modern Western dharma teachers, such as Jack Kornfield, or were influenced by the new wave of secular Buddhist teachers emphasizing democracy and openness in practice, such as Jason Siff and Stephen Batchelor. Therapists were often delighted to find there was a way to teach others the benefits they had discovered in their own meditation practices, and were relieved that it was now accepted as a legitimate evidence-based intervention.

Many who came later began their interest as a result of reading about the MBIs in scientific journals or hearing about them in professional conferences and trainings, so their pathway into teaching mindfulness was very different.

As a result, we have all the usual issues associated with passionate and dedicated meditation practitioners taking up this work, alongside of those offering mindfulness interventions with little training or experience of the practice.

As mirrored in the authors' own training pathways, it is not uncommon for those teaching MBSR to have been heavily influenced by Buddhist teachings and practices, and the work of Jon Kabat-Zinn and his colleagues at the Centre for Mindfulness. Some have even made the pilgrimage to the CFM and undertaken training there.

Those teaching MBCT are more likely to have been exposed to this approach through the research findings emerging from the work of Teasdale, Williams, and Segal (e.g., 2002) who developed this program in mental health settings. And as they were deeply influenced by Kabat-Zinn and the CFM, the connectedness of these two interventions becomes clear. However, this vital interconnectedness may get lost over time as mindfulness interventions move more and more into mainstream scientific literature and into various health care and other settings, which have their own beliefs, policies and structures that inevitably influence how mindfulness courses are offered and evaluated.

As connections with the MBIs' origins, intentions, and Buddhist underpinnings are lost, there is risk they will become diluted, thus ineffective, and soon passed over for the next emerging fashion or fad. Holding to the emphases on both long-term personal practice, and immersion in certain training and supervision experiences, is non-negotiable.

But of course, there are already a plethora of brief workshops that promise to rapidly train health professionals in mindfulness interventions for all sorts of conditions, with little respect for the fundamental concept that we need to teach from our own deep practice with authenticity and embodiment in order to convey an appreciation of what is possible (and not). Rigorous training is also required to assist in working with the complex paradoxes that arise as we both practice and teach—a rich topic that we expand on later in this chapter.

Indigenous peoples

In trying to capture something of the mindfulness context in Australia, it is clearly a work in progress, including finding a way to offer it to our indigenous peoples so that it resonates with them and their ways of seeing and being in the world. Yet the practice of non-doing has been known intuitively by those whose ancestors have lived close to the land for many thousands of years. One term for it is "dadirri" or deep listening. Aboriginal writer, Miriam-Rose Ungunmerr-Baumann, describes dadirri as an "….inner, deep listening and quiet, still awareness. Dadirri recognizes the deep spring that is inside us. We call on it and it calls to us. This is the gift that Australia is thirsting for. It is something like what you call 'contemplation'…" (Ungunmerr-Baumann, 2012).

Living Inside Paradox: The Necessary Quandary In Teaching Mindfulness

Everything changes

You can make a fresh start with your final breath.
But what has happened has happened.
And the water you have poured into the wine cannot be drained off again.
What has happened has happened.
And the water you have poured into the wine, cannot be drained off again.
But everything changes.
You can make a fresh start with your final breath.
—Bertolt Brecht (2013)

This poem offers a deeply optimistic view, and is also grounded in the reality of the moment. If we can see and hold a paradox lightly, act within its profound constraints and still know and breathe freedom in each breath, then here is a wholesome practice—but it takes some doing and some being. Here Brecht articulates something at the heart of the MBI process, and also at the heart of some of the wisdom traditions that inspired it: the discovery that things open up and moments of freedom and spaciousness arise when something is known and accepted as *neither this nor that*. This knowing involves an ongoing process of dissolving our conceptions about how things are as we keep on looking deeply.

A paradox is a statement that apparently contradicts itself—where both elements of the contradiction might be true, and not true. In the next part of this chapter, we will look at some of the paradoxes that emerge as we consider the origins of the MBIs, and in teaching and training in these processes.

* * *

We can clearly remember (and are frequently reminded when practicing, teaching, and training and supervising others), that the seemingly simple definitions and practices of mindfulness, and the leading of an MBI curriculum, are often quite perplexing and confounding.

Mindfulness can be understood as method, a process, an outcome, a trait and a state; as a form of awareness based on "non-doing" but involving a great deal of effort and commitment; a practice of abiding in the present moment, but which also opens us up to noticing patterns and making choices about how we live; and a practice which emphasizes the training of attention in a one-pointed way (concentration) but also offers a developing awareness of all phenomena and how they are conditioned (insight).

Mindfulness interventions span two powerful paradigms. One is the Western scientific approach with its emphasis on objectivity, cost-effectiveness, generalizability, and evidence-based practice outcomes. The other is the paradigm of Buddhist psychology with its emphasis on experiential, embodied and phenomenological learning, and on values such as wholeness, integrity, ethics, wisdom and compassion. These two different paradigms translate into different values about teaching and learning which the teacher is negotiating at any moment in the class.

The Early Vision of Jon Kabat-Zinn

Stepping back a little, perhaps this demanding pedagogy also lies in Jon Kabat Zinn's original vision in constructing an eight-week program so closely expressive of the "dharma" as he experienced it. Jon Kabat-Zinn writes that for him the word "mindfulness" is a placeholder for the whole of the "dharma" (Kabat-Zinn, 2011). His vision for Mindfulness-Based Stress Reduction was laid out in an early article in which he wrote a frighteningly long sentence about the choice he made in including both concentration and mindfulness (insight) in the MBSR program:

> "This has been the approach taken within the context of Mindfulness-based Stress Reduction, in part because the flexibility of attention characteristic of mindfulness lends itself to the immediate needs of people living highly complex lives within a secular rather

than a carefully controlled monastic society, and in part because the training can be made more interesting and more accessible to large numbers of people within the mainstream of society if the "wisdom" dimension characteristic of mindfulness (the capacity to discern differences non-judgmentally and to see relationships between objects of observation in a rapidly changing field of activity; and more traditionally, the cultivation of insight into the nature of suffering, into the impermanence of all phenomena, and into the question of what it means to be a "self" and a "self-in-relationship") is included from the very beginning of their exposure to meditation training." (Kabat-Zinn, 2011)

Hence, the approaches that have emerged from this vision can therefore be complex, rich and profound. But again, all depends on the depth and strength of the teacher's own practice, insight and capacity to communicate and embody this vision. We are teaching an application and view of mindfulness that will potentially alleviate immediate stress and distress but which also opens participants to a new way of living with the growing awareness of the three marks of existence: the nature of suffering, impermanence, and non-identification with the self.

In the MBIs, these realizations have sometimes been captured by the pithy phrase:

Life sucks!
Everything changes.
Don't take it personally!

To add to the challenge, much of this can only be communicated non-didactically. It is learned by facilitating experiences and relationships in which this can be discovered by participants in their own lives over time while we hold the paradoxes gently and with curiosity.

It is interesting to note that the most quoted operational rather than defintivie view of mindfulness from Jon Kabat-Zinn, is that mindfulness involves *"paying attention, on purpose, in the present moment and non-judgementally"* (Kabat-Zinn, 1996).

For many with little training or practice, this simple, succinct and iconic definition is taken as the sum of it. Armed with this kind of summary, people feel ready to teach others mindfulness in the context of therapy, coaching and corporate training, and even in mindfulness-based eight-week courses. In this way, by not examining and coming to know the rich and deep elements of this kind of "mindfulness," so much may be left out. And if no indication is given that difficulties (often rich in learning opportunity) can arise, then the potential for a deeper knowing is lost, or worse the participant is put off, feeling that they are failing to achieve some desirable state or are failing in the practice in some way or just failing again at something that promised to be a nonjudgmentally accepting refuge.

Central in the MBI pedagogy *is* the present moment focus where immediate experience in the here and now is both the starting place and the place to return, over and over again. Loud and clear, and seemingly unparadoxically, mindfulness is understood as an invitation to pay attention, in the present moment, nonjudgmentally. This attention to the present moment is how students in the classes are encouraged to approach their experience. This attention is also what teachers are invited to embody—a sense of deep trust in the present moment, a confidence that all the resources one needs are available in just being present to what is here, now.

Yet also central in the pedagogy is the structure and length of the eight-week program, and an openness to bringing the practice into the rest of one's life during and after the program has finished. This is a program that unfolds over time, involving significant home practice, and a deepening awareness (assisted by inquiry and reflection) of body reactions, hedonic tone, interpersonal communication patterns, various mind states and ways of thinking, feeling and reacting that cause or maintain or ameliorate suffering. This challenging and ongoing immersion may allow the capacity for insight and thereby give glimpses of the possibility of freedom from suffering. This investigation into the nature of things over time is needed in order to do so. So, with this slightly confusing message, it is little wonder that participants get perplexed and irritated at times, and hence want to "spit the dummy" with the whole project (Aussie for giving up in an exasperated way!)

What might be useful here is to draw on the perspectives of two authors who described two broad traditions of practice within Buddhism: the Innateist and the Constructivist paths of awakening.

Dunne, in "Non-dual mindfulness", writes of Jon Kabat-Zinn's deliberate choice to place the Innateist perspective (found in Zen and some forms of Tibetan and Indian Buddhism) centrally into the MBSR pedagogy. In this understanding of non-dual mindfulness, there is a seamless continuity between ordinary consciousness and a liberated state. Hence sudden realization is possible within present moment experience held with a non-evaluative and non-striving attitude (Dunne, 2011).

However, we would argue that also implicit in the pedagogy is the Constructivist view outlined by Dreyfus (Dreyfus, 2011) in his article "Is mindfulness present-centered and non-judgmental?". Here he argues against the non-dual understanding of mindfulness, saying that the main point of mindfulness:

> "is not to obtain a calm and focused state, however helpful such a state may be, but to use this state to gain a deeper understanding of the changing nature of one's bodily and mental states so as to free our mind from the habits and tendencies that bind us to suffering."

This understanding is also strikingly similar to Jon Kabat-Zinn's vision of what the eight-week program can offer. It is hopefully obvious to all who have a sustained practice but perhaps it is not so clear to those who have come to mindfulness interventions more recently. For without a longer immersion in the practice, familiarity with the patterns of the mind and body that give rise to insight is not known experientially, and therefore cannot be explored effectively with participants.

Dreyfus goes on to argue that it is a simplistic definition of mindfulness which has, to some extent, dominated the research into the therapeutic value of mindfulness. Grossman and Van Dam have also articulated the danger when researchers not immersed in a longer-term practice attempt to make operational definitions which therefore do not and cannot capture the ethical, cognitive, and affective processing aspects of this practice (Grossman and Van Damm, 2011).

An attempt to summarize these ideas in the table below likewise runs the risk of oversimplification, especially as there are many different schools of Buddhism with different emphases on practice and definitions of mindfulness (and as our expertise does not lie in Buddhist scholarship).

We have also borrowed the terms Innateist (or "Sudden") and Constructivist (or "Gradual") from Ruegg (1989), and Dunne (2011).

Present-moment focus	Cultivation-over-time focus
Innateist tradition (non-dual mindfulness)	Constructivist tradition
Tibetan and Zen practice	Theravadin practice
Sudden transformation is possible	Gradual development leads to transformation over time
All qualities of awakening are present in ordinary minds	Special qualities of mind are distinctive of the awakened state
Mindfulness involves present moment awareness	Mindfulness involves remembering and recollecting past experiences and deliberately shaping future experiences, i.e., discerning between wholesome and unwholesome states and making choices
Mindfulness involves a nonjudgmental quality of mind	Mindfulness involves discerning, comparing, analyzing, and reflecting on practice experience
Emphasis on nonconceptual knowing as a prerequisite to awakening	Emphasis on use of concepts to cultivate awakening

Teachers of MBIs may come with explicit experience in one or other, or both, or neither of these traditions. But inevitably they need to deal with the implicit tensions that exist in the program between these two ways of relating to practice, and to the emergent possibilities in the eight-week course.

The pedagogy again and again asks the student to keep looking into, and living into, present sensory experience of the moment, with an open curious mind rather than foreclosing the exploration through premature judgments. It also engages students in noticing patterns of thoughts, emotions, bodily reactions, and behaviors. Thereby, they begin to become able to disengage from unskillful states and to choose to engage with more skillful actions and responses as a way of looking after one's life, and the lives of others too.

Sustained practice is central in the course, whether it is underpinned by Innateist or Constructivist ideas.

The use of working memory is also implicitly and explicitly emphasized as students are invited to hold unpleasant experiences "in mind" and "in body" while bringing attitudes of acceptance, patience, compassion, trust, openness and curiosity to them.

Active cognitive and emotional processing is involved. This work involves a deep engagement with the body and affect in terms of body awareness as a central ground of investigation (Teasdale and Chaskalson, 2011).

Language is often invited to name, explicate and understand experience. Often through language, and the dance of language and silence, new meanings and possibilities are generated within the group. In this way, we can see that these meanings and possibilities are not just discovered as bare bodily experience in the present. A conceptual framework embodied by the teacher and sometimes brought alive with explicit teaching points at salient moments is necessary to facilitate and enable this emergence.

In the classes, thoughts can be extremely useful objects of exploration—seeing into how we construct ourselves with our thinking and how different ways of thinking can both open up or limit our next experience in the moment. And we use concepts from the realms of science, literature, and poetry to open to new experience and to relinquish old perceptual frameworks which may no longer serve us. Beginning teachers can often forget this in their enthusiasm for a body-based, non-judgmental focus on "how things are," and perhaps imply that thoughts and their historical origins are not important. Participants may also be confused by the relentless inquiry into "how is that in your body?" when a bridge to understanding why this inquiry is salient has not been provided.

In summary, inherent in the unfolding eight-week program there are both views: (1) a present moment emphasis with an understanding of transformative awakening as a capacity of each person and congruent with the kind of ordinary mind that ordinary people have (the Innateist view), *and* (2) the idea that awakening requires quite a lot of practice, learning, recollecting of experience, reflection and cultivation of different qualities of mind (the Constructivist view). It seems that both ways of understanding mindfulness are implicit in the pedagogy of the MBIs, and the tension between them may explain some of the tensions or paradoxes which emerge as teaching and learning dilemmas for participants and teachers.

Working with Paradox in the Class

While the previous section and its implications are challenging enough, we also encounter a wide range of paradoxical "teaching moment" dilemmas emerging in our own experience, and when training and supervising others. Some of these are outlined in Table 10.1.

The beginning teacher is often filled with a sense of responsibility for this precious offering, and wants to "get it right" so these questions are pressing. They arise as seeming oppositions as this is one way that a human mind tries to figure things out, and work out what to do next.

The attempt to find rules for "what to do next" can become a very constricting and dull way of relating to the moment, and can close down the possibility of encouraging our participants to approach these dilemmas in an engaged way on their own.

We would like to propose that the paradox in each of these moments is exactly what is skillfully held. The holding of these dilemmas, in collaboration with the group (as best they can), causes things to open up in a way that allows old constricted patterns to dissolve, with moments of freedom then arising. It also makes the exploration of these polarities something that participants and the group and the teacher can be engaged in.

Table 10.1 As teachers, do we …

Answer questions directly and fulsomely through stories, science, etc.	Inquire into the experience present in the question
Encourage practice (as this is the heart of the learning)	Encourage people to take their own authority in approaching the practice
Allow people freedom in the group to be as they are	Contain individuals to take care of the whole group process
Encourage acceptance of present moment experience	Encourage people to bring strong intentions and willingness to explore and make effort over time
Emphasize adult education aspects of the program	Explore "therapeutic" moments/responsibilities that may arise
See this as "pure" mindfulness	See this as a form of therapy
Explore a pattern to discover insights	See this as a phenomenological unpacking of present moment experience
Emphasize non-striving	Encourage making an effort
Use research outcomes to encourage practice and involvement	Accept and be open to outcomes (even uncomfortable ones for the teacher like people not practicing and not benefitting)
Explore process	Explore individual meanings
Encourage the concentration practice	Focus on open awareness practice
Approach this as an investigative practice	Encourage generative practices (e.g., the loving-kindness practice)
Contain our own personal experience	Employ skillful self-disclosure
Respond flexibly to different groups needs speak with one's own voice as a teacher	Offer a stable curriculum

The deep pull for all of us, but especially for beginning teachers, is to step out of paradox into having something definitive and "correct" to offer.

However, the likelihood is that the teacher has trodden this path for a while, and maybe does know something helpful about the practice and the beneficial and difficult experiences that arise. We do have responsibilities to open up the practice, to bring conceptual and affective understandings to the group so that they can continue to engage in a way that feels meaningful and manageable to them.

To offer the idea that the dilemma which is arising is not to be solved, nor even resolved, but rather lived inside of, will seem perplexing and frustrating, not only for the participants but also for the beginning teacher. These paradoxes need to be worked with inside the teacher's own practice.

Daniel Seigel points to the importance of ambiguity in helping the brain literally learn something new (Seigel, 2007). He outlines the idea that ambiguity offers the brain the best opportunity to engage and learn. The value of ambiguity is deeply present in the pedagogy of the eight-week MBI courses, and we need to bring this quality into the supervision and training of teachers too.

We need to make things workable and salient at the same time. How do we hold ourselves and participants in an exploratory space that is relevant to the moment and facilitative?

We are interested in what sort of conversations in supervision (and training) are helpful to allow space for both sides of these "teaching moment" dilemmas to be known and learned from? Some of these issues include:

Mindfulness or Therapy?

A common area of exploration for the beginning teacher, clinician or non-clinician, is the difference between "pure" mindfulness and therapy.

We have found that this either/or way of framing the dilemma is perhaps false. It is complicated further because Mindfulness-based Cognitive Therapy has the word therapy in clearly in its name and in its intention for preventing relapses of depression. Yet it still holds to most of the pedagogical ground of Mindfulness-Based Stress Reduction, which is based on the premise that "people are not broken and don't need to be fixed" (Kabat-Zinn, 1996).

Furthermore, there are many different kinds of "therapy," some of which occupy very similar ground to the MBI pedagogy, with an emphasis on investigation and "non-fixing," a non-reductionist cosmopolitanism regarding meanings, an attempt at a nonhierarchical relationship, an emphasis on present moment focus, and the sharing of such values as self-responsibility, empathy, compassion and the possibilities of growth and connectedness.

So beginning teachers often struggle with the distinction between mindfulness and therapy, and they make statements like: "I didn't want to go too deep, because it is not therapy." Or "I didn't want to ask too many questions about what was going on in the relationship, as it is not therapy." Or even, "I didn't want to ask about anything in the past, because it is not therapy."

We find that this kind of uncertainty is more likely to arise when teachers and their participants are working with strong emotions and accompanying distressing patterns of thought and impulses within the practices in the course.

Perhaps, rather than get caught in ideas of "depth" or areas of exploration that are out of bounds, it might be best to get more clarity about what we *are* offering in the MBIs: a method and practice of mindfulness grounded in a theory of how human suffering and transformation of that suffering works.

We are offering a well defined method of getting to know one's own body and mind in a vivid, rich and open-ended way, that enables one to recognize, accept, investigate and non-identify with our inner experiences in ways which are potentially liberating and even "symptom reducing" (Stahl and Goldstein, 2010).

As teachers immerse themselves in their own practice in a sustained way, and bring it to the fore when they are dealing with intensities in their own life, there grows a confidence that this practice can hold strong processes. And so they need not automatically revert to other models of "therapy" to help. It also clarifies that we need not fear that we are moving into "therapy," just because the material arising for processing in the practice pertains to developmental hurts, current painful relationships, and even trauma. When anxious or depressed participants are distressed and overwhelmed, something active may need to be offered which meets the needs of the present moment with discernment, kindness, and wisdom, yet which can allow the participant to continue with the course as well.

However, all of this needs to be held in a wider awareness that some people are struggling with mental states and conditions that may be inappropriate to be worked with within an MBI class at this stage of their journey, and that referral to a qualified health professional may be the wiser action. This particular dilemma underlines the need for high quality training of MBI teachers, as well as the importance of grounding their teaching in a robust and applied personal practice. Supervision is also important in helping with the ethical and professional decisions sometimes required during an MBI course.

Present Moment Experience vs. Learning About Patterns Over Time

When a participant with a history of recurrent depression notices a lot of negative thinking has appeared during a practice, a choice point arises for the teacher. We can choose to stay with investigation of this rumination experience: how this thinking arose; what else is here; and what happened next. We can leave it there, hoping that insight spontaneously occurs, and that skillful action follows that reduces the likelihood of further suffering. This option would be working within an Innateist approach.

From a Constructivist stance though, other possible questions arise—"Is this experience familiar to you?" or "Does this kind of thinking normally lead onto low mood or depression?" or "Is there anything you have learned in the course so far that suggests another approach?"

The latter questions are attempting to draw links between experiences that have occurred over time as a way to enhance insight and to prompt skillful action.

In this inquiry, there is tension between Innateist and Constructivist approaches. Some teachers might again experience this tension between "mindfulness" and "therapy", especially if they feel they must continually emphasize or adhere to the "present moment" as some special state that we from which we cannot stray.

Each moment needs to be met with awareness so that inquiry does not become formulaic but skillfully responds to where the individual and the group are in each moment and over the course of the 8 weeks. The approach in class 1 will be different from class 6, which can look contradictory to a new teacher. But the present moment in week 6 is different from the present moment in week 1 in many ways. One of these ways is the unfolding nature of the pedagogy. When viewed through the lens of intention, offering an MBCT course to people with recurrent depression is clearly about applying the knowledge gained through paying attention to the present moment, and then using that knowledge to prevent future relapses. The way we inquire into practice in the early weeks is grounded in drawing awareness to the immediate sensory experiences in the mind and body. Later in the course, there is a way of inquiring that brings memory and recollection into the field of awareness. This memory is used to cultivate wisdom and choice that may allow a more skillful way of responding in each moment. It can be confusing if spelled out didactically to participants, so it is best to let it unfold experientially so that this rich and complex process, with its seeming contradictions and paradoxes, actually becomes a useful approach to the different conditions that people are seeking relief from. For some, this experience will also become a transformative approach to the whole of life itself.

To Move or Not to Move

A "simple" question that often arises in an MBI group from a participant is about whether to move or not in the body scan. Of course, it depends. The participant might be asking a question about what is the "proper" technique. She might be suffering from chronic pain. She might be very anxious and feeling trapped about the assumed stillness of the practice.

So this question cannot be "answered" outside the person's experience. There are some fruitful lines of inquiry here: "What happened for you? What was it like to move? Or, What was it like not to move? What did that offer you? What happened then?". There is a tension, right away in week one, about self-agency and the freedom to respond to discomfort, and the freedom inherent in cultivating equanimity in the face of unpleasant stimuli. We can begin by holding the wisdom in both sides of the paradox that is inherent in the question to move or not to move.

There is good reason to make space for both kinds of freedoms. People are encouraged to do the best they can, stay curious, and work gently with their edges. Then, even over two weeks, there can be growth in equanimity towards strong intense sensations as they dance with the paradox and don't opt too quickly for one option over another.

This dilemma belongs to the participant, not to the teacher. It is an inquiry in which we can engage the whole group—an experiment which will unfold gradually anyway throughout the eight weeks. During and after the eight weeks, this experiment is their practice; they are finding their relationship to it, and to the possibility of responding more skillfully to pain of various kinds.

Meeting What Is Here in the Practice vs. Generating Compassion

A potential tension may be emerging in the MBIs related to the recent proliferation of courses that highlight compassion-based practices as a predominant way to reduce suffering.

Of course, the bringing of kindness and compassion is radically, implicitly present in the MBIs from the first phone call and in the way practices are led, poems offered, inquiries opened up, permissions given, and in the embodiment of the teacher. So, these qualities become qualities of the approach in quite a subterranean, yet powerful, way.

Within this context of *friendliness*, there is a strong emphasis in the MBIs of meeting, accepting and investigating experience in the moment without any attempt to change it too quickly through a generative compassion practice. Much can be learned from this investigative stance, especially opening up to the reality of constant change, and the possibility of not identifying so strongly with what is arising.

In being faced with the participant's pain, confusion, or struggle, sometimes the beginning teacher can feel uncomfortable, and prematurely offer a kindness or compassion practice instead of helping the person explore what is going on and hold it as gently as possible in awareness. We have found that this urge to immediately offer compassion practices in the face of someone's distress may be arising out of the teacher's own lack of understanding and confidence in investigating their own pain and difficulties, and therefore in assisting participants to approach and explore the difficulty in the moment without attempting to fix it.

Recognizing this avoidance is important. What may be missed is powerful: the power of becoming familiar with patterns of reactivity, and an opportunity to see and open to aversive moments with more ease and confidence. And also to see into how impasses, constrictions, and difficulties arise and dissolve depending on our relationships with them.

This is not to say that a very skillful response early in an MBI might be: "And are you able to bring some friendliness to that...?" The dance between the various categories of practice is part of the learning in an MBI (concentration, open awareness, insight, investigative, generative). This dance will, of course, become the territory of exploration and choice for the participants over time. But it is important that teachers see into their own patterns of attachment and avoidance in their relationships with these practices. They need to become clear about the rationale for both investigative and generative practices and what is called for in response to a participant's distress.

Non-striving vs. Strong Intention and Goals

Both new teachers and course participants may notice an apparent contradiction between the attitudinal foundations of non-striving and acceptance, and the demanding nature of the practice and the program. Gentle acceptance of each moment can seem quite at odds with the considerable planning, changes in schedule, and sheer effort involved in taking the course. Undertaking an "evidence-based" 8-week course also implies there will be a worthwhile outcome, which again can certainly seem at odds with letting go of any goals or special states to be attained (or positive findings in research trials!).

If the teacher holds too rigidly to some kind of stance about non-striving and acceptance, then he or she may be bringing an impotence to the discussions about home practice. If the teacher holds too rigidly to some ideal of a perfect regime of practice, then certainly the issue of failing at the practice can easily become an inhibition to participating in the group and the subtleties of the participants exploring this dilemma can be lost.

The challenge for the teacher is to hold both as a playpen of exploration in the group. A useful line of inquiry can be: "What would you have to tolerate and explore, if you were going to undertake the practice regularly this week?" The answers are wonderful and wide ranging: not being able to have a glass of wine when I get home, giving up my TV program, anxiety, boredom, loneliness, the lists in my head, feeling neglectful of my children and husband, feeling indulgent. Immediately, the relevance of the program and the practice is there in the moment, in the room, and a new possibility is there to "just do it" and tolerate these (unpleasant) thoughts, emotions, and sensations in the service of discovering something new.

Some people may find that they need to "loosen up" their striving attitudes, and some may find they could do well to "firm up" and bring some valuable discipline into their practices and their lives. It will vary for individuals over time as their mindfulness practice matures and changes.

The pedagogy asks that the teacher embodies a willingness to be with his or her own intentions and with a lightness and acceptance of whatever comes up in the group, including people not practicing and not benefitting. This requires a steady, kind and non-striving embodiment to be evident in the teacher, assisted by taking their own doubts and concerns to supervision and to the cushion.

Political and Social Paradoxes

Another dilemma arises as we bring this work into the world in our different contexts—the challenge of letting go of identifying with "I, me, and mine."

The very necessary work of making the MBIs accessible and effective means engaging with the active, sometimes entrepreneurial work of promotion of oneself and/or "the product." Whether one is teaching in the private sector, applying for research funding, implementing this in the public health system or attempting to establish an MBI within the workplace, it takes some capacity to "stand firm in that which you are" (Kabir, 1993) and to neither overpromise nor underplay the benefits.

It becomes a new part of one's mindfulness practice to ensure we are acting with power, authority and integrity, all the time working to undermine the tendencies of greed, hatred, and delusion with which we all have to live. These tensions cannot be avoided, however much we might like to. Unwanted issues of competition between colleagues can arise in these contexts too.

The same theme emerges in the development of mindfulness training organizations in different (and in the same!) countries across the world. There can be a sense of competition, and issues of inclusion and exclusion as we move towards a system of certification in local communities, and also move towards more regulation in the international community around standards and accreditation. We are in the flux of negotiating a sense of connectedness and community, and also in grappling with vivid experiences of the "I, me, my" configurations that constrict us.

Again, we must come back to our practices and the wider ethical space that it opens to us. Engaging in practice and mindful dialogue with our "competitors" may also assist with wiser responses within this rather challenging terrain.

Conclusion

We believe that opening these paradoxes in the training and supervision process can help cultivate embodiment in the teacher through:

- **Honoring the "dilemma" of the various paradoxes** as something not to be resolved, but to be explored with a gentle interest as part of one's practice and development.
- This framing can immediately relieve the teacher of the right/wrong split and more space is opened to see what is helpful and facilitative in the moment. These questions are often wisdom questions and depend on a fine level of listening at the time—to oneself and to participants—to find a path or a response that is salient. And of course, there may be many possible wise and workable responses.
- **Exploring the *experience*** of the pull of each "side" for the teacher.
- This exploration can be an interesting way to open up all kinds of theoretical and personal "knowings" and "unknowings" for the teacher. Teachers can begin to get to know their meditation habits, interests and beliefs, their personal strengths and weaknesses, as well as their assumptions about what will help, arising from their current and past roles as a "helper."
- **Examining the context** of the arising of the dilemma. Context is central and involves all manner of inquiries. As described in the MBI-TAC (Crane et al., 2013), it can be helpful to consider:
  What is happening right now for this person?
  What is happening for me now as the teacher?
  Where are we in the program?
  What is happening right now in the group?
  What has already happened in this group?
- **Drawing on the experience of the supervisor** who, when needed, can be relied on to take authority and hold firm to the curriculum and the spirit of the MBI peda- gogy. This experience is important as not everything goes in an MBI. Even with the best of intentions, we are blind to our blind spots. Having our teaching experi- ences listened to and observed carefully gives us the gift of another's perspective which can help steer the teacher and his or her group into calmer, clearer waters.

Coming back to the Australian context and the wisdom of the original people of this land, there is an inspiring Aboriginal educator, Chris Sara, who has worked in rural community schools to reduce absentee rates, and increase teacher, parent, and student engagement. His method is founded on the principle of "high challenge, high affection." When suffering is great, we need to make strong demands on people along with a great deal of *authentic* care, affection, and relationship (Sara, 2013).

His approach echoes the attitude we might bring to our own mindfulness practice, to our course participants, and to the way we train mindfulness teachers of the future, with the recognition of another paradox inherent in the word "challenge." For here, there is only the challenge of surrendering to the unfolding of each moment, and the challenge of letting go of the need to urgently achieve or resolve anything at all.

References

Brecht, B. (2003). *Sometimes in Poetry and Prose*. London, England: Continuum Press.

Cayoun, B. (2011). *MiCBT: principles and practice*. Chichester, England: Wiley-Blackwell.

Crane, R. S., Eames, C., Kuyken, W., Hastings, R. P., Williams, J. M. G., Bartley, T., … Surawy C. (2013). The Bangor, Exeter & Oxford mindfulness-based interventions teaching assessment criteria (MBI-TAC). *Assessment, 20*(6), 681–688.

Dreyfus, G. (2011). Is mindfulness present-centred and non-judgmental? A discussion of the cognitive dimensions of mindfulness. *Contemporary Buddhism, 12*(1), 41–54.

Dunne, J. (2011). Toward an understanding of non-dual mindfulness. *Contemporary Buddhism, 12*(1), 71–88.

Grossman, P., Dam, V., & Nicholas, T. (2011). Mindfulness, by any other name…: trials and tribulations of sati in western psychology and science. *Contemporary Buddhism, 12*(1), 219–239.

Hayes, S. C., Strosahl, K. D., & Wilson, K. G. (2011). *Acceptance and commitment therapy: the process and practice of mindful change* (2nd ed.). New York, NY: The Guilford Press.

Kabat-Zinn, J. (1994). *Wherever you go, there you are*. New York, NY: Hyperion.

Kabat-Zinn, J. (2011). Some reflections on the origins of MBSR, skillful means, and the trouble with maps. *Contemporary Buddhism, 12*(1), 281–306.

Kabat-Zinn, J. (2009). MBSR in Mind-Body Medicine: A seven day residential training and retreat, Sydney, Australia.

Kabat-Zinn, J. (1996). Mindfulness meditation: What it is, what it isn't and it's role in Health Care and Medicine. In Y. Haruki et al. (Eds.), *Comparative psychological study on meditation*. Delft, Netherlands: Eburon.

Kabir, B. (1993). *The Kabir Book: Forty four of the ecstatic poems of Kabir* (trans: Robert, B.). Boston, MA: Beacon Press.

Linehan, M. (2014). *DBT skills training manual* (2nd ed.). New York, NY: The Guilford Press.

McCown, D. (2013). *The ethical space of mindfulness in clinical practice*. London, England: Jessica Kingsley Press.

Ruegg, D. (1989). *Buddha nature, mind and the problem of gradualism in a comparative perspective: on the transmission and reception of Buddhism in India and Tibet*. London, England: School of Oriental and African Studies, University of London.

Sara, C. (2013). *Lecture at the Mind and its Potential Conference, Sydney*.

Siegel, D. J. (2007). *The mindful brain*. New York, NY: W.W. Norton.

Stahl, B., & Goldstein, E. (2010). *The mindfulness based stress reduction workbook*. Oakland, CA: New Harbinger.

Teasdale, J. D., & Chaskalson (Kulananda), M. (2011). How does mindfulness transform suffering? II: the transformation of dukkha. *Contemporary Buddhism, 12*(1), 103–124.

Ungunmerr-Baumann, M. Interview with Miriam-Rose Ungunmerr-Bauman, Eureka Street TV. Retrieved Jan 7, 2012, from http://www.youtube.com/watch?v=k2YMnmrmBg8.

Chapter 11
Teaching in South Africa

Simon Whitesman and Linda Sara Kantor

> *Never doubt that a small group of thoughtful committed citizens*
> *can change the world; indeed, it's the only thing that ever has.*
>
> (Margaret Mead)

Introduction

The snaking lines entering polling stations all over the country, the old man being brought in a wheelbarrow to vote, black and white standing together, chatting, sharing food and water, the excitement, expectation, and relief palpable. This was the miracle of the first democratic election held in South Africa in 1994. The ushering in of a new era. A bloodless revolution.

In the year following this seismic shift at the tip of the continent, the Springbok rugby team captured the World Cup at their first attempt on home soil. The iconic image of Nelson Mandela wearing the number 6 jersey of Captain Francois Pienaar being expressed so powerfully in the Clint Eastwood's film *Invictus*. In those heady and hopeful moments, Nobel Laureate Archbishop Emeritus Desmond Tutu dubbed South Africa the "Rainbow Nation," reflecting the sentiment that so many South Africans felt, that our diverse and previously fractured country might live together peacefully in all its multicolored uniqueness.

S. Whitesman, M.B.Ch.B. (✉)
Institute for Mindfulness South Africa, Christiaan Barnard Memorial Hospital,
Longmarket Street, Cape Town, South Africa
e-mail: simonw@lantic.net

L.S. Kantor, B.A. (HONS.), M.A. Psychology
Institute for Mindfulness South Africa, University of Cape Town Graduate School of
Business, Cape Town, South Africa

Faculty of Medicine and Health Sciences, University of Stellenbosch, 503 Rapallo,
292 Beach Road, Sea Point 8005, South Africa
e-mail: lindakantor@icloud.com

© Springer International Publishing Switzerland 2016
D. McCown et al., *Resources for Teaching Mindfulness*,
DOI 10.1007/978-3-319-30100-6_11

Postapartheid South Africa however was left with deep trauma, as described by Bishop Tutu at the opening ceremony of the first hearing of the Truth and Reconciliation Commission: "We are charged to unearth the truth about our dark past; to lay the ghosts of the past so that they will not return to haunt us. And that we will thereby contribute to the healing of a traumatised and wounded people—for all of us in South Africa are wounded people" (Tutu, 1999).

We are now 20 years into this democratic dispensation. The country is in many respects unrecognizable from what it was pre-1994. The freedoms for which lives were lost and for which many suffered are visible in so many ways but the reverberations of the Apartheid system are still part of the fabric of South African life.

We are living in a dynamic time in which the country founded on one of the most innovative constitutions anywhere in the world with a dynamic media, independent judiciary and vibrant civil society still faces enormous challenges of poverty, unemployment, violent crime, and a quadruple disease burden. In pockets there is a new level of integration, yet a tremendous sense of distrust still exists. One of the tragedies of Apartheid is that it was so effective, and that cause-and-effect still blows its way through all levels of society.

The Buddha's teachings on the Four Ennobling Truths center on recognizing both the universality of suffering and its causes as well as the capacities, attitudes, and qualities that can be developed to reduce it. Mindfulness is a significant element in this response. As Kabat-Zinn describes, the application of mindfulness is not a de-contextualization of these teachings but rather a recontextualizing in a postmodern, secular context (Kabat-Zinn, 2011). This fundamental trajectory lies at the heart of the diverse application and research of mindfulness-based interventions and approaches, which to a large degree, has occurred in developed countries.

One of the goals of the community of practitioners, teachers, and researchers in South Africa is to consider this "recontextualization" within the particularities and challenges of this country. We also need to consider further how this approach may serve to address suffering that is so pervasive on the African continent. The Buddha's Teaching on the Universal Truths is both conservative and radical; conservative in that the truths are perennial for all human beings in all contexts and radical in that the tone and texture of delivery changes and adapts according to the social context in which it is being absorbed and explored in order to be most effectively received. The "African Dharma" is in its infancy, certainly in terms of its use and application in a secular context, and as such, direct experience and research is limited. We have more questions than answers.

Interestingly and coincidentally we write this chapter in a South Africa that is grieving the loss of its beloved iconic leader Nelson Mandela. Mandela's presence was tangible; his love for his people and capacity to embody true presence, curiosity, and charisma allowed the most delicate state of transition to be turned into one of hope, peace, and potentiality. As the Father of the Nation, as the embodiment of what is best and possible for all South Africans—and for people everywhere for that matter—it is compelling to read Mandela's words of insight into the significance of the contemplative practices in his own journey:

"Incidentally, you may find that the cell is an ideal place to learn to know yourself, to search realistically and regularly the process of your own mind and feelings. In judging our progress as individuals we tend to concentrate on external factors such as one's social position, influence and popularity, wealth and standard of education. These are, of course, important in measuring one's success in material matters and it is perfectly understandable if many people exert themselves mainly to achieve all these. But internal factors may be even more crucial in assessing one's development as a human being. Honesty, sincerity, simplicity, humility, pure generosity, absence of vanity, readiness to serve others—qualities which are within easy reach of every soul—are the foundation of one's spiritual life. Development in matters of this nature is inconceivable without serious introspection, without knowing yourself, your weaknesses and mistakes. At least, if for nothing else, the cell gives you the opportunity to look daily into your entire conduct, to overcome the bad and develop whatever is good in you. Regular meditation, say about 15 minutes a day before you turn in, can be very fruitful in this regard. You may find it difficult at first to pinpoint the negative features in your life, but the 10th attempt may yield rich rewards. Never forget that a saint is a sinner who keeps on trying." (Sampson, 1999)

This compassionate and wise man is pointing towards, like all wise people before him, that which is shared and commonly held amongst all human beings. In a palpable way, the qualities that Madiba (his clan name) embodied and practiced in his life are the very antidotes to apartheid, to apartness, to separation, one of the primary causes of the suffering in this country. The sense of connection is a truth that is revealed in experience with deepening levels of Presence and heartfulness. As Mandela himself discovered, mindfulness or present moment awareness, developed through practice, will bring us into an awareness of what is fundamentally shared and as such, change the way we view our differences without negating or diminishing the beauty inherent in diversity.

To extend the symbology of Archbishop Tutu's image of the rainbow nation, it is worth considering that the diverse colors are actually refracted light, that the "light" is ultimately what is common, and the very foundation of a rainbow. Mandela's character and presence and Archbishop Tutu's symbol are compellingly bound together in the motto on the South African coat of arms: *!ke e: |xarra ǁke,* "Unity in Diversity."

One of the great challenges of dealing with diversity is the *felt experience* of difference. As often happens, in order to find common ground, attempts are made to homogenize the colors of the rainbow. This process dishonors the "eachness and suchness," which makes up our colorful nation. One of the fundamental questions that can and needs to be considered is whether and how a mindfulness-based approach affects the way of being in wise and compassionate relationship to the *experience of difference*, through both recognizing "other" and realizing the universal commonality of awareness itself. In Black South African Culture, this quality is referred to as Ubuntu: *I am because you are*: A beautiful concept and ideal, which is well served by exploring the incorporation of mindfulness-based approaches into diverse cultural contexts.

South Africa represents an ideal environment for exploring the pedagogy of mindfulness in diversity, a veritable "petri dish" to investigate, innovate, and collaborate over the value and applicability of this simple, universal capacity.

Mindfulness interventions were first introduced into this turbulent, powerful and exciting environment in 1998 in the form of Mindfulness-Based Stress Reduction (MBSR), while Mindfulness-Based Cognitive Therapy (MBCT) following 5 years later. Since then, various iterations of mindfulness-based interventions (MBI's) have emerged in a variety of contexts, including disordered eating, addiction, corporate leadership development, sports, tertiary education and in prisons.

Sixteen years on, the first national conference on the science and application of mindfulness was convened, while a postgraduate university-based training for health professionals is now being offered. South Africa is still some way behind the growth curve of Europe and North America in terms of research and programme availability.

With the growth and development of the current initiatives, knowledge and information about contemporary mindfulness in South Africa (and hopefully beyond into other African countries) is likely to increase rapidly over the next 5–10 years. In this context one of the primary challenges will be to widen accessibility, adapting MBIs in a culturally sensitive manner where necessary, without losing the "integrity of the approach" (Crane et al., 2012) and doing research into uptake and effectiveness of these innovative approaches in as many domains of our society as possible.

Context and Challenges

South Africa is a country of approximately 50 million people, with 11 official languages, diverse and beautiful habitats with significant natural resources. It is currently the second largest economy in Africa after Nigeria. Over 80 % of South Africans are of Black African ancestry, while the rest of the population is made up of European, Asian, and multiracial ancestry. The postapartheid dispensation is a constitutional democracy. Enshrined in it is a Bill of Rights akin to that of the United States with the majority party in Parliament—elected on a proportional representation basis—providing leadership of the government. Free speech and a vocal media along with an independent judiciary provide some of the "checks and balances" within the political system. South Africa is one of the countries spending the largest part of its GDP on social grants and social assistance, at 3.2 % (Only Norway, Sweden, and Denmark spend more).

The country often seems to stumble between fragmentation and cohesion, yet remains a vibrant and dynamic place to live for many citizens.

However, at certain levels of society the failure to deliver a "better life for all" (words derived from the African National Congress's Freedom Charter while still a banned organization) has led to social upheaval and anger where a large number of unemployed people live below the poverty line with little hope of improvement in socioeconomic status. While somewhat controversial, the Gini coefficient—a measure of relative inequality of wealth—is extremely high in South Africa and may be one of the factors driving social unrest.

The disparity in wealth is apparent than in the healthcare system. Private sector healthcare is mainly used by middle to high-income individuals and families and is comparable at all levels to many developed nations. The public system provides either free or low cost care to the majority of citizens (approximately 80 %) who cannot afford medical aid (medical insurance), but is often understaffed and under-resourced. The government is currently working to establish National Health Insurance supported by taxation, similar to the National Health Service in the United Kingdom, in order to improve access and services for the majority of people.

Of particular relevance is that South Africa faces an unprecedented quadruple burden of disease, viz., the *HIV/AIDS epidemic, communicable diseases* (tuberculosis, diarrheal disease, and pneumonia in particular) which interact in a negative feedback loop with malnutrition and HIV, *injuries* — many of which are non-accidental and related to interpersonal violence — and *diseases of lifestyle*.

Added to this dimension is the prevalence of mental health issues, many of which are deprioritized in the face of all the other health demands the country faces. A survey by a major national Sunday newspaper (Sunday Times, 2014) revealed that one-third of the population suffered from a mental illness and 75 % of them will not receive treatment, the most frequent diagnoses being depression, anxiety, bipolar disorder, substance abuse, and schizophrenia. In this context, only 4 % of the national health budget is spent on mental health.

Of course all of these factors — inequality, poverty, social upheaval, violence, and health crises — converge and reinforce each other in a complex web of interactions making clear the enormous challenges faced both by those who are suffering and those tasked with addressing these issues, none more so than health professionals. For example, three-quarters of the doctors in the Western Cape Province working in the state sector have symptoms of burnout while one-third are depressed, this being the *most* resourced of the nine provinces (Rossouw, Seedat, Emsley, Suliman, & Hagemeister, 2013).

South Africa, thus being a mix of both first and third world, has the challenge of dealing with the issues of chronic stress in its many guises and forms. Introducing, applying, adapting, and researching mindfulness-based interventions and approaches is a daunting prospect in this context, yet at the same time rich with possibilities for making tangible impact. As the poet David Whyte (Whyte, 2007) writes in his poem "Start Close In," we can only start with the ground we know, with the "pale ground beneath our feet, our own way of starting the conversation," a turning gently towards the difficult — one of the defining features of a mindfulness-based approach — and starting with where we are, as best as we can.

Creative Adaptations of Mindfulness-Based Approaches

We present some of the initial work that is being done and adaptations being made with mindfulness-based approaches. Given that we are just entering the third wave of teacher development in this country and quality peer-reviewed research is still limited, in the first iteration of this chapter we will use vignettes that represent some of the current initiatives in working with diversity.

We approached a few practitioners doing innovative work in the South African context with the following questions:

What was the experience of introducing mindfulness into your current context?
  What were the challenges and adaptations?
What have you learned from your teaching?
What have you understood and how have you grown?

Medicine in a Primary Care Setting in a Township

Srini Govender, Family Medicine Physician, Khayelitsha Day Hospital

Khayelitsha is a township in greater Cape Town. The name is Xhosa for "New Home" and it is one of the largest and fastest growing townships in South Africa. The name captures the irony and anguish of the Apartheid past. This "new home" was a result of the forced removal of black people from whites-only areas. Blacks found themselves living on arid soil, with no facilities, far away from their places of work. Although there have been changes in infrastructure since 1994, living conditions remain difficult with over 70 % of the population living in shacks and a 50 % unemployment rate. Crime and violence are endemic. Most residents do not have running water in their homes and are food insecure.

> Srini explains: "My clinical work as a Family Physician in Khayelitsha over the past 10 years has taught me that stress is common and often overwhelming. The levels of depression, anxiety and post-traumatic stress disorder are high. A brief personal survey in 2011, of patients in our Chronic Disease Club showed that almost 40 % of them tested positive when screened for depression and anxiety. And yet we compartmentalize care by focusing exclusively on their chronic disease, ignoring the elephant in the room. We need to be able to accept that our patients often experience extremely stressful lives. The challenge is to find ways to help both patients and health workers cope."

> Srini expands on how it is working in this context: "Working in Khayelitsha is stressful for me personally. The 40 kilometer drive there can be hazardous—negotiating potholes and taxis and sometimes cows and goats. The clinic is almost always busy and chaotic. Patients can present with anything from multi-drug resistant (MDR) TB to severe anxiety or schizophrenia. I am the senior doctor. The buck stops with me. So I have to keep calm and carry on—keeping a brave front for bewildered students, burnt out staff and sometimes critically ill or desperate patients. In short I work at a Dukkha factory—the suffering is ubiquitous."

Interestingly, in this context the issue of diversity is sometimes expressed most vividly through language, compounding the challenge of working in this environment. For example, Xhosa-speaking patients do not have a word for anxiety; the closest translation is: "I'm Thinking too much," while the closest word for Depression is: "Intliziyo yam u beata khanini—my Heart is beating softly."

Srini reports that he is often aware of feeling anxious, angry, and sometimes disgusted as he encounters all the Dukkha in his daily workspace and yet has to maintain a calm exterior for the benefit of his staff and patients. He sometimes takes flight to the local beach on his motorbike, where he recently was interrupted by an armed robbery.

> "The medical students, nurses and young doctors also feel stressed and may escape into alcohol, carbohydrate and coffee binges and our stressed and anxious patients may seek the dopamine rush of a sexual flirtation—while knowing that they are HIV positive or the Soothing High of a Carbohydrate fix—knowing that they are a poorly controlled Diabetic. In Indra's net we are all connected—all addicts."

In this high stress context, Srini has been able to introduce mindfulness into a weekly meeting. The joy of these practices is in the sharing.

> "We have started a Tuesday morning Yoga and Meditation session that is open to all—Doctors, nurses, cleaners and security guards. We all love these sessions, which includes mindful movement, meditation and lots of heartfelt compassion."

Postgraduate University-Based Professional Training in Mindfulness-Based Interventions

Simon Whitesman, Programme Coordinator, Faculty of Medicine and Health Sciences, University of Stellenbosch

2012 saw the launch of the first University-based training to build medium- and long-term capacity and career paths in MBIs in South Africa, housed at the Faculty of Medicine and Health Science at the University of Stellenbosch. The vision was to develop a new generation of teachers and facilitators and mainstream the practices, ethics, and applications of mindfulness-based approaches into healthcare and beyond that into education and business. The part-time course consists of four modules structured as series of short courses of 8–10 weeks duration, combining retreats and distance learning elements within each module.

Simon describes how one of the main motivations to offer a training of this nature in South Africa was to create a center of gravity which retains an affinity and alignment with the trends in the current pedagogy of MBIs, especially in the context of the proliferation of interest in mindfulness and the associated risk of dilution of the central themes and essence of the practice. Simon explains "It is an on-going challenge to understand how we can embrace diversity which is so complex and multilayered in this country within the context of limited resources. A central thread of the curriculum is to make clear what constitutes an MBI and support students to adapt their approach to suit the context in which they work. It wouldn't work in our country to use a one-size-fits-all training approach. However, the central mantra for all aspects of curriculum development is to maintain the integrity of the approach. We want to ensure that those who complete the programme are holding culturally relevant questions and issues in their own minds and hearts when they engage in their own exploration of teaching". One of the obvious and early challenges that is arising in offering a training programme of this nature is that there is a barrier to entry for many people in terms of both the costs involved for enrolling and the minimum level of education required, in addition to practical issues like having a computer and access to the Internet. "We are looking to build capacity to not simply offer it to middle-class professionals, but also to find ways to support and fund lay counselors, for example, who are already embedded and working within previously disadvantaged communities. This requires third-party funding as well as identifying uniquely positioned people who have an aptitude for teaching and an affinity for practice."

"It is still an experimental programme and as more people move through it there will be a feedback loop that helps us modify the curriculum in a way that serves both the MBIs teacher and the community they teach. There is a perception that the word *community* refers only to poor people, and whilst there are many communities that are impoverished, there are those that have material wealth, yet are highly stressed. We should not automatically make assumptions about where and for whom MBIs will be helpful. Rather we should hold the questions: Is it effective? Is it valuable? How do we need to adapt in order to optimize uptake and receptivity? What inner work do we need to do to be open and not presume to know what others need?"

It has been inspiring to teach people to teach and to feel how motivated and excited they are. It is a practice that speaks to them deeply and affords them a way to be in service to others whilst deepening their own self-knowledge. One of the great gifts is having this canvas to create something *de novo*, to draw on all previous experience in the field around the pedagogy of mindfulness and then allow the local influences to be infused." The challenge is learning on the job and keeping it relevant to the people enrolled, and always holding in mind the various communities that are being served and are yet to be served, in a way that is both compelling and relevant. "There is a rawness in this country, an immediacy of stress, poverty, and trauma that is impossible to escape, always in your face. It is impossible to live in this society without being influenced by these realities, whether one chooses to pay attention or not. This context, and the practice of mindfulness itself, repeatedly invites me to be affected by what is happening in its rawness and intensity and to work within myself to channel that energy into the curriculum content and process. I am beginning to see that there is no separation between my experience, others' experience, the curriculum, and a wider embrace of our beautiful, haunted, and fractured society."

Mindfulness in Leadership

Linda Kantor: Teaching Executive MBA Students at the University of Cape Town Graduate School of Business

South African activist and medical doctor, Mamphela Ramphele, writes: "Leadership in the transformation process must itself be transformative; it must embody the vision, values and principles of the society we aspire to become" (Ramphele, 2008, p. 295). In a nation where weakened leadership runs the risk of diminishing the energy and spirit of the nation, the role of leaders in South Africa is considerable. Turbulent times and the complexity of a country that is both first and third world necessitate leadership that is authentic and creative, a leadership of mind, body, heart, and spirit.

The University of Cape Town Graduate School of business offers a unique Executive MBA (EMBA) programme, where Mindful Leadership is taught to students as part of their 2-year journey. Set in one of the most picturesque parts of Cape Town close to the luxurious waterfront with backdrops of both sea and mountain, the genius of the building is that this is a converted prison, a symbol to me of how a true education is one that can break us out of the prison of limited thinking. The students come from diverse cultures, all walks of life, and all forms of leadership in education, health, government, and corporate. The logo of the school "full colour thinking" is testimony to the level of innovation and diversity that is valued there. For the EMBAs, mindfulness practice is an integral part of their course, and not just an elective.

Over their 2-year journey, students are taught a range of mindfulness practices and at the same time explore and reflect on how these practices might impact on their development as leaders. Daniel Goleman describes the need for leaders to manage high levels of distraction, and of the triple focus of awareness that is necessary to become a more effective leader, namely awareness of self, of other, and of the wider context (Goleman, 2013). In this light, students spend the first year cultivating self-awareness where they are required to engage in practices on a daily basis during and in between their modules (the course is part-time). They explore and develop concentration and open awareness practices, as well as some understanding of how stress might impact their choices, decisions, and relationships. In the second year they explore mindfulness in relationship to others and the wider world, and explore nonviolent communication as a modality of increased presence and clear communication.

Although there is resistance from some individuals and often confusion as to why a programme such as an MBA is encouraging participation at all in mindfulness, over the space of 2 years "I have observed that the students are more able to drop into silence."

The following student's comment demonstrates the potential of the practice:

The practice of mindfulness has also been a great tool … what I understand is that mindfulness allows self-compassion. If you can't practice self-compassion how can you lead or manage? There would be a number of people that might disagree with the statement but I consider the statement to be my awakening. The change that I have wanted to see and experience has had to come from within. Actually I couldn't be successful in implementing anything until I realized that.

As Sauer and Kohl observe: "Leadership … is being lived differently in different cultures. Hence mindfulness may be effective under certain conditions as opposed to others. Appropriate answers to the moderating role of cultural context in the mindfulness-leadership relation remain to be specified" (Sauer & Kohl, p. 303). These cultural influences are just now being considered through more substantive qualitative research within the mindfulness component of this EMBA programme. This study promises to reveal valuable data as to how best to adapt the teaching of mindfulness to leaders in this intensive educational environment.

Mindfulness in Disadvantaged Communities

Jamie Lachman-McLaren: Founder of Clowns without Borders, South Africa, and
the Sinovuyo Caring Families programme (violence prevention and positive parenting) and the Injabulo Family Programme (for grandparents or other caregivers with
children affected by HIV/AIDS).

Clowns without Borders, South Africa is an artist-led humanitarian organization
dedicated to uplifting communities in areas of crisis through laughter and play.
These are communities that have many orphans to the HIV epidemic, as well as
abused children, abused adults and other marginalized groups. Programmes are also
run in other African countries.

The story of how mindfulness was brought into these programmes is interesting.
In the middle of a programme, the news came in that a participant's house had burnt
down and another person in the group fainted. Recognizing the high level of emotional intensity and distress, Jamie led the group in a body scan, sensing that something was needed here to contain what was happening. It was a spontaneous and
intuitive decision, which catalyzed the further integration of mindfulness-based
approaches into these community programmes.

Sinovuyo means "caring friends" and in their Sinovuyo Caring Family Programme
for violence prevention and positive parenting, mindfulness is integrated in whatever
they do. Jamie explains: "The focus is that parenting can be seen as attentiveness to
one's child." Parents are taught to spend "special time" with their child 5 minutes
every day as a mindfulness practice. They are also taught how to describe what the
child is doing while they are doing it, as a form of connecting and staying present,
for example saying to them "I see you are working very hard on your maths."

Another practice is teaching them to name their feelings while also teaching
them to explore an "awareness of what your child is feeling" practice. They do the
body scan but the emphasis is on relaxation, often used by the parents as a sleep-aid
which is supportive in this high-stress environment. They discuss the ways in which
they deal with stress and although they do not do an awareness of thought *per se*,
they do an exercise where they look at their thoughts and consider question whether
their thoughts are always real. They are trained to be more self-aware and understand how children mirror their behavior.

For example, if they complain the child is swearing, to then consider where they
are doing the same thing. They share a day on the 10-day programme around finding
acceptance with where you are. They practice an exercise where everyone names
what stress they have in their life right now and everyone who has the same stress
says "Yebo" or "ewe" (meaning "yes" in Xhosa). Then they learn a breathing space.
The comments from participants are touching around this practice, "When I listen
to my breath, I feel good in my heart"—Nonthokozo Kama.

At the end of the programme they are given a thought-on-a-thread, a black brace-
let with a red bead representing blood, land, a red rose and a reminder of the whole
experience. The programme ends with a loving-kindness practice where they use
their bracelets to think about all the others from all over the world who have these
bracelets. As a parent reported after such a programme: "My body is feeling good,

fit and energetic, even emotionally I am feeling good. I have seen the change in my children and I will remember these 2 weeks with this bead."

The Injabulo Family Programme is geared specifically for grandparents. This is a phenomenon that arose out of the HIV epidemic where grandparents are often left to be the caregivers of their orphan grandchildren. Some of the heartfelt responses from the elders capture the essence of both the immense tragedy and challenge and the poignant, rich possibilities of this simple practice:

> Every day after the workshop, I feel like … my mind and soul gets peace. I am a person who is always thinking because my husband is not working and we have these children that are not ours as well as our own children. So for me, life it's very difficult because we don't have anything to eat. So every day I feel sick. But since I started coming here, I feel young, fresh, and well. At home we started playing, giving less time to think and when I go to sleep I do the relaxation exercise. It works wonders for me.

> I have been teaching my wife to do all the exercises we did here. To tell you a secret, before coming to this workshop, she used to wake up in the middle of the night and ask me to stretch her arms. But since I taught her all the exercises we are doing here, we have been sleeping in peace at home. Also, in these 2 weeks being together, I have realized the friendship that has been created in my house. Before, my grandchildren used to not come close to me but now I see the difference. We sit together sharing what was happening in the workshop and sing all the songs together. We thank you very much for all the knowledge you gave us hoping that even when you are not around we will continue doing them.

> I used to get very angry at my children because of the abuse I'm getting from my husband but since I started attending this programme a lot has changed in my home, the problems in my home won't go away that easy but now I know how to deal with them and I don't shout at my children anymore … we play together, share what we were doing here. I feel peace in my heart. Thank you so much for coming.

> I feel strong. I can even run. My body is fine and the day before today, I went to the doctor for my blood pressure treatment. My blood pressure was normal. They didn't want to give me my medication claiming that I'm okay. The physical movement helped me a lot. Even those pains in my knees are gone. There is also a change at home. Now children are not scared of us. They come home early from playing because they know that we will start a story time. We play and sing together even with their grandfather. We are happy. Thank you.

Jamie commented, "Our participants learn that although conditions are tough, and sometimes life is difficult, it is not all terrible and that there are the 10 000 joys as well as keeping awareness of the 10 000 sorrows."

Chrysalis Academy for Youth from Historically Disadvantaged Communities

CEO Lucille Meyer

In large areas of the Western Province, and throughout the country, the disruption to social and familial cohesion is substantial with the attendant issues that arise, placing youth at great risk from addiction, illness, and a great many other social ills. The

Chrysalis Academy is a 3-month programme initiated by the Western Cape Provincial government for youths aged 18–25, created as a means to prevent crime, support social upliftment, and contribute towards the empowerment of youth to ensure they become productive citizens of the Republic of South Africa. Many participants have been marginalized and dropped out of school. Others have passed matric, but simply cannot find work or do not know how to fully utilize their limited skills and experiences. Many of them have had substance abuse problems (alcohol, dagga/marijuana, tik/methamphetamine, mandrax), often to deal with inner turmoil, while many of the females have been traumatized, often in violent ways. A large number of these youth live with relatives and not with parents. With extreme levels of violence in the community a number of them have a family member in prison, or have witnessed loved ones being subjected to extreme violence.

The programme combines discipline, structure, and inner work. Students are up at 04:30 a.m. and in bed by 21:30 p.m. "We are about unleashing potential and leadership and in order to do that the foundation is awareness," describes Lucille. The first few weeks of the programme are about personal mastery and about having a sense of inner self. Chrysalis uses a range of interventions including a 24-hour solo ritual in nature. "We are learning a lot and discovering how little we know", she comments.

Lucille describes how "different modalities work for different people and the students are allowed to choose what they want to do." Half of the group so far chooses the yoga and mindfulness module where they meet for 2.5 hour a week. Another group may choose a modality such as TRE (trauma release exercises) in which physiological tremoring is elicited to discharge the accumulated tension and energy associated with the stress response. Many of the participants have lost family members and are filled with grief, anger or are victims of abuse, and for that reason sitting practices are kept shorter, with yoga and body scanning taking center stage. They also learn to work with developing intentions for their lives.

Here is some of what the students wrote about their experience of mindful yoga:

"Yoga has changed me emotionally and spiritually. My body is feeling different and I have grown out of my zone I was in. The love I have in myself now is much more powerful than before." (Tarren).

"For the first time I connected with my body. The dark clouds fell off and there was light. I felt a bright sunny sunshine over my life. I started to know my body and to become aware of very part of it." (Veronique).

Aphiwe wrote quite a lengthy poem; this is the final stanza:

> The load was lifted off my shoulder
> When I came across one thing
> So sharp like a razor blade
> So gentle like a mother's touch
> So mature like nature itself
> So authentic like genuine healing
> You took me places that I had never been
> You took my breathe to another level
> You took me to relaxation and mindfulness

Am no longer that overloaded person anymore
I think mindfully before I do things now
Yoga and Mindfulness you brought me back to ... Life

The students are also encouraged to write letters to future participants as to why they should do Yoga and Mindfulness. This is what Siposihle from Nyanga Township said:

Being in the Yoga and mindfulness class has helped me in a big way. It actually helped me become more mindful, to do things or say them with more awareness. Being alert is the best gift you can ever have. To actually notice your body's need to stretch in a flexible way with no harm, no pain. When you come to a class, you will notice how you will actually see things in a more different way and you will also think differently. And the other thing to remember whilst being in the class is not to let your mind wander around because the class is about being in the present.

After 8 weeks of mindfulness and yoga, Vuyiwe Mgijima, one of the top students at the academy, shared this inspiration for future students:

I never knew how unwinding and powerful connecting to mother earth can be, lying in a corpse pose on the ground, eyes shut and listening to your breathing. Now I am always present and aware of my surroundings and feelings and am able to control my thoughts. Ever since I started Yoga and Mindfulness, I have become a cool, calm, and collected person. I end off my day sitting quietly on the ground and reflect on my day. I choose the emotions I want to erase, the ones I want to embrace and set myself for bedtime. The biggest shift I have made on the programme is appreciating the smallest things in life.

In the context of the degree of upheaval and trauma from which these young men and women come, these insights and expressions of healing are truly extraordinary. As Lucille says: "It is about waking up." In all of these different expressions of exploring and utilizing mindfulness-based approaches in diverse settings, clearly this is exactly what is occurring, one person and one small step (and moment) at a time.

Possibilities

We hope these vignettes have given the reader a visceral sense of the South African context and the potential that mindfulness interventions offer a society still in need of deep healing.

At present access to mindfulness-based programmes is limited both by the number of well-trained teachers and facilitators as well as lack of knowledge and information about their impact and use amongst the broader population. However, because Mindfulness-Based Interventions and Approaches are effective, low-cost, nondogmatic, and participant-centered, they offer a potentially significant impact in a country in which resources—both material and social—are low while needs are high, as we have described.

The most creative and functional way forward is to focus attention on the development of teachers who can offer such programmes within their diverse spheres of influence and expertise—health, business/leadership, education and civil society—

and so availability will develop organically. The risk is that the training programme only attracts professionals working within specific sectors, especially the private sector.

Making the course available to professionals working within disadvantaged communities—especially within the public health sector—will require partnership with local and provincial state departments to support their employees to attend or for private corporations to fund their participation. Research into the uptake and effectiveness of MBIs is one of the factors that will drive such support. This will provide an evidence-base for their integration into multiple domains of our society.

The current university-based training programme is well positioned to continue this trajectory, and will need to take into account the particular nuances of cultural diversity within the curriculum content, for example, learning to adapt the length of formal mindfulness practices and choice of language to ensure that these issues are not barriers to entry.

Thus the circular interaction of training, research, and collaboration with organizations to fund training and research, while in its relative infancy, represents a rich opportunity for expanding the development of this field in South Africa, and further afield into other African countries.

We are still looking for ways for our growing mindfulness community to be more inclusive in terms of teachers and participants from diverse backgrounds. Creativity, sensitivity, and a deep understanding of the pain and trauma left by the legacy of apartheid remain crucial components as MBI's are integrated into this country. In certain communities for example, the levels of trauma are so high that almost everyone might have traumatic memories activated or would be in an ongoing traumatic environment beset by violence and crime. Here we still need to research the value of mindfulness-based approaches.

While there is a growing Westernization amongst many levels of this society, the prevailing worldview of many Black South Africans is that identity is collective as opposed to individual. The ancestors still play a role in maintaining harmony (health, relational, social), with well-delineated rituals used to maintain connection with them. In a country where traditional healing is the modality of choice for many of its inhabitants, how do we language mindfulness practice in a way that is congruent with these mindsets? How do we honor the cosmology that believes that illness can arise from G-d or the ancestors, intrusive spirits, pollution, witchcraft, and sorcery, and where the concept of Ubuntu embraces those alive and past, and ancestors hold a powerful place?

We need to hold a respect for these beliefs while developing research models— both psychological and neurobiological—to assess the relationship between cultural influences and uptake/effectiveness of mindfulness-based interventions. As Hans and Northoff observe: "To date there have been few examinations of the intercultural differences in the psychological and neurobiological processes of mindfulness … more recent neuroimaging studies provided evidence that the activity of the cortical midline structures that are thought to be related to self-referential processing is influenced by participants cultural backgrounds." (Hans & Northoff 2008, in Sauer & Kohls, 2011).

Conclusion

The echo of Nelson Mandela's words holds us steady in the ongoing work of healing and integration in our society: "No one is born hating another person because of the colour of his skin or his background or his religion. People must learn to hate and if they can learn to hate, they can be taught to love, for love comes more naturally to the human heart than its opposite." Mandela knew clearly what contemplative neuroscience has been pointing us towards in the last decade.

He not only embodied Ubuntu; he taught millions to find that truth within themselves. It took a man like Madiba to free not just the prisoner but the jailer as well; to show that you must trust others so that they may trust you; to teach that reconciliation is not a matter of ignoring a cruel past, but a means of confronting it with inclusion, generosity and truth. He changed not only laws but also hearts.

Bishop Desmond Tutu, when asked whether Mandela was an exception to the rule, points out that the spirit of greatness he personified resides in all of us.

As we write this, South Africa prepares to celebrate the first anniversary of the death of Nelson Mandela, with the beautiful invitation to gift sixty-seven minutes of service to others in need, one minute for every year he devoted to serving the people of this country. This practice is mindfulness in action, and in South Africa perhaps the most powerful mindfulness practice is that of *karma yoga* and the embodiment of engaged citizenship.

References

Crane, R. S., Kuyken, W., Williams, J. M. G., Hastings, R. P., Cooper, L., & Fennel, M. J. V. (2012). Competence in teaching mindfulness-based courses: Concepts, development and assessment. *Mindfulness, 3*(1), 76–84. doi:10.1007/s12671-011-0073-2.

Goleman, D. (2013). *Focus: The hidden driver of excellence.* London, England: Bloomsbury.

Kabat-Zinn, J. (2011). Some reflections on the origins of MBSR, skillful means and the trouble with maps. *Contemporary Buddhism, 12*(1), 281–306.

Ramphele, M. (2008). *Laying ghosts to rest: Dilemmas of the transformation in South Africa.* Cape Town, South Africa: Tafelberg.

Rossouw, L., Seedat, S., Emsley, R. A., Suliman, S., & Hagemeister, D. (2013). The prevalence of burnout and depression in medical doctors working in the Cape Town Metropolitan Municipality community healthcare clinics and district hospitals of the Provincial Government of the Western Cape: A cross-sectional study. *South African Family Practice, 55*(6), 567–573.

Sampson, A. (1999). *Mandela the authorised biography* (p. 252). London, England: Random House.

Sauer, S., & Kohls, N. (2011). Mindfulness in leadership: Does being mindful enhance leader's business success? In S. Han & E. Poppel (Eds.), *Cultural and neural frames of cognition and communication* (pp. 287–307). Berlin, Germany: Springer.

Sunday Times (2014, July 6) *South Africa's sick state of mental health.* Leader article.

Tutu, D. (1999). *No future without forgiveness.* London, England: Rider Press.

Whyte, D. (2007). *River flow.* Washington, DC: Many Rivers Press.

Chapter 12
Teaching Mindfulness with Mindfulness of Race and Other Forms of Diversity

Rhonda V. Magee

Introduction: A Brief Conversation

At a recent retreat for mindfulness teachers in Europe, one of my fellow attendees, a man whom, if asked, we would identify as white and who spoke with a European accent, noted that I was the only "Black woman" in the group of more than 200. "I imagine you're used to that, though," he said. I nodded, and we continued on without further reflection on these apparent facts. After all, he was right: in over 10 years of experience within a variety of communities focused on practicing and teaching mindfulness, I have more often than not been one of the few, if not the only Black woman in the room. Within and across a variety of mainstream, Western mindfulness communities, people of color across the spectrum remain significantly underrepresented (Kaleem, 2012).

This brief conversation with my colleague remained a source of reflection for me for days afterward, arising both in and out of formal meditations. Obviously, he had noticed the fact of my racial difference from nearly everyone in the group. He had noted it *to me*, while talking with me alone. He had mentioned it without any reference to the meanings he held himself regarding his own race and gender, or to any meanings he might attach to these differences between us. And yet, in so doing he had implicitly acknowledged some sense of relationship around the unspoken category of his own so-called race—White—among the large group of others who so identify, even given its historically troubling associations. At the same time, he was naming or acknowledging his awareness, of some dimensions of "lived experience" of the world that are, in some ways, different from mine.

In this chapter, I will discuss some of my experience as a woman of color through the lens of mindfulness. In the first few sections, I address and counter the belief

R.V. Magee, M.A., J.D. (✉)
University of San Francisco, School of Law, 2130 Fulton Street,
San Francisco, CA 94117, USA
e-mail: rvmagee@usfca.edu

© Springer International Publishing Switzerland 2016
D. McCown et al., *Resources for Teaching Mindfulness*,
DOI 10.1007/978-3-319-30100-6_12

among some mindfulness practitioners that we should strive for "colorblindness" in our communities. I then describe some of the ways that mindfulness is inherently available to us as a means of understanding racial- and social identity-based suffering more effectively, and call upon mindfulness teachers the world over to work on being more capable of working with bias through mindfulness practice and teaching.

Why Include Talk About Race in a Book for Teachers of Mindfulness?

Some of you may be wondering why this conversation should matter to me or to any of us at all. After all, "race" is an aspect of social identity which, like other aspects of embodied existence, may be seen through the eye of mindfulness as merely illusory. Thus, one of the ways that mindfulness practitioners and many in the Buddhist community have justified avoiding mention of the topic of race is to view it as a topic for the more or less unenlightened, or, to put it more euphemistically, for those at a lesser developmental stage along "the path." In addition, even when we are willing to examine these issues from the standpoint of embodied human experience, most of us believe that while race may be an issue for some folks out there, *we* are not biased by or infused with racial feeling or thinking. We are comfortable with the belief that bias isn't much of a problem, and that the demographics of our teaching settings, even if worthy of some note, are not really relevant to our experience of them.

Indeed, most of us appear to be confident that through the practices of mindfulness, and with the development that emerges from study and embodiment of the deeper teachings of Buddhism, bias based on social identity characteristics necessarily goes away—or at least, diminishes to the point that we need not give such aberrations any attention. Many may be of the view expressed by one mindfulness teacher from the United States in a recent conversation about my work in this area: that it isn't the fact of bias that is the problem, it's the fact that we (or I) talk about bias that is the problem. Otherwise, she seemed to believe, it would not exist. In twenty-first century discourse around the world, this is not an uncommon point of view.

As I discuss more fully later, there is certainly good reason for the belief that mindfulness practice can reduce some forms of bias. Over time, we may be either less prone to judge people on the basis of characteristics that we know to be part of the illusions of the material world, or we may be more quick to notice and work against the possibility that such biases will impact others. Indeed, recent research that suggests these outcomes are real in the world is one part of my own motivation to teach and to practice mindfulness. In a world of so much division based on perceived differences in race, culture, religion, and other socially created bases for identification and ranking, I am heartened by the nascent evidence that these practices may play a verifiable role in minimizing bias and its impacts in the lives of our children and others.

Nevertheless, I strongly disagree with the notion that focusing on race indicates some lesser level of development as a mindfulness practitioner. Race and related skin-tone-based social differences, as they have been shaped in each of our societies, are facets of our embodied experience as social beings. Though in some sense illusory—"socially constructed" as the sociologists would say—this aspect of our self-identity is no less a candidate for our awareness practice than the sense we have of having a separate body in itself.

Thus, we might turn with compassion toward that part of ourselves and of others that suggests that we don't need to talk about issues of social identity in a mindfulness-based teaching setting. Such thoughts may reveal more about the willingness, or not, of the thinker to bring awareness to the part of our communities and broader environments in which such biases are not merely present but are, in fact, sources of ongoing suffering. They reveal areas in which we have gone blind to a particular kind of suffering. What's more, they may also point toward some aspect of our own woundedness about these matters (or that of our practice mates) that itself is in need of gentle awareness and the healing that such loving attending may bring. In short, both race and our reactivity to it are worthy of being brought with skillful engagement into mindfulness practice. And they are worthy of compassionate responses.

So: About Race and Mindfulness in an MBSR Teaching

As the foregoing may suggest, I did not find my colleague's straightforward reference to the largely taboo subject of race in the midst of our MBSR retreat to be at all offensive. For one thing, I had already been identified to the group as someone interested in looking at race and other forms of bias through the lens of mindfulness. I had no way of knowing for sure, but I thought that this may have been the reason my fellow teacher felt free to speak to me about this issue that we so often avoid in mixed company. For another, this fact had not escaped my own awareness. Part of my experience of being taught to think of myself as a Black woman is that such conditions are in fact common in spaces marked by any degree of economic, educational, or other privileges. The typical MBSR learning and practice community is just such a space.

Thus, rather than cause concern, I felt somehow heartened by my colleague's mentioning of this obvious social fact. He'd taken the risk of raising this issue with me, when so many others had not mentioned it at all, and I appreciated that display of vulnerability and apparent willingness to connect on a more-than-surface level. And he'd done so in a tone of voice which conveyed empathy. Suddenly, this man I didn't know seemed a bit more trustworthy than other so-called strangers in the room. For a moment, it felt as if I were no longer carrying that part of my experience—a dimension that I must deal with virtually all day and everyday—entirely alone.

What this colleague was doing was noticing, recognizing the possible significance of, and speaking aloud about aspects of our experience of the world with which we inevitably relate every day. In doing so, he was accepting that race and skin-tone-based identity constitute one dimension of experience that we all know something about. It's an aspect which shapes our relationships with others, in often (if not mostly) unacknowledged and unspoken ways. It is the dimension of experience to which I refer sometimes as "racial." And however we might define it or name it, experience has shown that this dimension of experience has worldwide significance—as indicated by the United Nations' Convention for the Elimination of Racism, Discrimination and Xenophobia and its World Conferences Against Racism (one of which I had the privilege of attending—in Durban, South Africa in September 2001). Wherever we are in the world, it inescapably communicates something about our relationship to status and to power. It plays some role in how we *relate* to one another (whether explicitly or implicitly) along those dimensions as well. For one brief moment, then, my colleague at the retreat was naming, without judgment, an aspect of the world that might have significance beyond what we could name and or discuss in our short time together. In so doing, he was demonstrating a willingness to relate not merely to me, but to the context in which we found ourselves and its possible implications.

Relationality, as Jon Kabat-Zinn and other mindfulness teachers repeatedly remind us, is the heart of mindfulness. Though our definitions of it may differ, "mindfulness" practice may make us more aware of the ways in which "we," relate to everything else. This is true in my own experience. Whether I am sitting with awareness of breath, and noticing the relationship of body to breath; whether I am sensing the relationship of embodied breathing to *that which breathes,* and from there sensing and relating to the pool of mystery in which we all sit (that which we call things like "the earth" and "the environment"), choiceless awareness practice, like all practices, raises awareness of a never-ending variety of experience. I am made more aware of the interactions between what I call "me" and what is called, well, everything else. When breathing the air that I did not create, where does my body begin and the air end? Mindfulness practice is to me, then, a constant reawakening to the reality of lived interbeing between the so-called self and other. It is a constant waking up to nonduality or oneness, even as we live essentially differentiated lives. At the same time, on the plane of our relative, social relationships, mindfulness practice is a waking up to the ways that this sense of inclusive oneness is, may, or will be interrupted, again and again on any given day by experiences that are in some ways influenced by our socially constructed notions of race and its material consequences.

Thus, for years I have practiced bringing mindfulness to awareness of relationality in all of its manifestations—including, among other sometimes relevant aspects of my social identity, my own relationship with race and color. I bring mindful awareness not only to my own experience of race and color, but also to interactions between myself and those whose identities mark them as racially Other.

So while sitting during the retreat in Europe, I became aware of the arising of thoughts about the brief conversation I had about my being the only Black woman there. I sensed again the insight that "my race," and the race of others in even such seemingly stripped-down social settings, is relevant in ways that I do not fully understand. In such moments, I take a breath and open to inquiry about these questions: Why *are* Black women so rarely seen in Western mindfulness settings? *What did it mean* that my colleague and I, two seasoned members of the Western mindfulness teaching community, could see and acknowledge facts along these lines and then go on as if there might be nothing more to see, to be with, to do or to say about it? Was it enough simply to accept this reality and sit? And if so: how do my mindfulness practices assist in the ongoing work of racial justice?

In the remainder of this chapter, I explore questions like these and call on mindfulness teachers to be open to doing so for and with themselves and members of their practice communities. I not only discuss the specific issue of bias based on race and color, but I also issue a gentle challenge to teachers of Western mindfulness to commit to the work of bringing greater awareness to the specific issue of bias based on race and color into mindfulness, MBSR and other MBIs (Mindfulness-Based Interventions) teaching and learning communities. In the limited pages available to me here, I hope to make the case for rejecting our dominant culture's usual prescriptions of blindness, numbness, and muteness around these issues, and of blandly hoping that they will somehow get better over time. Instead, I hope to inspire the more heartful path of turning gently toward the particular and unnecessary suffering caused to so many and exacerbated by the very ways that we go blind to the operation of race and racism in our own lives and in those of our fellows in the world.

I place particular emphasis on race and color for two reasons. One is the fact of common difficulty seeing the deep yet often subtle infusions of race and racial meaning in contemporary cultures, the deep meaning, and effects that have led to and continue to lead to an inordinate amount of unevenly distributed suffering. Adding to that history, if we have been willing to look, we have each been reminded in recent months and years of the continuing significance of race and cultural difference in interactions between individuals in communities across the globe. And in America, at least, a stunning number have resulted in the absolutely senseless loss of life. For this reason, a particular focus on our awareness of the issue of race and its role in our lives and communities seems not merely worthwhile but in many ways urgently necessary.

The other reason is that, although it may be difficult at times to see, race is intimately bound up with literally *all* of our most socially relevant identities, whether they be labeled "gender," "sex orientation," or some other, and vice versa. "Race is lived through class," and through gender and sexual orientation, and so on, and vice versa (Bonilla-Silva, 1997; Nguyen, 2008). These claims point to very subtle social and psychological dynamics of the sort that typically elude common understanding, but for which understanding mindfulness practices may be particularly well suited to cultivate.

My hope, then, is that each of us separately and together will commit to inquiring more deeply into the ways that race and color play out in our own lives and in the lives of others in communities and in the broader world—however subtly and less prominently than other aspects of identity it may appear, at the moment, to be. If however race seems so much less relevant than other identity issues in your own life and communities that a focus on it seems unwarranted, then perhaps you will nevertheless read on. My hope for you is that this mindful meditation on race and on how this aspect of identity intersects with all others, operating subtly on all of us in different and nuanced ways, may assist you in exploring the bringing of mindfulness more fully to bear on the full range of identities and dynamics that arise in your experience or community—whether they are seen as religion, culture, or immigration status.

As a concrete support for this often difficult but essential work, I offer a few examples of the many ways we might experience and be with what we may begin to recognize more frequently as racial experience, within ourselves and in the lives of others. My goal is to support efforts intentionally to engage mindfully with lived experiences of racism—within ourselves and in the lives of others—through mindfulness-based awareness and compassion practices.

The continuing significance of race, ethnicity, and color, of these aspects of experience to which, together, we are gently turning our attention now, has recently been chronicled by other analysts both in and out of the mindfulness community (e.g., Alexander, 2012; Coates, 2015; Raiche, 2016). It is a pervasive if unacknowledged feature of our everyday lives. This is so despite the dominant embrace in America and in many other cultures, at least at the official and formal levels (if not in each of our hearts) of the ideal of colorblindness. Colorblindness is the idea that the best way of dealing with racial and other forms of perceived social identities is to be "blind" to them. As Dr. Martin Luther King, Jr. is believed by many to have suggested in his sea changing "I Have A Dream" speech, we are to see others not by the color of the skin but "by the content of our characters." In the United States, colorblindness as a political and social norm has been furthered by the Supreme Court, which has stated that "the way to get beyond race is to get beyond race," ushering in a new level of social commitment to policies and practices of colorblindness. Since then, cognitive scientists have questioned whether blindness to such relevant social facts is possible, while sociologists have noted that colorblindness may be deployed either for or against the cause of racial justice (Chow & Knowles, 2015).

Why "Colorblindness" Is Incompatible with Mindfulness and MBI Teaching

Given the deep entrenchment of the notion of colorblindness as the best way to reflect the lack of bias toward people of color, or at least to appear as what in America is called "politically correct" around the issue, contemplative inquiry into the notion and its implications is worthwhile.

We might begin by asking; What is the actual experience of colorblindness? Does it arise as a *literal* blindness, or complete lack of perception, of race? Are we completely unaware of racially differentiated bodies or of other aspects of our social and material worlds (neighborhoods, schools, music, etc.)?

A simple reflection on our experience everyday, including the brief story with which I began this Chapter, reveals that most often it does not. While colorblindness has been endorsed by many as the best way forward in the post-Civil Rights era, each of us is reminded daily that race still matters. In America and elsewhere around the globe, we still really do see race. We actually see race and other forms of social identity differences between ourselves and others all the time.

Depending on our own very personal experiences with racial identification and meaning-making in our lives, we each generally see race whenever we encounter another. Moreover, racial (and ethnic or cultural) identification has seeped into our understanding of various geographical and institutional spaces, such that neighborhoods, schools, and even retreat centers, for example, are often racially identified, in subtle or not-so-subtle ways in our minds.

And yet, despite some similarities among us, we also often see race very differently, one from another. So it is worthwhile to turn specifically toward the often difficult questions of *how* race and other identities appear and impact us *in each of our own lives*. What do our mindfulness practices tell us about our experiences of this? How can our awareness practices help assist us in opening up conversations about these issues that go beyond mere recognition and engage with effort to make the world more inclusive and just?

Each of us will have different answers to questions such as these. For example, for those racialized or trained to think of themselves as "White," and particularly for those conditioned to inhabiting traditionally white spaces, race may very often not be noticed at all unless or until a racial other appears in an otherwise unexpected place. For a person of color, on the other hand, the lack of diversity in the room or setting may indeed have a chilling effect. As one minority participant recently shared while in a conference where I was a publicized presenter: "I came because of who I saw in the promotions." Had all of the promoted speakers been white, she went on to clearly suggest, she would not have come. Indeed, there are some who will only be persuaded to come if people of color with whom they are familiar are listed. These people are not, as the Colorblind Thesis would hold, racist themselves. Mindful awareness and compassion practices can help us see that such quiet protestors are simply calling for acknowledgment of the pain and suffering of being in extremely minoritized positions.

The *racedness* of white experience (or any experience of a majority group with historically high political and cultural power)—the *Whiteness* of it, for example—is often perceived as raceless. Indeed, cognitive social psychologists have noted that a major dimension of the experience of Whiteness is its transparency or invisibility to those sharing the experience. Hence Whiteness, and the privileges or social and institutional benefits associated with it are often difficult to see (McIntosh, 1988). The issue isn't whether or not we *intend* to be privileged or racially biased. We are examining not merely our own emotional and cognitive experience, but the systems and structures that have evolved, for centuries, to privilege and to subordinate based on race and color. It is hard to see, as white privilege theorist Peggy McIntosh says, that we are in systems, and that systems are in us (Rothman, 2014).

Therefore, the work of examining the role and implications of race in the life of a person who has been racialized as White is often particularly challenging. A great deal of compassion and patience is required to do so, and most are seldom given the space and other necessary support. As an unfortunate result, we too often take comfort in the notion that through colorblindness, through ignoring racial difference as much as possible and leaving history aside, we stand a good chance of overcoming the legacies of racism without having to do much work.

Perhaps for these reasons it seems that despite various indications that race and color still matter very much in our lives, we have generally become less willing to turn toward the problem of race-based bias and racism.

Unfortunately, we have taken the largely well-intentioned point of view of color colorblindness too far. Somehow, in our efforts not to judge one another based on color, we have interpreted this powerfully encouraging rhetoric to mean that it would be best, and certainly less racist, not to recognize race or color *at all*. Since no one wants to be judged racist or racially biased, most of us have engrained in our minds the notion that the best indicator of that position is "blindness" to race, and to other potentially "divisive" factors. Moreover, against the backdrop of a much-conditioned colorblindness, the call to address these issues leads to what sociologists have called "white fragility": a hyper-sensitivity to discussing race that can lead to extreme reactivity and distress (DiAngele, 2011).

For those working for justice in the world, including many mindfulness teachers, such conditioned ways of avoiding this issue are more troubling than might be obvious. Research has shown again and again that colorblind framing does not support effective redress of public policy issues and debates related to equality and equity — instead, such framings may actually diminish the efficacy of efforts for reform (Mazzocco, 2006).

Despite all of these downsides, if colorblindness were, in fact, humanly possible, there might not be much call for a more mindful approach to this issue. However, research within the field of neuroscience provides fairly clear indications that the brain's functioning does not permit any of us to disregard what may turn out to be relevant information by the strength of our good intentions and strong will. As such, and as most of us know from simple, everyday experience, none of us is actually blind to race or color. Given the high stakes historically associated with color-based and racial line drawing, stakes that continue to permeate our lives today, social organization could ill function without efficient means of recognizing such differences, however silently or seamlessly in our social settings. So even when we try to be colorblind, we are brain-trained to fail.

So far, our efforts to control these dynamics with good intentions and strong will alone have not been particularly successful. For example, research confirms that most of us harbor race-based and other unconscious biases. Despite Dr. King's plea, we really do judge people based on race or on the color of their skin. As we try to behave as if we don't see race, we have developed elaborate ways of seeing while not seeing. In the U.S., we may use coded language, such as "urban welfare recipient" when we mean Black or Brown (Haney Lopez, 2015). Indeed, research indicates that those who have escaped the embrace of the *explicit* biases and forms of *explicit* racism of the sort that motivates terroristic hate killings in temples and churches even in the twenty-first century nevertheless hold *implicit* biases that, in cumulative, may be even more effective in perpetuating inequality (Staats, 2014). Research confirms common disconnects between our own, explicit belief in our ability to see beyond race and to resist bias, and our unconscious or implicit mental meaning-making around race and color (Kang, 2004). We are all searching for ways of living more effectively with these basic dynamics.

Thus, even if we try to adopt a colorblind view in the world, it doesn't work because our brains don't actually work that way. Cognitive, emotional, and behavioral dissonance results from implicit and explicit efforts to comply with social norms against recognizing race and color. Despite professing to be more or less colorblind, social psychologists have found that when confronted with a racial Other, anxieties cause us to, for example, arrange seats farther apart than we might otherwise, to overanticipate disagreement and conflict, and to avoid potentially charged topics that actually lead to enhanced understanding (Goff, Steele, & Davies, 2008). Research confirms common disconnects between our own, explicit belief in our ability to see beyond race and to resist bias, and our unconscious or implicit mental meaning-making around race and color. Professing to be colorblind amidst all such evidence to the contrary has been deemed by some to be a new form of racism—colorblind racism (Bonilla-Silva, 1997).

As indicated earlier, both insight and analysis suggest that both implicit bias and suffering across all backgrounds caused by our inability to work on issues of race may actually be heightened by the societal emphasis on colorblindness, a notion that dates to the nineteenth century, and which played an important role in the civil rights movement of the mid-twentieth. When embraced by conservatives in the late twentieth century, however, it became a basis for largely shutting down effective understanding of race and awareness of its impact in all our lives.

While the ideal of colorblindness (and other efforts to minimize awareness of social differences) has widespread appeal, mindfulness counsels something else. Indeed, at its core, mindfulness is about increasing awareness of often-underappreciated aspects of our daily lives. It might be that mindfulness is a radical waking up to one of the most hidden-in-plain-sight aspects of everyday life: the racial aspect and the ways that it has been and is continually being shaped by ideas and practices rooted in the ongoing construction of race and race-based hierarchies in the world.

By the way, some of us might be heartened to know that Martin Luther King would most likely wholeheartedly agree with the idea that we must focus on race to get beyond it. After all, in the oft-misunderstood passage of his famous speech, he counseled us not to be blind to color, but instead asked that we not *evaluate people* based on our inevitable recognition of such differences. He asked not that we *not see* color, but that we "judge … not by the color of [their] skin but by the content of [their] character" (King & Washington, 2003). Indeed, there is virtually nothing in the storied work and life of Martin Luther King that would suggest that he believed that the nonrecognition of race, in all circumstances, is necessary to effectuate racial justice.

And this is a good thing given that, as indicated earlier, when we examine our behavior and the operation of our institutions, we find much evidence to suggest that not only do we all continue to see race, but that race still impacts our lives and shapes our life chances. It may be our failure to see race and its implications that is the greatest of all our contemporary blind spots.

In sum, since it is a false model of how the mind actually functions, it increases suffering across all dimensions of racial experience, and it is ineffective if not detrimental as a matter of public policy supporting equality and equity, the time has come to recognize plainly that colorblindness is not the answer. Obviously, we might benefit from a new way of dealing with these dynamics in our lives. Could it be that the practices of mindfulness might be an important part of the solution?

How and Why Mindfulness Can Help

Addressing the challenges of racism and other forms of Othering in the context of mindfulness may not be easy for any of us. We may encounter any number of obstacles and objections—from a concern that doing so departs from the noninstrumental foundations of mindfulness, to, as noted above, a claim that as we simply practice—release attachments and release a view of the self or embrace oneness—problems such as these will naturally dissolve. I want to suggest that, like other teachers over the years, I view the question of instrumentalism versus noninstrumentalism through a lens large enough to contain and indeed merge the two. What we might call instrumentalism here or elsewhere (e.g., in the invocation of a loving-kindness meditation) may be better seen as a path to the noninstrumental. It may be that the greatest gift of mindfulness to the world is its capacity to help us see these patterns in our lives and in the world more clearly, to experience our inherent interconnectedness, and from there, to assist us in acting more effectively and compassionately in response to the race and other identity-related conflicts that plague our world.

So then, what, if anything, might we do to help minimize pervasive-biased reactions and reactivity to the racially, culturally, or otherwise "different"? Through more than 10 years of engaging with law students and mindfulness practitioners seeking greater understanding of race in our daily lives, I have been working to evolve a set of practices that support not only working with differences that may arise (and sometimes painfully), but also bringing greater understanding to bear on how they operate and impact experience in the world. I call these practices ColorInsight practices.

As we all know, as a general matter, mindfulness practices assist us in becoming aware. This state of awareness encompasses the multitude of feeling tones, thoughts, sensations, and perceptions by which we know the world, and the patterns and habits by which we have become conditioned to respond to these perceptions and stimuli. Naturally then, mindfulness may assist us in becoming aware of habits and patterns associated with the phenomenon of race in our lives.

As the experience of race is embodied and connected to thoughts, sensations, perceptions of likes and dislikes and so on, mindfulness practice provides limitless opportunities for enhancing awareness not merely of racial difference, which alone may mean nothing, but of the many, various, and mostly subtle ways in which we relate to these differences. Over time and with practice, mindfulness brought to bear on this field of experience in our everyday lives can lead to insights about how these perceptions shape our own actions and those of others in ways which reflect these subtle mental and social-interactional dynamics. This awareness is what I refer to as mindfulness-based ColorInsight. Mindfulness-based ColorInsight can assist us in seeing what there is to see in the realm of race and color in our own lives, acknowledging as my colleague did how these issues impact us. This insight leads us to compassionate action. Rather than merely noting their existence, we might bring compassionate inquiry to the question of what might be done to bring about more equity, even in spaces like mindfulness teaching and learning groups and to our broader world?

Why Mindfulness Alone Is Not Enough: The Work and the Joy of Mindful Awareness of the Racially Constructed Self

While mindfulness alone may reduce bias, there is more to the problem of racism than biased minds. Systemic patterns of injustice, patterns which routinely result in the privileging of many or most over the few, call out for the application of the particular expertise of mindfulness. In preparation for such work, as individuals on this journey, and as teachers responsible for serving others in a diverse world, we have an often underappreciated set of ethical obligations to members of our practice communities. Given the destructive nature of racism, the prevalence of its legacies, and the ways that these dynamics are difficult for many to understand, we must include among our ethical obligations, the obligation to consider the ways that our larger cultural contexts both do and do not engage us in experiences that sound in race and racialization, that give us body-based, first-person knowledge of what these concepts mean. We might engage the practices of mindfulness as support for becoming more aware of the nature and imprints of what we call race and of the practices of making race—that is, of racialization—in our own lives.

At the outset, we might reflect on two important dimensions of this work. Like all serious courses of study, the work of developing greater insight into race and its meaning in our lives will require learning that is not merely first person, or based on our own experience, but is primarily often focused on third-person epistemologies or ways of knowing—from recognized authorities dispensing information about concepts and phenomena (Varela, 1991).

As just one example, consider the concept at the heart of this section of the chapter, the concept of race. I use the word race, a word familiar to most everyone, but one which carries many different and often unexamined meanings. To better understand this and other terms that will arise as we reflect on these experiences together, we would first do well to consider third-person sources of information—definitions and discussions detailing how those words are defined by scholars in the area, subject to critical thinking and constructive thinking—individual and collaborative evaluation in the process we know as learning and thinking together (Thayer-Bacon, 2000).

However, to develop mindfulness-based insight into these words, we not only hold our third-person inquiry in a space of openness to critique and learning more, but we might also deepen our understanding of these terms by the inclusion of first-person ways of knowing using mindfulness practices developed specifically for this purpose, and second-person methods of deepening understanding in engagement with others. The multifaceted and layered work of developing our knowledge in this area through first-, second-, and third-person means of knowing is what I've called ColorInsight (Magee, 2016).

There are many ways to engage mindfulness in support of the study of a range of interdisciplinary social science dimensions of ColorInsight (historical, psychological, etc.). For our purposes, it would seem that this dimension of the work may be well served by contemplative inquiry grounded in the study of some of the most important definitions and insights of the field and then committing to building on these cursory understandings through ongoing study, criticism, and mindful inquiry over time. In the next few sections of this chapter, I present some of the ways of doing so. Here I draw on my own work and that of a body of interdisciplinary scholarship to provide a basis in contemplative inquiry focused on the relevant social sciences to foster common understanding about these issues going forward.

Similarly, there are many ways to use mindfulness to develop our innate and embodied capacities for deeper understanding in this area. Thus, in a section to follow, I explore some of the particular ways that the 8-week course in MBSR provides ample opportunities to explore the development of insight into the operation of race in our own experience, within our classrooms and within the communities in which we practice.

Teaching, Learning, and Meditating on Experiences of Race, Racism, and Other Biases

Just as many of us have come to see a sort of deep freedom as one of the benefits of mindfulness, available to any of us, we might inquire into whether mindfulness may assist us in experiencing a broader sense of social justice. My own experience is that indeed it does. By establishing ourselves in awareness that racial injustice is simply a particular kind of suffering, and yet a pervasive and under-acknowledged one in our world and within mindfulness communities, we may be guided toward a way of engaging mindfully with suffering based on the issue of race and/or color, wherever it arises.

The teachings upon which mindfulness is based provide ample indication of their usefulness for inquiring deeply into suffering of all kinds, knowing the causes, and developing a path toward freedom therefrom. One might suppose that, given the prevalence both of problems and conflicts around race, and the difficulties we have in addressing them well, we might have long ago thought specifically to bring mindfulness directly and explicitly to bear on such suffering in Western mindfulness circles.

And yet, this has most often not happened. Instead, we have most often experienced the typical patterns of silence around these issues in our teaching settings.

And when the effort is made to raise these issues in mixed dharma groups, failure often results.

This does not have to be so. Indeed, there are many ways that mindfulness may be skillfully brought to bear on issues of race and racism, using practices and lessons aimed at raising awareness at the personal, interpersonal, and systemic levels.

Developing skillfulness in this area should be considered important for teachers of mindfulness, not merely because we each have blind spots and unhealed wounds around these topics that cause us unnecessary suffering, or even because our failure to do so could very well interfere with the creation of safe spaces for the support of our participants. We should consider it important to do so to the degree that we see the interconnection, the interdependent coarising of each and all. Race-based suffering affects and is affected by each of us. Assisting others in becoming aware of this fact is a natural pathway for mindfulness into the world. In this way, we stand to relieve the suffering of individuals, communities, and a world in need of the compassionate support for healing that may be the greatest gift of our work.

For example, liberation theologist and educator Paolo Freire noted the power of teaching and learning to liberate those who are oppressed in communities and larger world. Oppressions based on identities vary from region to region, from community to community, but they exist everywhere. Mindfulness-based pedagogy, encompassing both *what* we are prepared to offer as appropriate, and *how* we address these issues in our teaching sessions, can assist us in bringing about a new dimension of liberation for ourselves and, more importantly, for those whose suffering consciously includes more intense forms of harm based on identity-based Othering.

Indeed, it bears repeating: most of us have suffered some form of this kind of injury. For various reasons, our injuries may be more or less intense, and may be more or less present in our field of awareness.

For me, I am aware that my brown skin and female features will likely give rise to stereotypes of the sort that abound about Black women. For another, a woman … the stereotypes abound about Black women. For another example, for a mindfulness practitioner, a woman with features often associated with Asian heritage living in America, Sweden, or in other Western cultures, it may be the subtle insult of not being seen or taken seriously, except as an object of exotic sexual desire.

Still another mindfulness practitioner, a man racialized as White, it may be the memory of having walked unknowingly into a neighborhood racialized as Black, and being surrounded by a group of young Black men who threatened to do him harm.

And yet another mindfulness practitioner, a woman whose racial features and coloring are not immediately recognizable as falling into any one expected category or another, it may be the subtle reminder of the presumption of difference and possible Outsider status that arises with the unintentionally harmful question, "No, I mean, where are you from?"

Finally, for a mindfulness practitioner, a man given to identify as Black and as American, it may be the deep fear of violent assault, physical or psychological, that he has come to see as possible for himself or any of his loved ones any time we are stopped by a police officer, or followed by an apparently white male with a baseball bat while rollerblading in a suburban park—regardless what we may be seeking to do to make ourselves acceptable, to fit in, to make our race "go away," to be seen as human beings (e.g., Steele, 2010).

Each of these moments of experience, when considered as a single moment or series of moments, may be more or less meaningful or worthy of reflection. But depending on the context—the time, the specific location in the country, and the demographics of the communities in which routinely we live and work—one's experiences may be more or less tilted in one way, or patterned. Such patterns have effects that may be seen as cumulative. And our classrooms are not immune or necessarily protected from instances of bias, stereotyping, or other examples of what experts call "identity threats" (Steele, 2010). Even if we manage never to bring any of these dynamics in, they may well be brought in by a participant.

Mindfulness practice is about making patterns of conditioned behavior more visible, and choosing a different response division. Thus, we may develop the intention to see more clearly the signs of racial or other identity-based exclusion. To do so, we must be willing, at least to some degree, to "read our classrooms" with a view toward identifying or "sleuthing" the person who might be feeling vulnerable to a sense of not belonging, and taking steps to make that person feel more welcome and identity safe (Steele, 2010).

To become aware of the ways that we have each suffered injury around these matters is not to endorse an identity of "the victim." Especially as mindfulness teachers, we strive to be open to all. In this case, this means openness to looking at such critical incidents in our own and in others' lives as examples of a particular kind of suffering, one associated directly with racism and its close associate colorism.

Recognition is the first step in mindful inquiry, and hence the first stage on the path toward deeper insight. We recognize that suffering along these dimensions exists—whether through attachment, aversion, or ignorance, according the to traditional teachings, or perhaps due to some other cause. We accept that this is what is happening in the present moment—without reacting in judgment, without fighting with reality. When we are ready, we may investigate or inquire more deeply into the nature of our suffering around this particular issue. And we may do so without identification, without making this experience another aspect of our limited sense of who we are.

As we practice working with bias and with the goal of enhancing inclusivity, we may find ourselves taking concrete steps to make our teaching and learning environments more safe and inclusive for all of our students. Thus, and with some degree of what traditional Buddhist teachings would call the Eightfold Path, we embrace Right View, Right Intention, Right Speech, Action and Livelihood, Right Mindfulness, and Right Concentration, applied specifically to the investigations of the causes and conditions of racism as it operates in specific ways in our time. In this way, we may bring the practice of mindfulness directly to bear on the work of relieving the racial dimension of our own suffering and the suffering of others.

Humility, Sensitivity to Context, and Love as Foundational Commitments

To begin to accept that the dislocations created by race are more pervasive than we might have been given to think—and that we've all suffered in some way around these matters—requires a great deal of insight and compassion. It requires understanding that seeing that all have suffered is by no means to suggest that we have all suffered *in the same way or to the same degree.* For each of us, suffering around these issues has varied depending on a great many things. Noting the relevant, particular context is critically important to understanding how and when these factors may be contributing to suffering in our world.

Because each of us may have had very different experiences of all of this, we are often not in a good position to guess what another has seen or lived around these issues. Thus, we need skillful assistance in examining our own experience more closely; in sharing those experiences with others; and, in learning from others about their experiences around the issue of race.

As the foregoing suggests, mindfulness can be a powerful tool for raising awareness of the limitations of our own experiences, and assisting us in communicating with others to learn more. Perhaps one of the biggest impediments to effectiveness in this area is the sense that we "already know" all that we need to know, and that we have already developed the sensitivity and awareness that we need. But like all aspects of our experience, the practices required to remain in awareness may indeed be ongoing. As demographics and social norms change, we may find ourselves differently challenged today than we were 10 years ago, despite 20 years of sitting! Our task is simply to practice coming to our senses in this area as in others (Kabat Zinn, 2006), to practice knowing ourselves, in this area as in others (Santorelli, 2011). We are practicing becoming aware of the dimensions of experience that signal bias, and working to shift into openness, in each moment. In this way, we may also find our way back to our sense of uplift, to aspects of our experience with so-called Others that bring us pleasure, and to what we have in common even when we may have very much that may be said to mark us as "different" from one another. Indeed, it can lead us to experience the joy that comes from recognition and connection, joy that may arise moment to moment throughout our days, increasing our overall well-being and health.

And yet there may be even more. Arthur Zajonc suggests that the deep basis of mindful contemplative inquiry is what might best be simply called love (Zajonc, 2008). Here, love might be defined as the desire to overcome *the sense* of separation that many feel between social identity groups—a sense of separation which many practitioners of mindfulness understand to be illusory (Tillich, 1960). Indeed, the Pali word, *metta,* or loving-kindness is an essential frame for this work, resting as it does in the unconditional friendliness that is at the heart of the work of compassionate justice.

The focus on possible links between knowing, deeper understanding, and love or loving-kindness seems particularly important as we turn specifically toward the work of inquiring more deeply into the nature of race, racism, and other forms of social identity-based bias in the twentieth century. More than anything else, we must bring to these efforts a sense of love, compassion, equanimity, and openness. We must bring the will, the intention at each moment, to work toward keeping our teaching spaces, and our own hearts, as inclusive as possible. And when we falter, as we inevitably will, we practice bringing ourselves back into alignment with our goals as soon as we notice that we have lost our way.

What Are Some Specific Teacher Preparations that Support Inclusive Teaching?

Experts in teaching and learning about diversity effectively note the importance of two dimensions of the work: both *how* we teach and *what* we teach. In mindfulness, as in teaching about diversity, the "teaching" is probably best thought of as facilitating. We seek to create environments in which traditional teaching and learning takes place, and information is shared from teacher to participant, but more critically, in which insights arise among participants as trust grows, risk-taking occurs and self-reflection leads to growth. I will focus on the question of how we teach in the following section. Here, I'll discuss some framing considerations regarding how we might better prepare to facilitate these discussions by being prepared to assist in our participants' examination of key concepts that may present themselves.

As we turn to some specifics of the teaching task, a caveat is in order: we should keep in mind that we do to continually raise our own levels of knowledge about the relevant identity issues in our environment is important. And yet, we should not expect ourselves, or any particular mindfulness teacher, to become "experts" on the teaching of race and racism, whether mindfully or otherwise. Instead, we might realistically aspire to become more familiar, over time, with the core teachings of racial formation and systemic racism by studying, and being prepared to discuss as necessary, three key categories of information. What follows are a few suggested considerations and practices:

- *History as Dharma*: As teachers, it is important that we (begin or) continue our own learning about the history of racism, sexism, sex-orientation bias, cultural racism, xenophobia, or other forms of bias in our particular communities. The recorded histories of oppression against people of color and other systematically subordinated groups provide the critical information necessary for deep understanding of the nature of problems that arise today. In addition, such records are themselves sources of contemplative inquiry (Young, 2014). There are numerous resources available to assist us in this ongoing aspect of our work. For example, in the United States, such organizations as Facing History and Ourselves provide free and concise resources for self-study across a broad range of the most common identity-based challenges to justice in that country. Wherever we are, you must be willing to engage in study about the fissures and histories that live on in the experiences and cultures of those most present in your environments. Reflect on the ways such matters may be present in mixed MBI settings. What results from such reflections may vary for each of us, and in some cases may lead us to new ways of being. For example, Insight Meditation teacher Jack Kornfield has stated that as a result of such examination of our history, he made a personal commitment to always include at least one reference to the suffering caused by racism in each of his public talks.

- *Key Concepts as Scaffolding*: Psychologists and other social scientists have developed deeper understanding of the dynamics by which race and racism are made and remade each generation, and given us new language for describing them. For example, such core terms as race and racism have been redefined to emphasize the constructed nature of each (Omi & Winant, 1994). Important concepts also help those who have suffered to name their injuries and particular vulnerabilities, and begin the process of healing from them. A few of the central concepts that have been researched extensively in the last decade (a number of which have been mentioned in this Chapter) include such notions as Privilege, Structural Racism, Colorism, Microaggression, and Stereotype Threat and White Fragility. Here, too, there are numerous resources available to support more effective cognitive understanding of the dynamics of bias today (see, e.g., Adams & Bell, 2007). Becoming familiar with these and other key terms in contemporary discussion of these issues may go a long way in establishing your comfort level with discussing and working with such dynamics as they arise, as well as your trustworthiness to students from a wide variety of backgrounds.
- *Lived Experience as Essential "Text"*: Sociologists agree that a key to understanding the operation of race and other identities in our lives is reflection on the lived experience of individuals, the lived experience of race in each of our lives. This instruction is highly compatible with mindfulness. Our own first-person experiences, reflecting the very processes by which race is made and remade in every generation, in each community, and in every institution must be reflected upon and examined as we would third-person texts. And we must see the importance of learning from one another's experiences in diverse community as well.

What Are Some Specific Practices that Support the Development of "ColorInsight"?

As teachers, each of us might focus with intention on developing a greater awareness of the role of mindfulness in our lives. As the opening story indicates, doing so may be essential to creating a sense of trust among participants from an increasingly wide background, to helping promote healing, and to increasing our capacities to dealing with whatever arises in group inquiry (Godsil & Goodale, 2013; Manuel, 2015).

Doing so may be more difficult for some than for others. Each of us must decide for ourselves where we are on the spectrum of capacity and comfort with all of these dimensions of experience, and rely on our practices to support us in deepening and moving forward.

Fortunately, the classical practices of mindfulness lend themselves to the cultivation of deep awareness that would encompasses the experience, process, and practices of racialization—the processes by which we make and remake meaning around race, and processes that often lead to various forms of race-based bias, whether on the individual, interpersonal, or institutional-systemic levels.

This is not easy work. Developing deeply in this area requires a deep commitment to doing so. For the reasons we've already uncovered together, I believe that such a level of commitment should be firmly encouraged among teachers of mindfulness in the twenty-first century. As a result, such teachers may be in a good position to work on healing around race and racism for ourselves. This is a necessary first step, an important obligation of teachers who wish to create spaces in which anyone, from any background, may feel welcome and may trust that their particular suffering will be met with understanding and love.

But there is more good news. If we commit to this dimension of the work, we may also ultimately live our way into the position of being able to support guided inquiry that facilitates individuals in experiencing freedom from their own experience of racial wounds and the fears that result from racial injury—a particularly valuable gift to those of us who have suffered racial subjugation over many years and in many places over the years, through which we who have actually been victimized may experience a measure of true freedom. Perhaps more importantly, we may support those more familiar with experiences of privilege to move through the emotions that accompany reckoning with our racial history, its present-day legacies, and the transformative implications of moving toward equity—including fear and the uncertainty that naturally arises from real change.

Thus, for example, a modified "mindfulness of everyday experience" practice, such as the mindful eating exercise (the classic "raisin meditation"), may be modified and deployed as a ColorInsight practice. Instead of bringing our attention to this object that we hold in our hands and examine through the senses, we bring the same level of awareness to a close examination of this outer layer of our embodied self … . What does it feel like? To the touch? From the inside? What about bringing the sense of hearing to it: what does this top layer of the "self" sound like? We might taste it, or not … If we decide *not* to or to do so, notice what thoughts arise from your decision-making process here … . And: what about the smell of it? What do we notice when we bring our eyes to focus on it? What thoughts, judgments arise?

Alternatively, a body scan meditation might be guided in such a way as to include a reflection on the skin. Weighing on an average about 8 lb, the skin is the largest organ of the body. Why is it not more commonly included as a point of focus in the traditional body scan instructions? I think this is because of the large extent to which we have been trained to ignore the skin, to behave as if we don't notice color, as it just "doesn't matter." Bringing awareness to the skin through a body scan can be a gentle reminder of the literal fact of the particular skin we are in, and open the door to deeper reflection on its impact on our experiences of the world every day.

Following exercises such as these, we reflect gently and with compassion on what came up. An open-ended prompt for group discussion might be used, such as the following: "What did you feel, notice or think about this exercise? Was there anything that surprised you?"

When I have done this exercise alone, so much comes up! I marvel at my own golden brown skin, which to me, seems to reflect the colors of the earth and sun, together. But I recall the time when I was dressed in one of my best little black dresses at a law school faculty-sponsored social, and a senior white male law professor on my faculty pulled me in for a one-on-one disclosure: "I hope you don't take this the wrong way," he said, putting me on notice of an upcoming offensive move, "but you remind me of a beautiful, perfectly fit *horse*." Was it my brown skin or some other feature that caused him to make such a statement? I will never know.

I wish I had sense of self to turn that comment into some sort of retort about how he must have seen some gorgeous horses in his day … . But instead, it left me feeling as if I've taken a punch. It felt like a veiled attack, a microinsult (Sue et al., 2007). I left the event soon after. And even now I sometimes wonder whether in the eyes of other Whites, I seem like some sort of animal because of my particular combination of skin tone and features. And even now, I am reluctant to say yes to invitations to join with Whites in relatively un-regulated, unvetted "social" spaces.

What comes up for those racialized as White, when reflecting on a story like this, or engaging in a racial awareness practice like this? For those racialized as Asian or Yellow? As Brown? As an "Indian?" Or for those racialized in any of the various other ways that we "do" race in the contexts in which we live? Once we acknowledge with compassion that bias does exist within ourselves and in our social settings, we have the opportunity to bring mindfulness to bear on our own experiences of bias—whether against others, or against ourselves. We might pause and ask: What specific sensations in the body accompany the sense that we've been treated disrespectfully because of our social identities? What thoughts and emotions arise? And reflecting on our own prejudices, what are the specific bodily sensations, thoughts, and emotions that accompany these? Bringing mindful awareness to these conditioned responses is the first step in undoing them. Alone, such awareness is not enough to change the world. But we most certainly cannot change the world without such awareness and the insights it may bring.

What Comes Up for You?

I offer these as just two of many practices that might be brought to bear within MBSR to deepen understanding of the nature of race in our lives. Similar practices could assist us in understanding the related and intersecting roles of gender, sex orientation, and class. This chapter, then, is a call for MBI and other mindfulness teachers to examine how social identity shows up in our lives, even despite our own "enlightened" thinking about the way that we are not defined by our identities! Our own experiences as teachers can give us some sense of the potential for exercises such as these to raise awareness of race in our own lives, of its subtle, often hidden meanings—and of the not so subtle or hidden meanings and continuing significance, to ourselves and to others. We can begin also to imagine some of the ways that we might mindfully deepen our own and others' understanding of these issues.

I complete this introductory overview of ColorInsight practices with a proposed addition to the teachings on perception. Mindfulness increases our ability not merely to be aware but to know something about our level of awareness and, whatever its state, about its incompleteness. So we might consider bringing particular attention to our conditioned habits of perception (or nonseeing) around race.

Finally, we might offer what might be called a "Critical Incidents Reflection," an invitation to identify and reflect on critical incidents, or particular moments when we (or our class participants) learned something new and important (for ourselves, if not for others) about the nature of race. This practice might be deepened by use of journaling or dyads, in which pairs of participants engage in mindful speaking communication about these important issues.

For example, participants might be instructed to sit in silence and with awareness of breath for a few minutes. The instructor would invite a shift from conscious sitting to a period of Focused Personal Inquiry into the topic of race in their own lives. Then, the instructor might offer one or more of the following prompts:

- When did *you* first learn something about the meaning of race? Reflect and recall at least one early memory of an incident in which you learned something that "stuck with you" about the meaning of racial or color-based differences in life.
- What is the race that is most often associated with you? With other people in your most frequent places of work or your fields of awareness?
- What thoughts, sensations, or emotions arise in you when you are asked to reflect on your own racial experience? On that of others?
- How might mindfulness and compassion practices support the work of social justice in your community?

Using Mindful Speaking and Listening in Dyads, and Guided Large Group Inquiry to follow, participants might be lovingly and compassionately supported in engaging in the practices of mindful awareness of one another's suffering, and of bearing witness to that which has wounded and may yet be healed. In this way, they may be gently supported in opening themselves to the experience of interconnected oneness—of the mosaic of human awareness—and to the experience of transformed consciousness that may and often does result.

Conclusion

Teaching mindfulness is a great privilege, providing the opportunity to connect with the full range of human experience. With it comes the call to make ethical commitments to meet each participant in our teaching and learning communities with as much sensitivity as possible. This is where loving-kindness and compassion thrive, and where sympathetic joy may be genuinely felt and equanimity genuinely challenged. Working together at this particular growing edge is often difficult. But the call to do so is at the heart of the work of bringing mindfulness into Western societies. Ultimately, it may be the greatest gift of Western mindfulness: the ennobling work of cocreating truly inclusive spaces for teaching and learning mindfulness and the mindful way of being, again and again.

At the time of this writing, Western mindfulness spaces tend to be predominantly White. Thus, experiences like the one I described at the outset of this Chapter—of people of color being alone, one of only a few, or otherwise feeling unsupported in their efforts to mindfully grapple with race, social identity, and related suffering—may be a feature of our practice and teaching settings for some time to come. A growing number of practice settings are being created by and for people of color. And in time, the Western mindfulness community will join the worldwide Dharma community in diversity and integration. To grow in skillfulness in ways that will support this evolution, we must each make "awareness of bias" practice central to our preparation for working with others, wherever we are. American history—indeed, world history itself—has been shaped in important and ongoing measure by the concept of race and by the patterns of distributed privilege and subordination that this concept has served to prefigure, justify, and legitimize. Turning toward the suffering caused by practices of racialization and of racism is but one way to experience the challenge and the joy of our inherent interconnectedness. Working to do so more effectively may be the radical heart of the mission of the contemporary Western mindfulness teacher, a mission that will be increasingly central to the work of mindfulness in the decades to come.

Acknowledgments Special thanks to Alexander J. Johnson (Class of 2018) for invaluable research assistance and to Indhumathi for patient editorial assistance.

References

Adams, M., & Bell, L. A. (2007). *Teaching for diversity and social justice.* New York, NY: Routledge.

Alexander, M. (2012). *The new Jim Crow: Mass incarceration in the age of colorblindness.* New York, NY: The New Press.

Bonilla-Silva, E. (1997). Rethinking racism: Toward a structural interpretation. *American Sociological Review, 62*(3), 465–480.

Chow, R., & Knowles, E. (2015). Taking race off the table: Agenda setting and support for color-blind public policy. *Pers. & Soc. Psych. Bull., 42*(1), 25–39.

Coates, T. (2015). *Between the world and me.* New York, NY: Bowker Books.

DiAngele, R. (2011). White fragility. *International Journal of Critical Pedagogy, 3*(3), 54–70.

Godsil, R., & Goodale, B. (2013). *Telling our own story: The role of narrative in racial healing.* Manhattan, NY: Institute for American Values.

Goff, P., Steele, C., & Davies, P. (2008). The space between us: Stereotype threat and distance in interracial context. *Journal of Personality and Social Psychology, 94*(1), 91–107.

Haney Lopez, I. (2015). *Dog whistle politics: How coded racial appeals have reinvented racism and wrecked the middle class.* Oxford, England: Oxford University Press.

Kabat Zinn, J. (2006). *Coming to our senses: Healing ourselves and the world through mindfulness*. London, England: Piatkus.

Kaleem, J. (2012). Buddhist 'people of color sanghas,' diversity efforts address conflicts about race among meditators. *Huffington Post*.

Kang, J. (2004) Trojan horses of race. *Yale Law Journal*.

King, M. L., Jr., & Washington, J. (Eds.). (2003). *A testament of hope: The essential writings and speeches of Martin Luther King Jr*. New York, NY: HarperOne.

Magee. (2016). The way of ColorInsight: Teaching race and law effectively through mindfulness-based ColorInsight practices. *Georgetown Journal of Law & Modern Critical Race Perspectives* (forthcoming).

Manuel, E. Z. (2015). *The way of tenderness*. Somerville, MA: Wisdom.

Mazzocco, P. (2006). *The dangers of not speaking about race*. Columbus, OH: Ohio State University.

McIntosh, P. (1988). *White privilege and male privilege: A personal account of coming to see the correspondences through work in women's studies*. Wellesley, MA: Wellesley College Center for Research on Women.

Nguyen, V. T. (2008). *At home with race*. New York, NY: Modern Language Association of America.

Omi, M., & Winant, H. (1994). *Racial formation in the United States*. New York, NY: Routledge.

Raiche, C. (2016). BlackLivesMatter and Living the Boddhisatva Vow. *Harvard Divinity School Bulletin, 44*(1&2).

Rothman, J. (2014). The origins of privilege. The New Yorker.

Santorelli, S. (2011). *Know thyself*. New York, NY: Bell Tower.

Staats, C. (2014). *State of the science: Implicit bias review 2014*. Columbus, OH: Kirwan Institute.

Steele, C. (2010). *Whistling vivaldi: How stereotypes affect us and what we can do*. New York, NY: Norton.

Sue, D. W., Capodilupo, C. M., Torino, G. C., Bucceri, J. M., Holder, A. M., Nadal, K. L., Esquilin, M. (2007). Racial microaggressions in everyday life: Implications for clinical practice. *American Psychologist, 62*(4), 271–286.

Thayer-Bacon, B. (2000). *Transforming critical thinking: Constructive thinking*. New York, NY: Teachers College Press.

Tillich, P. (1960). *Love, power, and justice: Ontological analyses and ethical applications*. Oxford, England: Oxford University Press.

Varela, F. (1991). *The embodied mind*. Cambridge, MA: MIT Press.

Young, E. (2014). *History as dharma: A contemplative practice model for teaching the middle east and Africa in contemplative learning and inquiry across the disciplines*. Westfield, MA: Westfield State University.

Zajonc, A. (2008). *Meditation as contemplative inquiry: When knowing becomes love*. Barrington, MA: Lindisfarne Books.

Part III
Teaching MBI Curricula to Everyone: Special Populations

Chapter 13
Teaching Inner City in Populations in the USA

Beth Robins Roth

Introduction and Overview

We are all tender, we are all brilliant, we all hunger for kindness.

Gregory Kramer (2007, p. 7)

In 1993, I founded the Stress Reduction Program (SRP) at The Community Health Center in Meriden, CT (CHC-Meriden). CHC-Meriden is part of The Community Health Center, Inc., a not-for-profit health care agency founded in 1972, that provides medical, mental health, prenatal, dental, substance abuse recovery, HIV care, school-based services, health care for the homeless, and community support services to medically underserved populations at sites throughout Connecticut.

The Stress Reduction Program (SRP) at CHC-Meriden is modeled on the MBSR program founded by Jon Kabat-Zinn, Ph.D., and has the same philosophy, structure, and format as the UMASS MBSR program. However, I have adapted the curriculum in a variety of ways for the CHC-Meriden population. The history, philosophy, and curriculum of this program have been previously described (Roth, 1994, 1997; Roth & Calle-Mesa, 2006) and research findings have been published (Roth & Creaser, 1997; Roth & Robbins, 2004; Roth & Stanley, 2002).

The CHC-Meriden SRP is a group intervention taught in either English or Spanish to adult patients. Groups are heterogeneous for medical and mental health diagnoses. Participants meet for a two-hour class once a week for eight consecutive weeks. The SRP does not include a Day of Mindfulness or extended weekend session. There are no individual meetings with patients prior to their enrollment in

---

B.R. Roth, A.P.R.N., S.E.P. (✉)
Hummingbird Trauma Resolution, L.L.C.
e-mail: bethroth@snet.net

© Springer International Publishing Switzerland 2016
D. McCown et al., *Resources for Teaching Mindfulness*,
DOI 10.1007/978-3-319-30100-6_13

the SRP. I rely on the medical record, and consultation with the patient's medical and/or mental health provider, to obtain information about SRP participants.

There is no set fee for participation in the SRP. As a Family Nurse Practitioner (FNP) and Advanced Practice Registered Nurse (APRN), I am a credentialed CHC Medical Provider. Therefore, each SRP class session a patient attends is a medical encounter. Using the patient's medical diagnosis code and a CPT code for "Health Behavior Assessment and Intervention" group intervention visit, CHC bills public and private health insurance companies, and accepts each insurance company's reimbursement rate for the visit. Patients who do not have medical insurance pay a sliding scale fee per session, based on their monthly income. I established a SRP scholarship fund to assist uninsured patients with the self-pay fee. Every attempt is made to ensure that no one is turned away for financial reasons.

Each weekly SRP session contains mindfulness meditation instruction and practice; didactic information related to health, illness, stress, and the mind–body relationship; group dialogue and inquiry; and discussion of the relevance of mindfulness to stress, pain, illness, and the quality of each moment of one's life. The mindfulness practices taught are the same as those of the UMASS MBSR program: breathing meditation, the body scan, gentle stretching (hatha yoga) done lying down and standing, eating meditation, and walking meditation. Daily home meditation practice is continuously encouraged and audio CDs are provided in English or Spanish. The first CD has 15- and 30-minute sessions of guided breathing meditation. The second CD has a 30-minute body scan and 30 minutes of gentle stretching done lying down.

The philosophy of the CHC-Meriden SRP is consistent with the original UMASS MBSR program. It rests on the premise that regardless of an individual's personal and family history, medical illness, or mental health disorder, there is more that is right and healthy with the person than what may be "wrong" or not well. The mindfulness practices, class activities, and group discussions are designed to help participants identify and nourish their internal resources to promote their health and well-being.

Mindfulness is explored conceptually and experientially throughout the SRP. I use a practical definition of mindfulness that emphasizes nonjudgmental, present moment awareness. This is consistent with definitions offered by Jon Kabat-Zinn (Kabat-Zinn, 1990, 2005) and employed by many teachers of MBIs (McCown, Reibel, & Micozzi, 2017). I introduce mindfulness in the first class and offer a definition.

Patients' level of interest in the SRP, combined with obstacles to class attendance, causes attrition during the early weeks of the program. The most common obstacles are conflicts with patients' or family members' other commitments, including medical, mental health, legal, and social service appointments; lack of child care or transportation; and the debilitating fatigue and associated low motivation engendered by chronic despair of health improvement. These factors contribute to fluctuating attendance and class composition during the first few weeks. I have learned to be flexible in my expectations and spontaneous in making on-the-spot decisions about what components of the curriculum to repeat, review, introduce, or postpone in each of the first weeks of the SRP, depending on which patients show up. Usually by the third week the SRP group is established, and the welcome shift toward greater comfort, trust, interpersonal resonance, and group cohesion occurs.

The educational background of the CHC-Meriden patient population varies from a third or fourth grade education to a university degree. Due to the wide range of literacy competency among SRP participants, I use few written materials. There are class discussions that include making written lists of participants' ideas, and activities that involve drawings (See Chap. 28).

I have not observed a relationship between SRP participants' formal education and their ability to readily grasp and utilize the concepts and practices of mindfulness. I emphasize the value of natural intelligence over educational achievement for the acquisition of mindfulness skills. Patients with little schooling have often internalized false and belittling beliefs about their intelligence and capabilities. I express unequivocal confidence that all SRP participants possess the innate intelligence to cultivate mindfulness and develop their inner resources, thereby actively engaging in their healing. Among the many joys of teaching the SRP is witnessing the growth of participants' dignity and self-worth as they are disabused, through their direct experience, of false and limiting self-concepts.

The SRP groups that I teach in Spanish are comprised of participants from the Caribbean, Mexico, and Central and South America. Some are functionally illiterate while others have a university degree, and some have taught at the university level in their native country. Although there are differences in pronunciation, vocabulary, and grammar among Spanish speakers of different nationalities and educational backgrounds, common ground is easily found. With the publication of "Vivir Con Plenitud Las Crisis" (Kabat-Zinn, 2004), the Spanish translation of Jon Kabat-Zinn's book "Full Catastrophe Living," the Spanish equivalent of MBSR terms have become more standardized. I use "la atención plena" for "mindfulness," and "estiramientos suaves" for the hatha yoga gentle stretching. With the Spanish-speaking SRP participants I experiment to find best translations of other key terms such as presence, body scan, embodiment, and loving-kindness. The SRP instructor, whether a native or non-native Spanish speaker, must possess exceptional Spanish language skills, as well as the commitment to learn whatever new vocabulary, grammar, and conceptual expression is needed to effectively teach in Spanish.

The majority of SRP participants have multiple medical and mental health diagnoses. Common medical problems include diabetes, hypertension, asthma, migraine and tension headaches, obesity, digestive disorders, chronic kidney disease, substance abuse, and chronic physical pain. The most common mental health conditions are depression, anxiety, panic attacks, insomnia, bipolar disorder, and post-traumatic stress disorder (PTSD).

Unresolved Trauma and PTSD: Teaching MBSR from a Somatic Experiencing Perspective

Most of the patients diagnosed with PTSD have survived some form of childhood abuse, and/or have experienced a shock trauma, such as a severe motor vehicle accident, war combat, or adult sexual or physical assault. However, as is made clear from the clinical literature on Somatic Experiencing, many people who do not have a diagnosis of PTSD have experienced significant trauma and are suffering from its debilitating effects. Due to unresolved trauma, many CHC-Meriden SRP patients are unable to engage with or benefit from mindfulness practices. This observation has resulted in my modifying the process and content of the CHC-Meriden SRP. It is noteworthy that Jack Kornfield, Ph.D., a renowned meditation teacher, clinical psychologist and author, requires his Vipassana teacher trainees to have one year of professional training in Somatic Experiencing.

Somatic Experiencing (SE), developed by Peter Levine, Ph.D., recognizes that trauma may result from any experience perceived by the individual as life threatening, and that occurs under circumstances of helplessness. Framed in this way, trauma is understood to be much larger than childhood abuse and shock trauma. Many ordinary experiences are traumatic for some of the people who experience them (Levine, 1997; Scaer, 2014). Examples include medical surgery, dental procedures, falls, minor motor vehicle accidents, incarceration, death of a loved one, serious illness, chronic physical pain, natural disasters, fires, birth trauma, chronic psychosocial stress (marital, parenting, job related), and witnessing violence or death. Members of minority groups may be at higher risk for trauma and PTSD as a result of experiencing prejudice, discrimination, and harassment (Ford, 2008; Ponds, 2013). Trauma and PTSD may also result from what has been termed "microaggressions" commonly endured by members of minority groups (Schoulte, Schultz, & Atmaier, 2011). Low socioeconomic status is associated with increased vulnerability to PTSD following a potentially traumatic event (DiGangi et al., 2013; Ozer, Best, Lipsey, & Weiss, 2008; Ruglass, 2014).

From the SE perspective, PTSD is primarily the result of physiologic injury to the autonomic nervous system that, over time, can cause a variety of psychological problems and medical illnesses (Scaer, 2014). In response to a traumatic event, the instinctual Fight-or-Flight Response produces vast amounts of neurochemical and hormonal energy designed to enable the organism to physically overpower or successfully flee the threat. When it is not possible to fight or escape, or when attempts to fight or flee fail, human beings engage the physiologic response of last resort: freeze immobility (Levine, 1997). If the massive physical energy of the freeze response is not released from the body when the person survives the threatening event, the autonomic nervous system sustains physiologic damage that negatively impacts an individual's physical and mental health, personal relationships, and ability to engage effectively with life (Levine, 1997; Ogden et al., 2006; Scaer, 2005; Van der Kolk, 2014).

The hallmark PTSD symptoms of heightened arousal, hypervigilance, flashbacks, nightmares, and avoidance of stimuli reminiscent of the trauma may appear. Anxiety, panic attacks, insomnia, depression, chronic physical pain, and a variety of medical ailments may develop (Scaer, 2014). SE trauma resolution facilitates the gradual release of the bound energy from the body in ways that are manageable and fully conscious, based on somatic mindfulness coupled with awareness of present moment thought, emotion, and meaning (Levine, 2010; Payne, Levine, & Crane-Godreaun, 2015). A thorough discussion of SE is beyond the scope of this chapter, and can be found in resources listed in the references (Levine, 1997, 2008, 2010; Levine & Phillips, 2012; Payne, Levine, & Crane-Godreaun, 2015). The SE approach to understanding and healing trauma and chronic stress is very compatible with MBIs, allowing for a natural integration of SE didactic information and somatic awareness exercises into the SRP.

The Person of the Teacher

This intimate dance between healer and client is the essence of the therapeutic relationship...this dance is intimate in the most nonphysical but existentially most meaningful ways we can be as human beings together on the planet.

Daniel Siegel (2010, p. 246)

It is difficult to convey in words the essence of the "person aspect" of the SRP instructor. I am certain that presence and love are important characteristics. Daniel Siegel (2010, p. 245) describes a "professional form of love" that is distinct from romantic love and respectful of professional boundaries. This description feels resonant, and is compatible with the characteristics of friendship, authority, and authenticity attributed to the effective MBI instructor by McCown et al. (2017). As a SRP instructor I consider myself an artist engaged in a vital art form: meeting others' full and imperfect humanity with my own, for the explicit purpose of growth and healing.

There is general agreement among MBI instructors and researchers that the person of the teacher is essential to every mindfulness-based intervention. The instructor's very being, separate from her knowledge base, skill set, and professional experience, is important for the effectiveness of the MBI (McCown et al., 2017). The totality of my education, training, and work experience, along with my life experience, enable me to teach the SRP at CHC-Meriden. SRP participants arrive with assumptions about me as the instructor, and about the professional distance that will exist between us, a distance to which they are accustomed and to which they have learned to acquiesce. It is in our roles as patients and health care professional that SRP participants and I come together. These roles are both respected and transcended by the "face-to-face and soul-to-soul contact" (Levine, 2010, p. 108) of authentic human relationship intrinsic to the SRP.

When I introduce myself to participants in the first SRP session, I share that I have been practicing for decades the same mindfulness meditation techniques that I teach in the SRP. I add that I came to these practices for the same reason that participants enter the SRP: to decrease stress and suffering. I bring to this work my own life experience: the joys, sorrows, successes, and failures, great and small. I have an unshakable confidence in the healing power of mindfulness, and a resolute faith in the capacity of every human being to engage with mindfulness in the service of their healing. These beliefs form the foundation upon which I meet participants and together create the SRP experience.

The Skills of the Teacher

Stewardship of the Group

The greatest gift that a guide can offer to participants is the opportunity to listen to themselves and each other. And when they really do that, so much caring and wisdom emerge that the participants become each other's teachers.

Joanna Macy and Molly Young Brown (1998, p. 73)

Just as a knowledgeable guide facilitates travel to an unfamiliar country, the MBSR instructor facilitates each participant's journey into their own inner territory. Poet Deena Metzger writes, "The inner world is always, by its very nature, every moment, for one's entire life, new territory" (1992, p. 6). And while a guide must know the map of the terrain, the map is not the territory. My knowledge of MBSR history, philosophy, and curricula are my maps. These maps are rich and reliable, and serve me well. Yet it is my meditation practice, silent retreat experience, personal history, experience teaching mindfulness, and connection to the people I teach, that enable me to guide individual participants, and the group as a whole, along our shared SRP journey.

The moment-to-moment flow of SRP group work is dynamic and ever changing. The instructor's stewardship skills support this flow, allowing the participants' innate wisdom and compassion to unselfconsciously come forth as they truly become one another's teachers. The non-pathologizing focus of the SRP sustains this process, as it is based on creative exploration of human health and well-being. I make this focus explicit in the first session of the SRP. With the chairs prearranged in a circle, I welcome participants as they arrive. I ask everyone to please sign in, make a name tag, and take any available seat. I introduce myself and give a brief overview of the SRP philosophy, the rationale of the CHC-Meriden SRP, and the curriculum, including the importance of home meditation practice. Years ago, I asked participants to introduce themselves, and perhaps say something about their reason for attending the SRP. I learned that this way of doing introductions was rigid, time consuming, and inherently flawed. Many SRP participants live with significant social anxiety. They are uncomfortable in a room with other people, and their discomfort is exacerbated if the chairs are placed too close together or if the classroom door is closed. Participants often enter the SRP feeling isolated, alone, and uncertain of how to interact with others. Some are prone to share excessive detail about their personal difficulties and health problems, while others are quiet and withdrawn. Few participants are able to sustain attention for the duration of multiple individual introductions. These introductions emphasize personal problems and illness rather than the universal aspect of human suffering, and rarely bring forth mindfulness or touch into the uniquely non-pathologizing focus of the SRP. Therefore, I developed a different way of managing introductions.

I used to ask everyone to introduce themselves at this point in the first class. I learned that almost every person in every class shared two things in common. So I thought it might be possible for me to introduce all of you to one another. I'm going to give it a try. Please let me know what you think.

I pause to scan the group, and then continue.

I believe that each person here is experiencing some kind of personal stress, family problem, medical illness, or physical pain. Am I right so far? I say this because I've never met anyone, myself included, who does not have any problem, difficulty, illness or pain.

Participants are starting to nod their heads and there is greater stillness in the room.

Since each of you has walked through the door to the Stress Reduction Program, I believe that everyone here has a desire to feel better and enjoy life more. I trust it is this beautiful human desire to move towards greater health and happiness that brought you here today. Is that right?

Attention is riveted on my face and my words. In naming aloud these universal characteristics of the human condition, and claiming them as our own, we feel the power that accompanies every profound truth. This particular truth establishes the tone of the SRP, and sets the precedent for honesty and open interaction within the group. There is a shift in the room. Everyone seems more present and more real. I see pain, hope, smiles, and tears on the faces of participants.

After pausing to allow this to settle, I explain other important aspects of the SRP.

I want to clarify that I am not a therapist and this is not group therapy. I am a Nurse Practitioner. The SRP is an educational program. Coming to this program is like attending a course at a community center or college. We are here to learn how to become healthier, and we practice specific techniques that can help us. When we speak in this class, it's for the purpose of sharing our experiences with the mindfulness practices we are learning, and talking about how mindfulness is relevant to everyday life situations. It can be very useful to talk about one's childhood, personal problems and illnesses, and there are places to do this. If anyone would like to find a therapist to help in these ways, please let me know and I can direct you to an appropriate person or service.

Another aspect of my stewardship role is establishing an environment of *relative* safety, defined as "an atmosphere that conveys refuge, hope and possibility" (Levine, 2010, p. 75). Chronic stress and unresolved trauma alter brain structure and function in a variety of ways (Scaer, 2005; Van der Kolk, 2014). Thus, it is difficult for many SRP participants to correctly perceive safety, and their altered physiology may cause them to sense danger and threat where none exist. I attend to details of the physical environment, and to verbal and nonverbal interpersonal interactions, with the intention of creating a strong sense of safety for all. This involves monitoring signals from within myself, as well as from participants, and intervening to restore safety as needed. I try to maintain a relaxed manner, use kind and gentle speech, demonstrate interest and acceptance of group members, and facilitate class activities so that each session unfolds at a slow and manageable pace. I encourage participants to carefully look around the room, notice details of the physical space, and become aware of one another. This orienting response helps participants to accurately perceive safety in the present moment.

Individuals living with chronic stress or unresolved trauma have experienced profound helplessness and loss of control. Thus, it is important to offer participants choices about whatever aspects of the SRP experience are amenable to their control.

I seek opportunities for participants to make decisions and have their decisions honored. I ask participants to choose between the different types of chairs in the room, and I solicit their input when adjusting the lighting and the temperature. Participants decide if they want to lie down or remain seated for the body scan, and whether they want to cover themselves with small fleece blankets, which can strengthen their sense of personal boundaries.

It is often appropriate for participants to focus their attention on what I am saying or doing. It is also important for participants to turn toward one another, and I create many opportunities for them to do so. When we are having a whole group discussion or activity, I ask whoever is speaking to please address all participants, and I use my eye contact and nonverbal cues to remain connected with the entire group. When I divide the group into dyads or triads for short structured activities, I look for nonverbal cues about which participants would be likely to work well together. When I present small "chunks" of didactic information, I notice that some participants seem to quickly understand what I am saying, while others appear uncertain or confused. I ask those who seem to understand if they would be willing to rephrase what I have said for the benefit of the whole group. I listen carefully to the explanation, both to make sure it accurately represents what I said, and also to learn ways of phrasing concepts that may be more resonant with the language and learning styles of participants.

Homiletics: Talking with the Group

> *Dialogue is a horizontal relationship. It is fed by love, humility, hope, faith, and confidence.*
>
> Paulo Freire (In Gadotti, 1994, p. 50)

As the revolutionary Brazilian educator Paulo Freire articulated, the predominant "banking system" of education, where learners are treated as empty vessels into which the teacher deposits ideas and factual information, is a debasement of teachers and learners alike (Freire, 1976). Freire promoted a problem-posing education wherein teachers are also learners, and learners are also teachers. Together teacher and learners co-create an active and participatory process of dialogue and inquiry. This educational process is designed to bring about the inner transformation of learners, enabling them to claim their rightful dignity, authenticity, and authority.

The basic tenets of Freire's pedagogy are resonant with the MBI approach. Both promote a nonhierarchical relationship of mutual respect between teacher and learners, and posit authentic education to be an unfolding process cocreated by teacher and learners. Both describe dialogue, inquiry, and exploration of lived experience as hallmarks of the educational process, and both recognize personal transformation through clear comprehension of reality as the remedy for suffering. The explicit purpose of Freire's model is empowerment of oppressed people, enabling them to take action to end poverty and oppression. The individual transformation effected by Freire's educational process prepares oppressed people to create a society where all people are equal, thereby gaining true liberation for both oppressed and oppressors. While the curriculum content and meditation practices of MBIs direct participants' attention primarily to their inner subjective world rather than the circumstances of their social and political reality, Freire's pedagogy is a useful theoretical framework for MBI work with impoverished, marginalized, and oppressed populations.

Encouraged by Freire's educational model, I seek ways to explore didactic information that are participatory and draw directly upon participants' life experiences. Participants intuitively know, or are in the process of discovering, most of the conceptual and factual information of the SRP. My responsibility is to facilitate activities, discussions, and meditations that encourage participants to articulate their intuitive understandings in ways that support and clarify the SRP curriculum. I use participants' lists of causes of stress in their lives to discuss how mindfulness helps us move along a continuum from habitual stress reactivity to more consciously chosen, health promoting stress responses. I repeat anecdotes shared by participants to demonstrate that group members are already using mindfulness skills to increase choice and freedom during everyday difficulties. Self-efficacy grows as participants recognize how their own intelligence and efforts are creating positive change.

Everyone's participation in discussions is invited and valued, and I emphasize that no one is obligated to speak. We often use the process of Council Circle, passing around a talking piece, giving each participant the opportunity to share a comment, question, or observation. Anyone who chooses not to speak simply passes the talking piece to the next person in the circle.

I pause at transition points between class activities, inviting reflection, questions, and comments, which may be directed to me or to the group. Ultimately, my intention and efforts are to create an environment where participants discover themselves to be skilled learners: engaged with one another, enjoying themselves, and incorporating with relative ease onto their existent internal scaffolding the new information, ideas, and experiences arising in the SRP.

Guidance: Not Performance but Connection

> *Therapists should recognize the power of facial recognition and social engagement in calming their clients, and in meeting people's deepest emotional needs and motivating many behaviors, both conscious and unconscious...Along with facial recognition, the sound, intonation and rhythm of the human voice...have an equally calming effect.*
>
> Peter Levine (2010, p. 108)

Connection is vital to growth and healing. When I guide the meditation practices, I am aware of connection on a variety of levels. First, I connect with my deepest beliefs about this work and explicitly state these beliefs in the meditation instructions. There is connection between the instructions I am speaking and the mindfulness arising in me. There is connection between participants and me, and intrapersonal and interpersonal connections as participants hear my guidance and cultivate their mindfulness skills.

...Please take a moment to remember the reason you came to class today...recognizing your motivation to learn about mindfulness...This motivation is your personal variation of the very beautiful human desire to experience greater health and happiness in our life... connecting with this motivation is important, as it provides the energy to fuel your meditation practice...And remind yourself that you have everything it takes to practice mindfulness... you are completely capable of using your inner resources to participate in your healing...

I want to be sensitive to how my words and phrases are "landing" inside of participants. I try to gauge the receptivity of the participants to the meditation instructions, and assess their capacity to be present with whatever inner experiences the practices evoke. I also take into account the pacing, volume, intonation and rhythm of my voice, periods of silence, offering variations of instructions for persons with severe physical pain or anxiety, posing questions instead of statements, naming possible examples of what might be noted, and acknowledging distractions in the environment.

Clearly, guiding mindfulness meditation is a practice in itself. When done well, the exquisite presence offered by the instructor is matched by participants' presence to their own inner experience, and by extension, in their resonance with one another. Conditions are ripe for individual growth and healing in a group setting.

Inquiring: Curiosity About Participants' Experiences

Curiosity is an openness and a "not knowing" that functions as an antidote to our judgments, fixed ideas, and rigid, distorted identifications.

Laurence Heller and Aline LaPierre (2012, p. 206)

Inquiry is delicate. The mindfulness meditation practices and the topics of discussion are completely new to most SRP participants. These are not everyday experiences and conversations. Everyone is feeling their way, into their own internal world, and into group discussions. Due to past conditioning, participants may be reluctant to share their direct experiences with the group. Participants may not yet have the words needed to express what they encounter during meditation practice, or the phrases to articulate the thoughts that SRP activities stimulate in their minds. They may assume that there is always a right answer, and they don't want to be wrong. They might think they are the only one in the group who has a certain experience, feels a certain way, or holds a certain belief. They may wonder if an open-ended question has some special answer that would please me or other group members. They may regard speaking in a group to be a performance, and feel anxious about how their performance will be judged. They may have had relationships in which other people denigrated or dismissed their subjective reality, and they learned to mistrust their perceptions and distance themselves from their inner world.

Many SRP participants have consciously or unconsciously internalized powerful destructive beliefs from our society and its institutions. To be a member of a racial, ethnic, or religious minority group; to not speak the language of the dominant class; to be a woman; to be lesbian, gay, bisexual, or transgender; to have been abused or neglected in childhood; to be a recovering addict; to be uneducated; to have served time in prison; to be an alcoholic; to have been abused or abusive in an adult relationship; to be living in poverty; to be homeless; to be an immigrant; to be defined by a stigmatized medical illness or mental health disorder; to feel like a "living dead person" due to unresolved trauma—there are so many reasons to believe that the human right to know one's inner reality and speak of it to others is a right that cannot be claimed.

Inquiry into one's inner world, or in a shared verbal process with others, requires curiosity. Curiosity cannot coexist psychophysiologically with trauma or fear (Levine, 2010, p. 218). Thus, to free up curiosity and inquiry, participants need a strong sense of safety. I approach inquiry by explicitly encouraging SRP participants to identify a reliable personal resource of safety. I introduce this in the first or second SRP class by conducting a guided Resourcing Visualization.

As you hear the sound of the bells, please take a moment to settle ... feeling your body in contact with the chair, noticing the sensation of the breath... See if you can remember an experience where you felt safe and protected, relaxed and loved ... this experience may have occurred in childhood or adulthood, perhaps with a family member, a friend, a pet, or a stuffed animal ... your special moment may have been in someone's home, in a church or community gathering, or at a place in nature ... whatever the experience was, seeing it in your mind as clearly as you can right now ... and if no such experience comes to mind, please use your imagination to create an experience of safety and security right now ... Seeing the scene in your mind, noticing where you are, what you are wearing, who else is there, what the environment looks like, what you are thinking or feeling or saying ... seeing it in color and detail, like a photograph in your mind ... and perhaps adding one more sense to the visual scene, maybe a sound, or smell, or taste, or physical sensation ... whatever might make the image feel more alive, more real to you in this moment ... if your attention wanders, gently return to your image, allowing yourself to experience the safety, security, love or connection that is available to you ... and noticing now how your body feels right now ... areas of softness, ease, or tension ... your heartbeat and your breathing ... your arms, legs, neck and shoulders, your jaw, your back, your belly ... noticing whatever physical sensations are present in this moment ... and exploring if there might be someplace in your body where your mental image can go right now, where your inner resource can comfortably stay ... if there is, invite the image to enter that place and feel it settling there ... if not, simply noticing the image in your mind ... knowing that this inner resource is truly yours to connect with at any time, as often as you like ... resting with yourself and your Resource ...

When participants complete this exercise and return attention outward, I invite people to speak about their experience without necessarily sharing what their resource was. This exercise yields powerful and rich exchange among group members. Once participants are familiar with this Resourcing Visualization, a shorter variation can be integrated into any mindfulness practice, or done as a mini-meditation at the beginning or end of class. I also encourage participants to practice resourcing in daily life.

The capacity to resource oneself in this way is a strong support for mindfulness meditation. During meditation practice, participants can move attention back and forth between painful sensations or emotions and the Resource. This increases tolerance for difficulties and builds confidence in the ability to manage whatever may arise. Participants discover true refuge.

Intentions of Teaching

The intentions of teaching, eloquently described by McCown et al. (2017), illustrate how the person of the teacher and the skills of the teacher connect to the teaching practices that unfold in the MBI classroom. What follows are some of the ways that the Intentions of Teaching manifest in the CHC-Meriden SRP.

Experiencing New Possibilities

Learning is the process of becoming open to more and more possibilities.

Russell Delman (2008)

From the first moments in the SRP, participants encounter novelty. The universalities of the human experience are emphasized over fixed individual identities. Intrapersonal and interpersonal relationships begin to shift. Participants' conditioned roles as patients change as they establish relationships with me, the SRP instructor. Participants discover the wisdom of the body and experientially redefine the mind–body relationship. They observe the breath and body sensations, and notice the habitual and incessant activities of the mind. They look within at existent inner resources, and find their natural intelligence poised to support mindfulness and healing. The conceptual and the experiential begin to converge within their own being. Participants sense they have entered an experiment of sea change, where identities, habits, beliefs, assumptions, and capacities may all be questioned.

Experiencing new possibilities requires presence, and presence requires safety. The container of relative safety includes the physical environment, use of space, comfort of seating, control of temperature and lighting, as well as the energetic ambience of kindness, curiosity and acceptance towards each person and whatever arises in the group. Experiencing New Possibilities is a teaching intention that applies to the instructor as well. I remind myself that every SRP group is unique, and each moment with every group is new. I am guiding and facilitating, and I can never know what will happen next.

Entering the world of physical sensation is full of new possibilities. Turning toward sensation brings participants into proximity with their thoughts and emotions. I guide a series of short discussions and mini-meditations in preparation for introducing breathing meditation in the first session, and the body scan in the second session. The Stressed Body Drawing activity (see Chapter 23 G) reveals that the ability to monitor and modify physical sensations enhances our capacity to modulate reactions to stress. Participants recognize the importance of becoming fluent in the language of the body. This means learning to direct attention to the body, perceive sensations that are present, and name the sensations. I guide participants to feel their feet against the floor, their backs touching the back of the chair, the air touching the skin of the face, and we begin a list of sensation words: contact, pressure, heavy, light, cool, warm, vibration, tightness, softness, flow.

I guide the first body scan as a partner exercise. With participants seated in pairs facing each other, I ask everyone to greet their partner, and then shift attention inward. I guide the group to one area of the body at a time, beginning with the feet, to identify and name sensation(s) there. We pause after each area of the body for participant dyads to name what each person felt in that body region. I ask for new sensation words to add to our list. We continue, moving to the legs, torso, arms and hands, neck, face, and head. Participants briefly bring attention to each body region, and then turn attention outward to interact with their partner again, describing what sensations they noticed. Because connecting with the internal felt sense may initially feel alien or frightening, I invite participants to lightly tap or press into the different body areas with their fingertips. This contact with the body's outer layers of skin and musculature can counteract habits of dissociation from the body, and build confidence in accessing the more internal felt sense. As we move through the body, I suggest that participants steady their attention for a few more seconds in each region, noticing what happens next. Do the sensations stay the same, disappear, or change into other sensations? Tracking sensations in this way, paying more attention to beginnings and endings of sensations, builds tolerance for unpleasant sensations, appreciation for pleasant sensations, and awareness of change and impermanence.

Participants leave this second SRP session with the second CD to do the body scan at home as a silent individual meditation practice. The following week I guide the body scan as an individual practice, moving sequentially from the feet to the head, with a group discussion afterwards.

Discovering Embodiment

Physical sensations are the very foundation of human consciousness.
    Peter Levine (2010, p. 133)

The vast majority of participants enter the SRP with little somatic awareness and minimal appreciation of its value. They regard the mind–body connection with suspicion and confusion, often because of health care providers' overt comments or covert attitudes that participants' ailments are "all in their head." People living with severe stress, unresolved trauma, or chronic physical pain often experience the body as a formidable enemy. Areas of pain or dysfunction demand constant attention. The capacity to perceive pleasant or neutral sensations is diminished, and regions of the body that are symptom free disappear from conscious awareness. Sensations associated with physical pain, anxiety, and unresolved trauma are coupled with emotions of rage, fear, helplessness, and shame, causing distortion of perception and reaction. Attempting to tame, avoid, or escape unpleasant sensations and their associated emotions and thoughts is physically draining and mentally exhausting. Distraction and dissociation become the norm. The body is viewed as alien, unexplored, and foreboding. The mere thought of focusing attention on the body can provoke fear and resistance. The default strategy to prevent overwhelm is conscious or unconscious avoidance of present moment embodiment.

Learning to perceive, tolerate, and appreciate sensation is vital to living in the present. In the SRP, we "touch into" the world of sensation through tactile awareness, noting what parts of the body are in contact with the floor, chair, clothing, or air. Gradually I guide participants' attention further within the body, developing the felt sense while continuing to practice slowly alternating between feeling the breath, noticing objects in the visual field, and hearing sounds in the environment. We also move attention between the breath and the Resource, offering participants more skill building in preparation for turning the attention inward for sustained periods of formal meditation practice. In contrast to the sitting posture, the standing position engages more interoceptive activity (i.e., kinesthetic, proprioceptive, and visceral) and provides greater integration of these different aspects of somatic experience. To afford participants a more powerful experience of embodiment, I guide a somatic awareness exercise, experiencing standing, grounding, and breathing. Many participants say they were surprised by this short and simple practice. They report increased physical relaxation and mental calm. They have accessed their capacity to more fully inhabit the physical body, and discovered the clarity and stability of embodiment.

Cultivating Observation

> On a planet that seems so busy and distracted, a clear awareness of what is true is a priceless gift that we give ourselves, others, and our world.
>   Gavin Harrison (1994, p. 17)

Observation is one of the primary methods of learning in the SRP. Participants are cultivating new objects of observation as well as new strategies for observation. In preparation for formal mindfulness practices, I introduce a series of short exercises to help participants trust their capacity to direct attention to different objects in ways that are successful and manageable. This direct experience strengthens participants' confidence that they can turn toward the inner world of sensation, thought, and emotion, with less apprehension about becoming lost, overwhelmed, or shutdown.

Participants need a safe and gentle "way in" to the internal world, and an effective and reliable "way out." We start by focusing attention on objects likely to be neutral, thus titrating both duration of mindful awareness and intensity of possible emotional reaction to the object of attention. I guide the group to look outside the windows and choose one thing to observe in some detail: a tree, a building, the sky, a parked car. Then I ask everyone to direct their attention back inside the classroom and focus on one object: a light fixture, the door, a window, or the carpet.

We do this a few times at a slow pace, feeling the intention to direct attention to a specific object, feeling the attention connected to the object, and discovering it's possible to know where the attention is and to move it both away from and back to the chosen object. We repeat the exercise a few times, moving the attention back and forth between the chosen objects outdoors and inside the room.

After inviting participants to share their experiences with this first set of exercises, I direct everyone's attention to a neutral body sensation, perhaps the sensation of the feet against the floor or the back touching the back of the chair. We go back and forth between the physical sensation and the chosen object outdoors, and later, alternating physical sensation with a chosen object inside the classroom. After inviting inquiry and dialogue about what participants are experiencing, I generally sense that the group is ready to bring attention to the breath.

Moving Towards Acceptance

Accepting is to the mind what relaxation is to the body. It is how the mind relaxes.
   Gregory Kramer (2007, pp. 123–124)

Acceptance is integral to mindfulness. I have dedicated much time and effort to understanding what acceptance actually is, and how one goes about moving towards it and inviting others to do the same. SRP participants often demonstrate common misunderstandings about the meaning of acceptance. Acceptance is most often mistaken for either approval or resignation. When mistaken for approval, the belief is that to accept is to condone who or what one accepts. Naturally, there is willingness to accept what is agreeable and pleasant, and resistance towards accepting what is disagreeable or unpleasant. When confused with resignation, the assumption is that acceptance endorses disempowerment by promoting passivity towards the circumstances, relationships, or personal habits that are contributing to one's suffering.

When SRP participants equate acceptance with either approval or resignation, they understandably reject acceptance as unattractive, illogical, dangerous, or unwise. These assumptions about acceptance are very tenacious. I share that the word "accept" is related to the Latin verb *accipere,* which means "to receive," and the definition of accept is "to receive willingly" (Merriam-Webster's Dictionary, 2015). To receive unwillingly would be to resist what is true, what is present. It takes tremendous energy to resist what is present, but because we are so used to doing this, we rarely feel the energy being expended. I also suggest that participants "try on" other words that might feel more resonant than acceptance. Possibilities include acknowledge, allow, recognize, or receive. I describe acceptance as "the practice of nonresistance."

Like any practice, acceptance requires both conceptual understanding and much repetition. I clarify that acceptance takes place inside of us, for the purpose of changing perspective and meaning about ourselves, other people, or our life experiences. And while acceptance may give rise to a new action or behavior, it does not require any outward change. The best motivation to engage in the practice of acceptance is a clear awareness of the physical and psychological suffering caused by the unwillingness or inability to accept what has happened in our lives. Ultimately, I return to direct experience and invite further exploration, guiding a meditation inspired by Tara Brach (2003, p. 87).

Growing Compassion

Compassion is our deepest nature. It arises from our interconnection with all things.
Jack Kornfield (2008, p. 23)

Kindness and compassion are inherent to mindfulness, and naturally arise with dedicated mindfulness practice. By consciously bringing compassion to the foreground of the SRP, its growth can be strengthened and deepened within individual participants and in the group as a whole. The literal translation of "karuna," the Pali word for compassion, is "experiencing a trembling or quivering of the heart in response to a being's pain" (Salzberg, 1995, p. 104). Compassion is the love that responds to pain or suffering. This experience of love is neither conceptual nor intellectual. The heart "trembling or quivering" describes an alive, visceral experience that the giver, (and often the receiver), can feel as sensation in the body. Responding to the presence of pain or suffering with avoidance, denial, pity, or indifference obstructs the arising of compassion, and shuts down the aliveness, flow, and expansiveness of the physical, visceral experience of compassion.

Given that each one of us is "a being," compassion by definition includes self-compassion. Compassion for others and compassion for oneself mutually support each other. SRP participants recognize compassion as a component of human nature, and appreciate the ethical value of relating to others with compassion. The importance of self-compassion tends to be less apparent. The realization that cruelty, rather than compassion, is often directed towards oneself may come as a great surprise.

In the first session I introduce the breathing meditation, which includes affirming the inevitability of the attention wandering. I describe the attitude of patience and kindness toward oneself and one's mind that mindfulness meditation requires, and how the way we return to the breath establishes the tone of our practice. I guide 10 minutes of breathing meditation. In the discussion that follows, I offer the following example to emphasize the practical, moment-by-moment practice of compassion for oneself.

Has anyone ever taught a child to ride a bicycle? Maybe it was your child, or a grandchild, or a neighbor's child?
Many participants raise their hands.
And what happens if the child has difficulty balancing, or falls and scrapes her knee? What if the child gets frustrated and says, "I'll never learn to ride a bike. I'm an idiot?" Do you say, "That's right, you're an idiot. You'll never learn to ride a bike?"
Participants look at me in disbelief and shake their heads "No." Some laugh at the ridiculousness of my statement.
What would you say to the child?
A participant replies, "You're doing fine. Of course you'll learn to ride a bike."

I explain that if we get frustrated and criticize ourselves or our mind when we practice meditation, the practice won't be enjoyable, and our mind will feel reprimanded and judged. I emphasize that the attention wandering during meditation is not a problem, and urge participants to treat themselves the same way they would treat the child learning to ride a bicycle: with encouragement, patience, and kindness. When we are gentle and friendly with ourselves we facilitate the learning process, and our meditation practice will be enjoyable.

Throughout the SRP we return frequently to the theme of compassion. Participants demonstrate increasing capacity to meet their own and others' painful experiences with compassion.

Conclusion

There is growing awareness around the world of the benefits of mindfulness for physical and mental health and happiness. There is also increasing recognition that mindfulness can positively influence interpersonal relationships, productivity and satisfaction in the workplace, communal well-being, and ultimately peace on our planet. For mindfulness to move steadily toward fulfilling its great potential, MBIs must be offered equally to all. Bringing mindfulness training to minority, low income, and underserved communities will require sincerity of intention, effort, and allocation of resources. Additionally, creativity and experimentation are needed to develop and evaluate effective practices for training teachers, publicizing programs, and adapting the curriculum to best meet the needs of specific populations and of the unique individuals who comprise each MBI group. It will be the collaboration of the hearts and minds of many people that will move this great endeavor towards fruition.

References

Brach, T. (2003). *Radical acceptance: Embracing your life with the heart of a Buddha*. New York: Bantam Books.

Delman, R. (2008). www.russelldelman.com/writings

DiGangi, J. A., Gomez, D., Mendoza, L., Jason, L. A., Keys, C. B., & Koenen, K. C. (2013). Pretrauma risk factors for posttraumatic stress disorder: A systematic review of the literature. *Clinical Psychology Review, 33*(6), 728–744.

Ford, J. (2008). Trauma, posttraumatic stress disorder, and ethnoracial minorities: Toward diversity and cultural competence in principles and practices. *Clinical Psychology, 15*(1), 62–67.

Freire, P. (1976). *Education: The practice of freedom* (1st ed.). London, England: Writers and Readers Publishing Cooperative.

Kabat-Zinn, J. (1990). *Full catastrophe living: Using the wisdom of your body and mind to face stress, pain, and illness* (1st ed.). New York, NY: Dell Publishing.

Kabat-Zinn, J. (2004). *Vivir Con Plenitud Las Crisis: Cómo utilizar la sabiduría del cuerpo y de la mente para afrontar el estrés, el dolor y la enfermedad* (A. de Satrústegui, Trans. 2nd ed.). Barcelona, Spain: Editorial Kairós.

Kabat-Zinn, J. (2005). *Coming to our senses* (1st ed.). New York, NY: Hyperion.

Levine, P. A. (1997). *Waking the tiger* (1st ed.). Berkeley, CA: North Atlantic Books.

Levine, P. A. (2008). *Healing trauma: A pioneering program for restoring the wisdom of your body*. Boulder, CO: Sounds True.

Levine, P. A. (2010). *In an unspoken voice: How the body releases trauma and restores goodness*. Berkeley: North Atlantic Books.

Levine, P. A., & Phillips, M. (2012). *Freedom from pain: Discover your body's power to overcome physical pain*. Boulder, CO: Sounds True.

McCown, D., Reibel, D., & Micozzi, M. S. (2017). *Teaching mindfulness: A practical guide for clinicians and educators*. New York: Springer.

Merriam-Webster's Dictionary. (2015). Retrieved from http://www.m-w.com/dictionary/acceptance

Metzger, D. (1992). *Writing for your life: A guide and companion to the inner worlds*. San Francisco: HarperSanFrancisco.

Ogden, P., Minton, K., & Pain, C. (2006). *Trauma and the body: A sensorimotor approach to psychotherapy*. New York: W.W. Norton.

Ozer, E. J., Best, S. R., Lipsey, T. L., & Weiss, D. S. (2008). Predictors of posttraumatic stress disorder and symptoms in adults: A meta-analytic review. *Psychological Trauma, S*(1), 3–36.

Payne, P., Levine, P. A., & Crane-Godreau, M. A. (2015). Somatic experiencing: Using interoception and proprioception as core elements of trauma therapy. *Frontiers in Psychology, 6*. doi:10.3389/fpsyg.2015.00093.

Ponds, K. (2013). The trauma of racism: America's original sin. *Reclaiming Children and Youth, 22*(2), 22–24. Retrieved from www.reclaimingjournal.com.

Roth, B. (1994). Anchoring in the present moment: Meditation in the inner city. *Nurse Practitioner News, 2*(5), 12–14.

Roth, B. (1997). Mindfulness-based stress reduction in the inner city. *Advances: The Journal of Mind-Body Health, 13*(4), 50–59.

Roth, B., & Calle-Mesa, L. (2006). Mindfulness-based stress reduction (MBSR) with Spanish- and English-speaking inner-city medical patients. In R. A. Baer (Ed.), *Mindfulness-based treatment approach* (1st ed.). Amsterdam: Elsevier.

Roth, B., & Creaser, T. (1997). Mindfulness meditation-based stress reduction: Experience with a bilingual inner city program. *The Nurse Practitioner, 22*(3), 150–176.

Roth, B., & Robbins, D. (2004). Mindfulness-based stress reduction and health-related quality of life: Findings from a bilingual inner-city patient population. *Psychosomatic Medicine, 66*, 113–123.

Roth, B., & Stanley, T.-W. (2002). Mindfulness-based stress reduction and health care utilization in the inner city: Preliminary findings. *Alternative Therapies in Health and Medicine, 8*(1), 60–62.

Ruglass, L. (2014). *Screening and assessment of psychological trauma and PTSD*. Jenkintown, PA: HealthForum.

Salzberg, S. (1995). *Lovingkindness: The revolutionary art of happiness*. Boston: Shambhala.

Scaer, R. C. (2005). *The trauma spectrum* (1st ed.). New York, NY: W. W. Norton.

Scaer, R. C. (2014). *The body bears the burden trauma, dissociation, and disease* (3rd ed.). New York: Rutledge.

Schoulte, J., Schultz, J., & Atmaier, E. (2011). Forgiveness in response to cultural microaggressions. *Counseling Psychology Quarterly, 24*(4), 291–300.

Siegel, D. J. (2010). *The mindful therapist: A clinician's guide to mindsight and neural integration*. New York: W.W. Norton & Company.

Van der Kolk, B. A. (2014). *The body keeps the score: Brain, mind, and body in the healing of trauma*. New York, NY: Viking.

Chapter 14
Teaching Frail Elders and Caregivers

Lucia McBee

Look at Me

What do you see, nurses? What do you see?
    Are you thinking when you look at me?
    A crabby old woman, not very wise,
    Uncertain of habit, with far away eyes,

Who dribbles her food and makes no reply
    When you say in a loud voice- "I do wish you'd try."
    Who seems not to notice, The things that you do,
    And forever is losing a sock or a shoe.

Who unresisting or not, lets you do as you will,
    With bathing and feeding, the long day to fill.
    Is that what you think, is that what you see?
    Open your eyes, nurse, you're not looking at me…

But inside this old carcass a young girl still dwells,
    And now and again, my battered heart swells,
    I remember the joys and I remember the pain,
    And I'm living and loving life over again,

I think of the years all too few- gone too fast,
    And accept the stark fact that nothing can last.
    Open your eyes, nurse open and see.
    Not an empty old women, look closer- see ME.

L. McBee, L.C.S.W., M.P.H., C.Y.I. (✉)
207 West 106th Street, Apartment 12C, New York, NY 10025, USA
e-mail: lucia@luciamcbee.com

© Springer International Publishing Switzerland 2016
D. McCown et al., *Resources for Teaching Mindfulness*,
DOI 10.1007/978-3-319-30100-6_14

This poem has been attributed, variously, to an old woman who died in a geriatric ward in England, to Phyllis McCormick (an English nurse), and to an old man who died in a nursing home in Tampa Florida.

Full version: www.agingcare.com/Articles/cranky-old-man-legend-157110.htm. Or video: www.youtube.com/watch?v=LDP83gejkoE.

Mindfulness for Frail Elders and Their Caregivers

Mindfulness is widely conceptualized and taught grounded in the model of mindfulness-based stress reduction (MBSR). As MBSR has been adapted for various specific populations, the basic structure of the program and its practices have often been maintained, while population-specific materials have been integrated.

Teaching mindfulness to frail elders, however, may require a more comprehensive range of adaptations to the basic structure of the MBSR program. An appreciation of the complex and varied nature of this population is an important start. Frail elders are characterized by a physical and cognitive decline in function often requiring assistance. Caregivers for frail elders are the essential component of life for them. These caregivers may also be elders, requiring their own stress reduction and modification of programs. Further, some of the standard curricular components are more physically and cognitively rigorous than may be useful or safe for frail elders, requiring significant, sensitive adjustments. This chapter, therefore, will, describe some ways in which mindfulness may be taught to frail elders and caregivers.

Mindfulness instruction comes from the teacher's authenticity and personal practice. Teaching special populations requires deep saturation in the experiences of the population, as well as self-reflection and understanding of the effect of such experiences on the teacher herself. It is both common and human to deny the presence of our own frailty and the inevitability of our own demise. This denial is nurtured by a culture focused on youth and life extension. We are, in fact, living longer but with more loss and impairment. In order to work with elders and caregivers, it is crucial to understand the emotional impact of aging.

Most frail elders and their caregivers face the reality of aging, loss, illness, pain, and mortality daily. To teach mindfulness effectively with this population requires the teacher to be intimately comfortable with the knowledge that she, too, is subject to these realities. Together, then, teacher and participants may cultivate fearlessness and compassion in awareness of life's most challenging lessons. Formal and informal practices, skills, homiletics, and inquiry may be adapted and modified for those with differing abilities. Most important, however, is connecting with the person in front of us: "Look at me."

Definitions

Elder

Among special populations, "elder" is not so special, being inclusive of everyone who lives to a certain age. In the USA, for AARP, the age is 50; for Medicare, 65; and for Social Security, 66 and rising. Unique to this generation, the population is living longer worldwide. The range of ability and disability associated with aging also includes a spectrum from active, well elders, to those needing care for physical and cognitive disability, to those at the end of life.

Frail Elder

As the world's population ages, acute medical interventions increasingly prevent early death. While some age without disabling chronic conditions, others experience aging with added pain, loss, illness, and disability, often described as "frailty." Frailty is a medical term used to describe complex conditions that affect the ability to function independently. Most commonly associated with elders, frailty includes at least three of the following: low physical activity, muscle weakness, slowed performance, fatigue or poor endurance, and unintentional weight loss (Torpy, Lynm, & Glass, 2006). These conditions reflect a range of disability but often lead to illness, infection, hospitalization, and initiating a spiral of increasing problems. Nonphysical losses are often the most devastating: loss of dear ones, homes, jobs, roles, and sense of self. Mild cognitive impairment (MCI) often leads to cognitive impairment that is more serious, including Alzheimer's disease (AD), now increasing in epidemic proportions. Physical and cognitive disabilities often cause physical, emotional, mental, and spiritual pain for elders and their families and friends.

Caregivers

The nature of frailty requires assistance. Medication, equipment, and therapy offer partial support for frail elders, but direct, personal caregiving, from shopping and bill paying to feeding, toileting, and bathing, is crucial. This caregiving is often provided by informal caregivers, such as family and friends, and paid professional (formal) caregivers. And these arrangements are often combined. The nature of these care relationships is physically, mentally, and emotionally challenging. It is an intimate interaction, with a potential for strong emotions on both sides. Introducing mindfulness practices to frail elders may reduce their suffering, while teaching mindfulness to caregivers potentially impacts the entire situation.

Teaching Mindfulness to Frail Elders and Their Caregivers

Increasing evidence supports the protective and healing qualities of mindfulness on the immune system, the brain, aging, and chronic conditions. (Davidson et al., 2003; Epel et al., 2004; Hölzel et al., 2011). In addition, research on the unique effects and benefits of MBIs for elders is growing. Trait mindfulness has been shown to buffer the effects of stress and positively affect the mental health of older adults (de Frias & Whyne, 2014). MBSR programs are shown to have small yet positive effect on depression, anxiety, and psychological distress linked to chronic conditions for adults (Bohlmeijer, Prenger, Taal, & Cuijpers, 2010). In a 2014 review of the literature, Prakash and colleagues found that mindfulness practices potentially benefit older adults by improving attention, emotion regulation, and overall well-being and targeting the general tendency toward cognitive decline in aging. A smaller recent study of an adapted MBSR program for relatively intact elders over 80 years of age in a long-term community care facility quantitatively found MBSR participants showed improved acceptance of age- and health-related limitations. In qualitative interviews, the MBSR participants reported increased awareness, less judgment, and greater self-compassion (Moss et al., 2014). A review by Larouche, Hudon, and Goulet (2014) summarizes the literature and points to a connection between stress, depression, and inflammatory conditions with MCI and AD.

Thus, evidence shows that MBIs can benefit older adults and the chronic conditions that disproportionally affect them. The teachability of mindfulness practices to elders with cognitive loss is less studied. Previous MBI interventions for elders exclude those with cognitive loss, but important new findings show benefits for those with MCI and diagnosis of AD. In a randomized, double-blind clinical trial conducted in the Canary Islands, Spain, Quintana-Hernandez and colleagues compared three interventions (mindfulness based, cognitive stimulation, and progressive relaxation groups) to treatment as usual (TAU) for 127 community dwelling elders with a diagnosis of probable early AD. Participants in the mindfulness-based group remained stable for the 2 years in global cognitive function, functionality, and behavioral disorders measures, while participants from the control group as well as the other experimental groups showed a mild but significant worsening of their mental capacities (2013). Wells et al. (2013) reported initial fMRI results from a small MBSR controlled study targeting adults with MCI. This MBSR group was slightly modified in time requirements for class and homework length. While both control and experimental groups evidenced brain atrophy post group as expected, participants in the MBSR class group showed less hippocampal atrophy and also increased functional connectivity.

Mindfulness-based interventions engage participants in exercises that enhance ability to be *with* difficulty while respecting and trusting what is right for each in the moment. Through supported group and individual experience and discussion, participants may increase their comfort level with discomfort. Many report that MBSR provides skills that allow them to learn to trust and care for themselves in more helpful ways. In a sense, they learn to access their inner wisdom. This can be available at any age.

In the spectrum of aging, mindfulness practices may need to be adapted to provide appropriate challenges and support. Younger, more able elders have the capacities to participate in mindfulness-based interventions that have little or no adaptation. For the more frail populations, however, the difficulties of daily life may be challenge enough, and mindfulness teaching and practice may be best focused on supporting and enhancing the abilities of participants, including compassion, kindness, and spirituality. Quality of life is also significantly enhanced for all concerned when caregivers are also trained in and practice mindfulness.

Caregiver stress is well documented, as well as the challenges of recruiting caregivers for groups targeting self-care. (Schulz & Beach, 1999). MBSR and modified MBI groups have shown benefits of teaching mindfulness to this needy and growing population. (McBee, 2008; Whitebird et al., 2013). Modifications for time, location and inclusion of those who receive care with the caregivers will increase participation. In *Mindfulness Base Elder Care,* many of the modifications are described; the most promising was a group that included nursing home residents, staff and informal caregivers (McBee, 2008). The restrictions of providing care often are cited as the major obstacle for group attendance by caregivers. Groups including both caregivers and care receivers offer many benefits and are recently the focus of some studies including Paller et al. (2014). In this program, persons with cognitive loss and their caregivers who participated together in an 8-week group with modified group length and exercises. Participants reported better sleep, increased quality-of-life ratings, and fewer depressive symptoms post group.

This chapter will focus on adaptations for frail elders and their caregivers. Adaptations of curriculum and teaching practices are fluid and flexible, to match participants' needs and abilities. Key characteristics of adapted programs for frail elders and caregivers may include:

- Short class sessions, from 15 to 90 minutes each
- Short meditations, with high levels of guidance
- Ongoing groups rather than time-limited ones
- More directive, concrete, and specific instructions, with attention to nonverbal as well as verbal cueing
- Slow pace, allowing more time for response and for more repetition
- Focus on informal homework
- No retreat/all-day session
- Adapted mindful movement practices (e.g., walking meditation and yoga adapted to physical limitation)
- Limited group discussion and use of dyads
- Monitoring of group by Instructor for comprehension and modification as needed
- Inclusion of caregivers, either separately or jointly with frail elders

The Context for Teaching

Mindfulness may be taught to frail elders within institutions and assisted living settings, in the elder's homes, and in adult day-care/senior centers. Mindfulness may be taught to informal caregivers in community programs or within the institutional settings. Mindfulness for staff/formal caregivers may be taught at the workplace/ institution.

Teachers of mindfulness are frequently also staff members of the institution or community program. This situation brings benefits and potential complications. Mindfulness programs in these settings may be shorter in length but ongoing or more integrated into the environment. The teacher who is also staff will have continued input and opportunity to hone their teaching skills and to refine curricular adaptations.

Mindfulness teachers who are also staff will develop expertise in modifying communications, physical expectations, and adaptations for this population. Yet the staff position may present role conflicts, as well. Teaching mindfulness requires a stance toward the participants that is non-pathologizing, nonhierarchical, and noninstrumental (McCown, 2013), which differs significantly from the problem-solving mode that is an integral component of health-care training and work expectations. For the teacher, it may require differential monitoring for the appropriate "hat" to don in each situation.

For mindfulness teachers from outside the institution or community program who wish to offer these practices, it may be helpful to team up with someone who is familiar with the needs of frail elders and their caregivers.

Supportive Environments

Frail elders may be cared for at home with support, but as their needs and/or the caregiver's limitations increase, a congregate setting may be safer and more appropriate. It is especially true for those with dementia, behavioral problems, poor safety awareness, and/or limited income and social support. Congregate living also reflects a range of options from supported housing, assisted living, temporary rehabilitation facilities, skilled nursing homes, and special care units. For many elders without financial resources, the only option is a nursing home or wait list for senior housing. Institutional living usually requires routine, dependency, and conformity, which may reinforce feelings of limitation, disability, and low self-worth for elders. As a result, institutionalized elders are at high risk for depression and behavioral problems, impacting their caregivers. Most institutional settings are noisy, routinized, and based on the medical, pathological model of care. Teaching mindfulness in this context may feel like fighting the waves, unless the teacher learns to surf. At the same time, teaching mindfulness within congregate settings is meaningful and rewarding for all.

Adapting the Curriculum: Teaching Awareness and Compassion

Teaching mindfulness to frail elders and caregivers is possible, rewarding, and valuable. Programs require transmitting the core mindfulness teachings of *awareness* and *compassion* in ways that are challenging without excluding any of the participants. Teaching modifications will be unique to each individual and group; thus, it is impossible to describe the range and articulations. They may include adjusting standard content, guiding inquiry, improvising one-on-one teaching, and creating unique content.

Essentially, the teacher of the class emphasizes opportunity not limitation and what is available not what must be changed. The fundamentals of mindfulness are not only understandable to frail elders; they offer relief from suffering. This chapter will offer some suggested adaptations; many more are possible.

Three Essentials for This Work

There are three essentials for working with frail elders and caregivers: connection, communication, and caring for caregivers. As with all mindfulness teachings, the skills are only fingers pointing to the moon, not the moon itself.

Connection

Authentically connecting with frail elders means seeing the person, not the disability, as illustrated by the poem above. Often, fear and denial of our own aging causes an inability to recognize ourselves in the elder in front of us. But we are not different except in age and ability. The basic tenets of mindfulness are that there is always more right with us than wrong with us and that anyone can practice some form of mindfulness as long as they are breathing and conscious. Can we apply these precepts to the frail, deaf, demented person in front of us? The first step is the hardest for many. This communication and belief will be transmitted to the frail elder, whether verbally or nonverbally. *It is the teacher's embodiment of mindfulness that makes this connection.*

Communication

If we believe we can transmit mindfulness to frail elders, our next step is to consider adaptations or modifications of the practice best suited for the particular setting and person(s). Frail elders may require adaptations for visual, hearing, and other sensory differences, as well as physical and cognitive loss, and the teacher will need to investigate a variety of approaches for each situation. For community dwelling, homebound elders, interaction can be via the telephone or the web. Teaching mindfulness in congregate living or senior centers may require environmental considerations.

Caring for the Caregivers

Caregivers often have difficulty caring for themselves. Family/friend (informal) caregivers, often women, rarely even consider it a job. Undervaluing the importance of this responsibility, often combined with tending a household and/ or working, also underestimates the toll of stress. Yet family and friend caregivers are at high risk for illness and death related to these pressures. Paraprofessional and professional (formal) caregivers are the health providers in facilities and homes. At highest risk for emotional and physical problems are the underpaid, paraprofessional caregivers, often female minorities without their own health benefits. Formal caregivers are also less likely to care for themselves. Caregivers who are stressed will transmit this stress to their care receivers. Most will agree that we are impacted by the affect and behaviors of those around us. Stress is contagious! Caring for the caregivers benefits not only the caregiver but also the care receiver.

Four Skills of the Teacher

As described in more detail elsewhere in this book, the four skills in common, yet uniquely expressed among MBSR teachers, are stewardship, homiletics, guidance, and inquiry. Stewardship denotes the distinctive qualities of MBSR leadership best described as encouraging *co-creation* of the group. Homiletics points to an engaged rather than didactic method of conveying the principles and practices of mindfulness. Mindfulness teachers interact with class participants in a particular way, using guidance and inquiry to demonstrate, or embody, mindfulness teaching. These core teaching skills provide a framework that also allows for individual teacher qualities and also differential applications for student abilities, age, and life circumstances. Illustrated below are the differential adaptations of these skills for frail elders and their caregivers.

Stewardship

Stewardship, the art of creating and holding a space conducive to mindfulness, requires the teacher's attention to both psychodynamic and environmental issues. As described above, some general adaptations apply to groups for frail elders and caregivers. Since these groups may be shorter and not consistently attended by the same participants, the traditional trajectory of group formation and cohesion may not apply. Conceptualizing the groups as a single session rather than a time-limited series may be helpful for the instructor. Each group, or mini-session, can be designed to stand alone but in the context of ongoing mindfulness teaching for the population or institution. In addition, elders and caregivers may be taught in a variety of environments, from individual homes to institutional and congregate living settings. Each of these also requires specific adaptations to create a space conducive to learning mindfulness.

For Frail Elders

Holding the space in which participants can discover and work with their own skills and knowledge may itself be an empowering message for a traditionally disempowered population. Cultural attitudes toward aging, dependency, and the medicalization/pathologizing of chronic conditions all contribute to the disempowerment of frail elders. Nursing and assisted living homes often employ a medical model that reinforces the hierarchical and pathological approach. If the mindfulness teacher is also an employee, it will be important to shift his/her approach in order to adopt the collaborative model of mindfulness groups.

Engaging a group of frail elders is a multifaceted endeavor for the teacher. There may be a range of abilities within any group. The teacher's sensitivity to individuals and the group as a whole requires flexibility and co-creation. Group contributions may be verbal or nonverbal, and the mindfulness teacher may play a more active role than traditional training requires. For example, if one participant is hard of hearing and another speaks softly, the teacher may repeat the comments or perhaps articulate nonverbal communication for a participant with vision limitations. Facial expression can offer nonverbal cues, yet processing time for elders is often slow, and the flat facial affect of those with Parkinson's disease may be taken as disinterest. It is helpful for the teacher to be knowledgeable on the common geriatric medical conditions and symptoms and/or have expert resources. In addition, the teacher's awareness of his/her own internalized aging bias and fears is essential. While actively assisting in communication, the teacher also speaks from his/her experience and authentic respect for the personhood of all group members.

Environmental Issues

Elders needing assistance may be supported by a range of housing options and will benefit mostly from on-site or in home MBI programs. Some elders live in their own home with family or professional caregivers. These elders may also make use of community programs such as senior centers and adult day programs. Some elders, however, require special housing to meet their needs. Specialized housing is often congregate and can include assisted living for more independent elders, to institutional living for those requiring the most assistance. Mindfulness teaching for frail elders and caregivers may take place in a wide range of settings, all with unique challenges and opportunities.

Elders in congregate housing and institutions may not easily connect due to communication challenges. The mindfulness teacher can facilitate connection with encouragement and concrete support. In groups I ran for institutionalized elders, members reported that they found the group experience to be very important. As one elder remarked, "I realize we all have pain." An adapted mindfulness program for low-income minority elders, ELDERSHINE, reported similar results. Elders in this program were co-housed but initially isolated. They reported that mindfulness skills not only improved coping with stress but also increased a sense of community within the assisted living building where the program was taught. ""[ELDERSHINE] brings people together and they feel comfortable talking about different things in life because they get to know the people in the circle" (Szanton, Wenzel, Connolly, & Piferi, 2011).

Dyads, or small group discussion, are generally inappropriate for frail elders. Small groups (total of 5–10 participants) are optimal, allowing the teacher to be more active and to ensure connection and communication with all members. Working with a partnered teacher can also be helpful for larger groups.

Groups for frail elders may also be held in a community program site, assisted living facility, or long-term care. Elders and caregivers may also benefit from individual mindfulness teaching in certain circumstances, when secluded due to infection, extreme frailty, or at the end of life, for example. Individual teaching can be in the resident's room or home. Optimally, the elder and caregiver can both participate, and recorded practices can be utilized between sessions. Mindfulness can also be taught by telephone or internet. A telephone group for homebound elders that I taught was very well received, with both participants and instructors feeling a sense of connection despite the lack of physical presence.

Community centers and assisted living sites may have dedicated space; however, many institutions will not. Groups may need to be held in dining areas or other public space where noise and interruptions occur. The teacher can make some adaptations to create a group milieu in this often semi-chaotic environment. Soft music can be used as a "white noise" to reduce intrusive sounds, and aromatherapy can help define a healing space that residents may come to associate with mindfulness practice. While modifying the environment may seem contrary to the mindfulness approach of "being with what is," I liken this kind of adaptation to closing a door to minimize distractions. Still, it may be impossible to prevent completely a confused and agitated resident from walking into the groups' space or a nurse from coming in with medications for a resident. In one group, I even had a doctor come in and, without a word, wheel a resident out of the group for an appointment! In these circumstances, the instructor has the opportunity to model the practice of equanimity.

Other requirements of the environment may include making space for wheelchairs and walkers. Logistically, to make ongoing classes work, forgetful elders may need reminders of the group time and location, and some may require an escort. Stewardship of the group will vary according to the specific environmental issues. For all frail elders, the attitude of acceptance, support, flexibility, and compassion should be modeled and conveyed by the instructor.

For Caregivers

For both formal and informal caregivers in mindfulness groups, the teacher may redirect the caregiver group expectation from a complaint session to self-care. Caregivers often focus on unhelpful worrying about the care receiver. To keep the participants engaged, the teacher will need to be sensitive to all of the reasons a caregiver may have difficulty with self-care.

Despite acknowledgment of stress, distress, and low life satisfaction, informal and formal caregivers are generally unlikely to utilize support services even when available and affordable. Most informal caregivers assume caregiving responsibilities as a natural extension of their connection to the family or friend care receiver. The care receiver is the center of attention and concern. Many informal caregivers do not self-identify as a "caregiver." Other reasons caregivers are reluctant to accept support are lack of free time and denial of need for assistance. Respite care may assist in some cases, allowing the caregiver time for self-care. Modifying the time of day a class is offered, group length, location, and course requirements may improve participation. Thus, the biggest challenge for caregivers may be to get them into the room.

Formal caregivers may participate in stress reduction classes if offered relief from their job responsibilities. Teaching mindfulness to frail elders and formal and informal caregivers within an institution may offer the opportunity for stewardship if the teacher is also an employee. The institution may become the "group" and the participants may reinforce the practices among themselves. During a mindfulness class I taught for staff, participants were able to remind each other to take a breath or eat mindfully when not in class, expanding the teaching from classroom to workplace. One private nursing home in Manchester, UK, has incorporated mindfulness training for all staff as a condition of service. The length of the working day has been extended to incorporate individual/team sitting meditation. Staff receive mindfulness training via daylong workshops provided by a dedicated team and distance learning and supervision as well as a "Buddy system" to provide ongoing peer support. Despite the interesting oxymoron of "mandated mindfulness," the trainers note that there has been "no objection to attend and support a Mindfulness based philosophy in the care of Elders" (Email correspondence, Henderson, 10 November, 2014). Without institutional support, however, it may be difficult to recruit professional caregivers in stress reduction training despite acknowledgment of high stress levels.

A group that includes formal and informal caregivers and care receivers allows caregivers relief from the guilt of taking a break and serves as an activity for both. More importantly, such a group emphasizes their essential sameness, denying the artificial separation between those who give care and those who receive it. Group members here are all breathing, stretching, and paying attention.

Homiletics or Delivery of Didactic Material

Content of mindfulness teaching is both didactic and experiential, learning from the outside and from our own internal experiences. Homiletics refers to the instruction of didactic material, less like a lecture and more like a dialogue. Elders may have communication challenges, such as hearing and vision loss, as well as cognitive changes requiring the teacher to adapt teaching methods. At the same time, mindfulness teaching conveys respect for the abilities of each individual.

For Frail Elders

The experiences of aging and caregiving offer rich material for teaching. The group will have similar experiences and stressors that resonate for all. For the teacher, reframing the elder's current life experiences may prove the richest work. In the context of a society that does not value aging, a medical system that often views aging as a disease, and institutions based on treating illness, frail elders may internalize these views. By connecting with the whole person and continually focusing on ability rather than disability, the teacher is able to reframe unhelpful perceptions. For example, frail institutionalized elders may express distress when their basic needs are not met in a timely way. Without discounting the pain this situation causes, a teacher may remind an elder of options to practice deep breathing, simple stretches, or guided imagery. This redirection also requires the teacher to avoid the "helper" mode, based on dependency, and step into co-creation with the participants.

Finding the appropriate learning edge for each participant requires connection and communication. In cognitively intact populations, the teacher is able to encourage and inspire the participants to increase their comfort level with discomfort. When the teacher is unable verbally to communicate encouragement and inspiration, the nonverbal alliance established with elders may serve. Make sure those with hearing limitations sit as close as possible to the instructor. Ask everyone to raise a hand if it's hard to hear the instructor's voice. Elders who are not able to articulate may often register responses through physical expression or behaviors. The teacher's mindful awareness will guide when to adapt and step in and when to allow and step back. With frail elders and elderly caregivers, adjustment to the practices as described above increases access. On the other hand, the mindful teacher will be aware when her desire to protect frail elders circumvents mindfulness practice. The verbal and nonverbal message continuously communicates/reinforces the message of working with adversity with acceptance and compassion.

As suggested above, elders display a wide range of abilities. In addition, frail elders may vary from day to day or even within the context of a single group. Parkinson's disease (PD) often presents in this way. Pickut et al. (2013) have pioneered a group for persons with PD and report: "PD symptoms may impact participation and function during training. Medication timing is important in order to help minimize motor and cognitive off's. Anticipating that people will have off's (sometimes sudden and unpredictable) within the time frame of the session maybe helpful" (Email communication, Pickut, August 18, 2014).

Isolated elders and caregivers may be taught individually or via internet and phone. Despite the distance, elders in one phone group reported benefits (McBee, 2008). Meditation instruction was given verbally with time for discussion and questions. The yoga poses were pre-mailed in handouts with visual information. Participants were given verbal instruction and then asked to put down the phone (some participants did not have a speakerphone at the time) and try the pose. Following this exercise, participants were able to discuss, ask questions, and report back.

For Frail Elders with Dementia

Teaching is generally associated with cognition, yet teaching mindfulness includes elements of transmission. The nature of mindfulness necessitates the use of experiential practice, group exercises, questions without answers, and stories and poetry to convey meaning. Rather than instructing, the mindfulness teacher creates an environment and the conditions for learning from within. In Eastern spiritual traditions, this may be referred to as the *transmission* of the teacher. This could also be described as co-creation, the learning created when a teacher engages a student with a beginner's (open) mind. Clearly, those with dementia have a beginner's mind, open to the present moment, giving the mindfulness instructor a unique opportunity. Of course working with a demented population is not this simple; there are often communication, emotional, and behavioral conditions that impede. Yet those with dementia may be highly attuned to affect and connection, allowing the teacher's embodiment of mindfulness practice to become the transmission. Connecting with the person beyond or behind this condition called dementia is the first step.

This connection is a felt sense on the part of the instructor and conveyed via eye contact, tone of voice, perhaps a touch on the hand, and/or body language. In a group, this becomes almost a dance, with the instructor moving from one participant to another, offering verbal encouragement, physical guidance, and eye contact to assess comprehension and inclusion. The teacher's awareness of potential communication differences, and her/his adjustment to each individual, requires both acute assessment skills and a general knowledge of the range of potential issues for elders. For some elders, the teacher may learn whether the right or left ear is less hard of hearing. For others, the teacher may know that even though they seem unengaged, they benefit from the group. Some agitated elders may disrupt the group initially but seem to settle in when patiently encouraged by the teacher. In these circumstances, the teacher may choose to sit with this elder, holding his/her hand. If the disruptive behavior continues and is causing other group members to become agitated, the elder may be moved slightly away from the group or even out or the group room by a staff member.

In the group setting on a dementia unit, I found it helpful to establish a routine structure. Each weekly class included deep breathing, simple stretches, and guided body scan, followed by simple discussion or comments. At the same time, I remained open to the unpredictable nature of a dementia unit. For example, one day, a resident wandered into the group carrying a plate of cookies during the meditation. This attracted everyone's interest, so we did an eating meditation. During another group, one member could not stay seated despite my encouragement due to physical agitation. So, while leading the meditation, I held her in my arms and walked in the center of the group.

For Caregivers

Both formal and informal caregivers face considerable stressors and often focus on their challenges during groups. This real-life experience is an excellent opportunity to explore the concept of our perception. One family member participating in a 10-week course modeled on MBSR described sitting outside with her mother, listening to a bird, and enjoying spring weather. She noted that in the past, she would have been worrying about her mother's declining health, but on this day, she could enjoy sharing the moment. Staff caregivers frequently reported taking a deep breath before difficult situations and finding this shifted their perception and their handling of the situation.

Many formal caregivers comment that the effects of stress reduction are counteracted when they return and feel overwhelmed by their workload again. I have found staff receptive to mindfulness skills when offered in 15-minute breaks, on the unit where staff are working. Teaching mindfulness in shorter and more accessible intervals may mean coming to where the caregiver is, at convenient times for them. It could include 10–15 minutes of deep breathing or stretches for professional caregivers in institutional settings during charting time or staff transition or meeting with informal caregivers individually for stress reduction.

Guidance of Formal Practices or Informal Group Experiences

An essential aspect of teaching mindfulness is guidance: the use of mindfulness practices and nonverbal instruction to facilitate participants' connection to their own inner experience and wisdom. Appreciating the value of all inner experience is key. While often not able to articulate feelings, frail elders remain feeling beings.

For Frail Elders

In a group setting, formal practices may be offered with adaptation, including the general guidelines suggested above. Co-creation of the group experience may require more active engagement by the teacher. During meditation or movement practices, the teacher may visually monitor participants to ensure communication is received and understood by all. During movement practices, the teacher may interact with individual members to demonstrate physically or hands-on assist for physical safety and maximum benefit.

The core of formal mindfulness practice is meditation, specifically awareness of the breath. Clearly, elders are breathing, and this pre-qualification for mindfulness is open to all. Articulating this baseline for participation conveys the fundamental intention of acceptance to all elders who are able to understand. Teaching awareness of breath may be problematic for those with cognitive impairment. For elders, often in wheelchairs or semi-slumped, the act of opening their front body and breathing deeply may begin to activate the parasympathetic nervous system or relaxation response, introducing the elder to the concept nonverbally. For the quiet sitting group experience, redirection is often required. For example, if I rhetorically ask, "what are you feeling?" an elder may reply out loud!

Meditations such as the body scan, sitting meditation with awareness of breath, and mindful movement may all be performed in a chair; walking meditation may be altered to wheeling meditation, or other mindful movement such as adapted chair yoga may be substituted.

Eating meditations may be adapted for those with special dietary needs. For some, soft foods or thickened liquids are appropriate. For those who can no longer eat by mouth, another mindful activity may be used. Elana Rosenbaum developed pioneering practices to introduce mindfulness in intensive care units. She uses ice chips for mindful mouth awareness and gentle movement in the bed for those with restrictions and frailty (Rosenbaum, 2012).

Gentle movement/yoga may be the best modality for teaching didactic material to elders with physical, cognitive, and communication loss. The essence of mindfulness teachings such as "there is more right with you than wrong with you," "abilities not disabilities," "non-judgmental awareness," and "being present in our bodies" may all be conveyed through mindful movement. For a clear description of basic postural and sensory adaptations for elders with moderate physical frailty and communication challenges, see Morone and Greco (2014). Mindfulness teachers concerned about safety in teaching movement for frail elders are encouraged to consult a specialist such as a physical or occupational therapist about contraindications for specific conditions. On the other hand, the medical model, focused on safety, often limits and disempowers elders from listening to their own body's wisdom.

Encouraging slow, mindful body awareness in the elders is helpful. Rather than focusing on the external representation of a particular pose, elders can be encouraged to move into the pose until they first feel a physical sensation. Staying at this point for a moment, the elder may notice some release that allows them to stretch a little further or not. Most importantly, the teacher encourages participants to back off if there is pain. Specific adaptations include poses for the chair or bed and the use of props such as pillows and blankets. The internet offers instruction on adapting yoga for the chair or bed. For inspiration, read *Waking*, by Matthew Sanford, who became a paraplegic at age 13 and later, a yoga teacher. Sanford describes how, despite being unable to move or feel his lower body, he still experiences sensations, such as "tingling, surges and even a mild burning" (2006, p. 82), and works with them in his yoga practice and teaching.

When giving basic sitting and yoga instructions, don't assume everyone can see. Be careful to describe movements thoroughly in words. The poses are generally held for short periods. The teacher may offer more assistance; a gentle hand may help the elder into a stretch without pushing or pulling. The overall practice may offer elders a renewed way of inhabiting their body and ultimately embodying life.

The Value of Homework

Frail elders may find it difficult to establish a daily formal practice without assistance. The use of computers, CD or MP3 players, written assignments, and journaling requires physical skills, memory, and executive function often no longer available. Caregivers may have limited time and inclination for rigorous homework assignments. Yet, elders and caregivers have many opportunities to practice interpersonal and other skills informally. It is helpful for the teacher to encourage this homework and use it as a basis for dialogue in group or individual settings. When an elder or caregiver describes a difficult situation, the teacher can discuss ways to use mindfulness practices when confronted with the distress or difficulties of daily life.

For Caregivers

Skills taught to caregivers may be most well received when taught in short and accessible stretches, as a caregiver/frail elder dyad and/or as skills that are usable while caregiving or performing related caregiving tasks. Respite care for the frail elder may increase caregiver participation. Groups taught to caregiver/frail elder dyads require teacher flexibility and creativity. While caregivers may understand didactic content, frail elders may better understand nonverbal content. Caregivers may be able to get on the floor for the body scan, while frail elders may need to stay seated. Ensuring inclusion of all group members with awareness of different levels of ability and understanding, the teacher also reinforces a sense of connection and similarity.

In addition to practicing formal skills, elders and caregivers may more likely practice informally with concrete suggestions. For example, before coping with a challenging caregiving experience, caregivers might be encouraged to take a deep slow belly breath. Mountain pose, seated or standing, simple stretches, deep breathing, and short meditations may all be practiced in the context of the busy caregiver's life. For example, caregivers I worked with responded well to Segal, Williams, and Teasdale's *Three Minute Breathing Space* (2008, p. 184) or the acronym *STOP* [stop, take a breath, observe, and proceed with what you were doing]. While longer, formal practice may offer more benefits, the shorter, as needed practices may also benefit and perhaps serve as an introduction to deeper formal practice.

Inquiry into Participants' Direct Experience

In MBSR teaching, dynamic inquiry is the cultivated format in which the teacher and the taught mutually explore their direct experience. The following quote from Rumi may best describe this engagement. "Beyond our ideas of right-doing and wrong-doing, there is a field. I'll meet you there."

(For an online video of this quote by translator Coleman Barks, see https://www.youtube.com/watch?v=a-AX6_YrsWM.)

For Elders

For those with cognitive loss or communication deficits, inquiry may be limited and more directive; nonverbal response may take a larger role. Elders' capacity to participate may be uneven or unpredictable. I have run groups in which elders only engage with their eyes or seem to be dozing, only to surprise me with a comment or response. Never underestimate a participant's ability to rise to the occasion, as illustrated below.

The story of *The Don't Hate Me Because I'm Beautiful Club*

It was at the end of our group and we were discussing what makes us feel proud and joyful. I went around the group, there were about 10 of us, and asked, "what are you proud of that makes you feel joy when you think of it?" Many responded the love of family, particularly, parents, and some talked about qualities that they possess including warmth, humor, and always doing their best. We somehow got on the topic of loving ourselves, which brought on lots of laughter, rolled eyes and conversation. It was during this time that I noticed a woman, who had been sleeping during our time together, woke up and wanted to contribute to the discussion. This woman, I'll call her Mary, had become more and more isolated from her community in the time that I had known her (about 8 months). When we first met I was struck by her wonderful sense of humor and wit. As time passed, she became more withdrawn and extremely anxious, and struggled with increasing difficulty with word-finding. It was clear that the conversation that we were having sparked something in Mary! I could see the twinkle in her eye. I inquired, "is here something that you would like to say?" Her response, "I can't help that I am beautiful!" Delivered with sardonic wit…beautiful! I asked the group if they heard what Mary had said, and most responded no, so I repeated it. At this point Mary was belly laughing, and the group responded in kind! Mary was generally not accepted by the others; her agitation and frequent outbursts made people uncomfortable, so they tended not to engage with her, and yet, in this moment, everyone reveled in her perfectly timed humor! It was beautiful and the beginning of *The Don't Hate Me Because I'm Beautiful Club*, to which I give Mary all the credit at the beginning of each group. (Email communication, Ellen Dimille, July 7, 2014)

This inquiry led to a group connection through laughter!

For Caregivers

Caregivers may learn mindfulness skills in traditional MBSR groups, with similar or more general populations. Many caregivers, however, will not participate in ongoing longer groups with expectations of home practice. Mindfulness groups for caregiver populations frequently offer shorter (1.5–2 hour) classes, shorter series length (5–7 classes), shorter (4 hour) retreats, and modified or no homework assignments. Clearly, these modifications may reduce the benefits found in the traditional MBSR format, and yet caregivers may learn via experiential exercises that they gain tools for self-care during their busy lives. Integrating yoga or mindful movement into daily activities, awareness of activities of daily living, and even using mindful caregiving may all be powerful and important for caregivers. At the same time, when caregivers engage in longer and more formal mindful practices, they may become increasingly aware of the emotional, physical, and psychological costs of caregiving. Inquiry in this context may reveal the grief, fear, guilt, and anger underlying the compulsive busyness for some caregivers. The instructor's ability to stay present may also help caregivers with difficult decisions as described below:

> Jane attended the class in her wheelchair. Her goal was to manage the stress of caregiving for her husband, who was suffering the late stages of dementia. He had asked her to agree that he be allowed to decline without employing measures that would prolong his life. She found this request agonizing. Meditation practice helped her to make peace with his decision, as well as difficult behavior not in keeping with his usual conduct. (Email communication, Laura Peters, May 28, 2014)

The forgiveness meditation, in which we offer forgiveness to ourselves and others, may be very meaningful in these circumstances.

Introductory mindfulness sessions may be a helpful way of engaging both family and professional caregivers. These groups may be offered as a workshop, 1 hour or more. I have also taught sessions as short as 15 minutes to caregivers. In short, single-session groups, inquiry with caregivers seeks to encourage self-care as an extension of caring for others. It may be done verbally, with discussions of the contagious nature of stress and also the effects of long-term stress. Frequently, I have found these mini-sessions well received and utilized, often leading to longer and more regular self-care.

The Practice of Living with Illness, Loss, and Dying

For elders and their caregivers, illness, loss, and death are not concepts but realities of daily life. Chronic and acute medical illness, pain, facing their death, or the death of friends and spouses may create a sense of immediacy and presence for these populations, making simulated exercises less relevant. During a mindfulness group series, a member may experience an illness with significant and obvious changes, and the group will also be faced with this loss, as well as the knowledge that they, too, may become more impaired. During a family caregiver group series, it is entirely possible that a one or more participants may lose their family member, and the other members will not only mourn this loss and also their own impending loss. Formal caregivers frequently experience sadness about the decline or loss of a patient.

A mindfulness instructor working with frail elders and caregivers also always remembers and nurtures the resiliency, wisdom, individuality, and humor of this population. Opportunities to hold discomfort and be with life's most challenging moments are presented within group or individual mindfulness teaching. Regardless of the group context or circumstances, the instructor serves as witness, acknowledging difficult changes in ways appropriate to the group or individual. Elders and caregivers are often responded to with medical solutions aimed at fixing a problem. As a mindfulness teacher, I often found the most helpful intervention was to be with, to be present, and to witness and acknowledge, verbally and nonverbally, all that cannot be fixed or changed.

Conclusion

Teaching mindfulness to frail elders and caregivers is not only feasible but also crucial. Aging, death, illness, and loss are inevitable, the one "special" category we all face. As teachers, we can learn from our own relationship to this inevitability. In my experience, it is the essential quality needed for teaching mindfulness to frail elders and caregivers, seeing that we are all alike in this quality of being human.

Sonnet LXXIII
That time of year thou mayst in me behold
When yellow leaves, or none, or few, do hang
Upon those boughs which shake against the cold,
Bare ruined choirs, where late the sweet birds sang.
In me thou see'st the twilight of such day
As after sunset fadeth in the west;
Which by and by black night doth take away,
Death's second self, that seals up all in rest.
In me thou see'st the glowing of such fire,
That on the ashes of his youth doth lie,
As the death-bed, whereon it must expire,
Consumed with that which it was nourish'd by.
This thou perceiv'st, which makes thy love more strong,
To love that well, which thou must leave ere long.
… William Shakespeare

Acknowledgments With gratitude for the contributions and support from my editor, Victoria Weill-Hagai, and all who bring mindfulness to frail elders and caregivers. I received teaching suggestions and contributions from Laura Peters, Human Resources Development and Learning Manager, Kendal (assisted living) at Ithaca, NY; Peter and Mo Henderson, mindfulness teachers, Manchester, UK; Ellen Dimille, volunteer, Converse Home, Burlington VT.; and Barbara Pickut, MD, Parkinson's Movement Disorders Program, Mercy Health Hauenstein Neurosciences, Grand Rapids, MI. For teaching mindfulness in the community to low-income elders, Amy Connelly and ELDERSHINE offer a guiding light. And my dear Elana (Rosenbaum) who brings mindfulness to everything and everybody, teacher, and colleague. I bow to you all and to the elders and caregivers whose patience allows us to learn and grow!

References

Bohlmeijer, E., Prenger, R., Taal, E., & Cuijpers, P. (2010). The effects of mindfulness-based stress reduction therapy on mental health of adults with a chronic medical disease: A meta-analysis. *Journal of Psychosomatic Research, 68*(6), 539–544.

Davidson, R. J., Kabat-Zinn, J., Schumacher, J., Rosenkranz, M., Muller, D., Santorelli, S. F., … Sheridan, J. F. (2003). Alterations in brain and immune function produced by mindfulness meditation. *Psychosomatic Medicine, 65*(4), 564–570.

de Frias, C. M., & Whyne, E. (2014). Stress on health-related quality of life in older adults: The protective nature of mindfulness. *Aging & Mental Health, 19*(3), 201–206. doi:10.1080/13607 863.2014.924090.

Epel, E. S., Blackburn, E. H., Lin, J., Dhabhar, F. S., Adler, N. E., Morrow, J. D., & Cawthon, R. M. (2004). Accelerated telomere shortening in response to life stress. *Proceedings of the National Academy of Sciences of the United States of America, 101*(49), 17312–17315.

Hölzel, B. K., Carmody, J., Vangel, M., Congleton, C., Yerramsetti, S. M., Gard, T., & Lazar, S. W. (2011). Mindfulness practice leads to increases in regional brain gray matter density. *Psychiatry Research, 191*(1), 36–43.

Larouche, E., Hudon, E., & Goulet, S. (2014). Potential benefits of mindfulness-based interventions in mild cognitive impairment and Alzheimer's disease: An interdisciplinary perspective. *Behavioural Brain Research, 276*, 199–212. doi:10.1016/j.bbr.2014.05.058.

McBee, L. (2008). *Mindfulness based elder care*. New York, NY: Springer.

McCown, D. (2013). *The ethical space of mindfulness in clinical practice*. London, England: Jessica Kingsley.

Morone, N. E., & Greco, C. M. (2014). Adapting mindfulness meditation for the older adult. *Mindfulness, 5*, 610–612. doi:10.1007/s12671-014-0297-z.

Moss, A., Reibel, D., Greeson, J., Thapar, A., Bubb, R., Salmon, J., & Newberg, A. (2014). An adapted mindfulness-based stress reduction program for elders in a continuing care retirement community: Quantitative and qualitative results from a pilot randomized controlled trial. *Journal of Applied Gerontology, 34*(4), 518–538. doi:10.1177/0733464814559411.

Paller, K. A., Creery, J. D., Florczak, S. M., Weintraub, S., Mesulam, M. M., Reber, P. J., … Maslar, M. (2014). Benefits of mindfulness training for patients with progressive cognitive decline and their caregivers. *American Journal of Alzheimer's Disease and Other Dementias, 30*(3), 257–267. doi:10.1177/1533317514545377.

Pickut, B. A., Van Hecke, W., Kerckhofs, E., Marien, P., Vanneste, S., Cras, P., & Parizel, P. M. (2013). Mindfulness based intervention in Parkinson's disease leads to structural brain changes on MRI: A randomized controlled longitudinal trial. *Clinical Neurology and Neurosurgery, 115*(12), 2419–2425.

Prakash, R. S., De Leon, A. A., Patterson, B., Schrida, B. L., & Janssen, A. L. (2014). Mindfulness and the aging brain: A proposed paradigm shift. *Frontiers in Aging Neuroscience, 6*, 120. doi:10.3389/fnagi.2014.00120.

Quintana Hernandez, D. J., Miro Barrachina, M. T., Fernandez, I. I., del Pino, A. S., Rodriguez, J. G., & Hernandez, J. R. (2013). Effects of a neuropsychology program based on mindfulness on Alzheimer's disease: Randomized double-blind clinical study. *Revista Española de Geriatría y Gerontología, 49*(4), 165–172.

Rosenbaum, E. (2012). *Being well (Even when you are sick)*. Boston, MA: Shambala.

Sanford, M. (2006). *Waking: A memoir of trauma and transcendence*. Emmaus, PA: Rodale.

Schulz, R., & Beach, S. R. (1999). Caregiving as a risk factor for mortality: The caregiver health effects study. *JAMA, 282*, 2215–2219.

Segal, Z., Williams, M., & Teasdale, J. (2008). *Mindfulness based cognitive therapy*. New York, NY: Guilford Press.

Szanton, S. L., Wenzel, J., Connolly, A. B., & Piferi, R. L. (2011). Examining mindfulness-based stress reduction: Perceptions from minority older adults residing in a low-income housing facility. *BMC Complementary and Alternative Medicine, 11*, 44. http://www.biomedcentral.com/1472-6882/11/44.

Torpy, J. M., Lynm, C., & Glass, R. M. (2006). Frailty in older adults. *JAMA, 296*(18), 2280. doi:10.1001/jama.296.18.2280.

Wells, R. E., Yeh, G. Y., Kerr, C. E., Wolkin, J., Davis, R. B., Tan, Y., … Kong, J. (2013). Meditation's impact on default mode network and hippocampus in mild cognitive impairment: a pilot study. *Neuroscience Letters, 556*, 15–19.

Whitebird, R. R., Kreitzer, M. J., Crain, A. L., Lewis, B. A., Hanson, L. R., & Enstad, C. J. (2013). Mindfulness-based stress reduction for family caregivers: A randomized controlled trial. *The Gerontologist, 53*(4), 676–686.

Chapter 15
Teaching Individuals with Developmental and Intellectual Disabilities

Nirbhay N. Singh and Monica Moore Jackman

Introduction

Intellectual and developmental disabilities are essentially lifelong chronic conditions, and psychological therapies are directed at preventing or reducing social, emotional, and behavioral problems often exhibited by individuals with these disabilities. Intervention efforts begin almost from birth (e.g., early intervention, special education) and continue throughout the life span to enhance adaptive behaviors (e.g., communication, daily living skills, and vocational activities) and to reduce maladaptive behaviors (e.g., aggression, property destruction, self-injury, pica, and rumination). Maladaptive behaviors have received most attention in the research literature, as well as in clinical practice, because of negative educational, vocational, and social consequences for individuals with intellectual and developmental disabilities (Singh, Lancioni, Winton, & Singh, 2011). In addition, severe and persistent maladaptive behaviors often significantly impair the quality of life not only of the individuals but also of their caregivers (Hastings, 2002).

A number of approaches have been taken to manage or treat the maladaptive behaviors of individuals with intellectual and developmental disabilities, including psychopharmacological, behavioral, and cognitive-behavioral strategies (Singh, Lancioni, Winton & Singh, 2011). Psychopharmacological approaches, although shown to be reasonably effective in managing maladaptive behaviors, have been gradually losing ground to other approaches because of the potential risks posed by the medicines on the health of the individuals. Behavioral approaches have proven

N.N. Singh, Ph.D. (✉)
Medical College of Georgia, Augusta University, Augusta, GA 30912, USA
e-mail: nisingh@augusta.edu

M.M. Jackman, O.T.D., M.H.S., O.T.R./L.
Little Lotus Therapy, 3242 SW Fillmore Street, Port Saint Lucie, FL 34953, USA
e-mail: mjackman2317@gmail.com

© Springer International Publishing Switzerland 2016
D. McCown et al., *Resources for Teaching Mindfulness*,
DOI 10.1007/978-3-319-30100-6_15

to be effective, but the approach does not lend itself to the individuals being able to effectively control their own maladaptive behaviors. Cognitive-behavioral strategies have emerged as the approach of choice because they enable the individuals to learn adaptive ways of managing or eliminating their maladaptive behaviors. Furthermore, they also enable the individuals to exercise self-control with overt and covert behaviors, thoughts, and feelings in multiple settings in the absence of their caregivers.

Recently, several mindfulness-based interventions have been used in the field of intellectual and developmental disabilities, attesting to the utility of these interventions with individuals with these disabilities, as well as with their caregivers (Harper, Webb, & Rayner, 2013; Hwang & Kearney, 2013, 2014; Myers, Winton, Lancioni, & Singh, 2014; Whittingham, 2014). Therapists can use a majority of these mindfulness-based interventions when working with caregivers—parents, paid caregivers, teachers, or clinical staff—of individuals with intellectual and developmental disabilities or directly with higher-functioning individuals with intellectual and developmental disabilities. One method, *Meditation on the Soles of the Feet* (SoF), was initially designed to be used with such individuals, but therapists have found it to be generally useful across various populations as an effective way of regulating one's emotional state when faced with an emotionally arousing situation.

In the first part of this chapter, we briefly discuss the SoF meditation and provide brief instructions for therapists (the term includes teachers). In addition, we suggest that therapists and their clients learn and use *Samatha*, a physiologically calming meditation, to enhance the utility of the SoF meditation during emotionally arousing situations in their life. In the lexicon of mindfulness-based interventions, mindfulness is integral to maintaining concentration during *Samatha* meditation, but the two terms (i.e., mindfulness and Samatha) are not interchangeable. For the purposes of this chapter, *Samatha* is understood to mean resting awareness on the chosen object of meditation (such as the breath) and using mindfulness in a regulatory capacity to ensure that concentration does not deviate from the object of meditative placement. In the second part, we present ways that therapists can support mindful engagement in individuals with intellectual and developmental disabilities to improve their quality of life.

Meditation on the Soles of the Feet

The SoF meditation is a simple procedure that therapists can use with clients who wish to control their arising anger, angry outbursts, or physical aggression. The meditation requires the practitioner to focus his (or her) awareness on the first noticeable physical and/or emotional changes that occur as anger arises. The practitioner rests his awareness on the perceived changes and then swiftly moves the awareness to a neutral part of the body, the soles of the feet. Finally, the practitioner uses mindfulness in a regulatory capacity to support concentration on the soles of the feet for a few minutes. This meditation provides a skillful means of dealing with arising anger by shifting attention and awareness from the anger-producing situation and any subsequent perceptions of the situation, to a neutral point on the body, the soles of the feet.

The SoF training manual provides detailed, step-by-step instructions for teaching an individual to learn the SoF meditation (Singh, Singh, Singh, Singh, & Winton, 2011). Here we provide an overview of the training steps, but therapists should note that these steps serve as a flexible guide rather than a static protocol. Therapists should individualize the training to maximize their client's potential to become an effective user of SoF. (An example of a soles of the feet script can be found in Section IV, Chapter 23, H.)

Step 1: Preliminaries (note: these preliminary teaching steps should be initiated when the individual is in a calm and alert state and is open to learning):

(a) *Goal and rationale.* Briefly discuss the nature of anger and how it leads to aggression and how aggressive behavior can cause problems for the individual in terms of injury to self and others, as well as in social relationships. Ascertain the methods the individual currently uses to control anger and how well these methods work. Then ask the individual if he would like to learn a new method that may help control anger a little better than the ones currently being used. Proceed if the individual agrees.

(b) *Introduce the SoF meditation.* Briefly provide an overview of the SoF meditation. Ascertain that the individual knows where the soles of the feet are and can identify the toes, arches, and heels of the feet. Ensure that the individual can fully focus attention on them without having to touch them.

Step 2: Practice SoF with a happy situation:

(a) Introduce the SoF meditation by having the individual recall a happy situation and be in that situation. Then instruct the individual to shift the focus of attention from the happy situation to the soles of the feet. SoF is best experienced initially if it is linked to a happy situation, because most of us can think of a happy situation very readily and can recreate specific instances of it in our minds.

(b) Work with the individual's sitting or standing posture and breathing during the training.

(c) Lead the individual through the SoF meditation based on the instructions provided in the manual.

Step 3: Practice SoF with an anger-producing situation:

(a) Inform the individual that you will repeat the SoF instructions with a situation that made the person angry.

(b) Repeat Step 2 with an anger-producing situation.

Step 4: Practice SoF with the trigger to the anger:

(a) Discuss with the individual the various triggers to anger-producing situations that the individual typically encounters.

(b) Take the individual through an anger-producing situation up to the point when the trigger occurred and observe closely for any nonverbal signs of rising anger—changes in the face, breathing, movements, and so on.
(c) Lead the individual through the SoF meditation with one of these triggers.

Step 5: Using SoF in daily life:

(a) Emphasize that the reason for learning the SoF meditation is to be able to use it, when needed, in daily life.
(b) Discuss the need to practice the SoF meditation and then to use it when needed.

The training manual provides instructions on how to assess a therapist's competency in teaching SoF, as well as forms for measuring progress.

Therapists may find that the SoF meditation works best if the client first learns to practice *Samatha* meditation, because it assists the individual to develop resting awareness on the object of meditation, usually the breath. This skill is used in the initial stages of the SoF meditation when the individual learns to rest his awareness on the physical and/or emotional changes noticed at the first inkling of arising anger. In addition, the practice of *Samatha* meditation requires the client to use mindfulness to maintain concentration on the chosen object of meditation (i.e., breathing). The same skill is required in SoF, when the client uses mindfulness to engage in unwavering concentration on the soles of the feet. Thus, the client is able to use both aspects of the *Samatha* meditation in the SoF meditation, which provides a skillful means of controlling arising anger and subsequent aggression. We see SoF as a stabilizing meditation (Dalai Lama, 2002) that shifts the focus of attention from the anger or emotionally arousing thought, event, or situation, to a neutral part of the body. This shift in attention leads to the fading of the anger or rapid deescalating of the emotionally arousing situation because the mind cannot fully concentrate on two non-habitual processes simultaneously (Foerde, Knowlton, & Poldrack, 2006).

A number of research studies have attested to the effectiveness of the SoF meditation in changing the behavior of individuals using it. In the initial study, a young man who functioned at the mild level of intellectual disabilities and had mental illness used SoF to effectively self-regulate his verbal and physical aggression in multiple contexts (Singh, Wahler, Adkins, & Myers, 2003). Prior to SoF training, his aggressive behaviors had precluded successful community placement several times, and community providers had mandated he must remain aggression-free for 6 months before being accepted in one of their group homes. Following baseline observations, the individual was taught the SoF meditation twice a day for 5 days, followed by a week of homework practice assignments. He was then instructed to use this meditation to regulate his emotion during rising anger in an effort to preempt the anger from manifesting as aggression. Results showed that, as his use of SoF progressed, there were substantial decreases in physical and verbal aggression, use of emergency medication, physical restraints, and staff and resident injuries, accompanied by considerable increases in self-control and physically and socially integrated activities in the community. These improvements resulted in his successful transition to the community without readmission to a facility, and he displayed no aggressive behavior during the 1-year follow-up after his community placement.

Effectiveness of the SoF meditation for emotion regulation has been confirmed in a series of subsequent experimental studies. For example, SoF has been shown to enable individuals who function at moderate levels of intellectual disabilities to control their anger and aggression, although the training procedure needed to be modified to enable individuals who function at this ability level to be able to learn and use it in daily life (Singh et al., 2007). Other studies have reported similar outcomes for male offenders with mild intellectual disabilities and adolescents with autism spectrum disorder, including Asperger syndrome (Myers et al., 2014). In a randomized control trial, the outcome for individuals with intellectual and developmental disabilities resulting from the use of SoF to control their aggressive behavior was found to be statistically and clinically significant when compared to a waiting list control (Singh et al., 2013). Other researchers have reported similar outcomes for SoF with different populations (e.g., Felver, Frank, & McEachern, 2014; Shababi-Shad, 2014; Wilson, Kasson, Gratz, & Guercio, 2015). In sum, the research data show much support for the use of the SoF meditation by individuals with intellectual and developmental disabilities.

Meditation Training for the Therapist for Using SoF

Our usual requirement for the therapist is to have a personal meditation practice that will inform the teaching of the meditation to clients, including individuals with intellectual and developmental disabilities and their caregivers. At a minimum, the therapist should have extensive experience with the basic *Samatha* meditation. In addition, the therapist should have learned and practiced the SoF meditation, as specified in the SoF training manual (Singh, Singh, Singh, Singh & Winton, 2011).

There are many reasons why a therapist needs to have a personal meditation practice. The therapist, much like any teacher of meditation, needs to be able to demonstrate how to sit with the proper posture and meditate. When a therapist meditates with his or her clients, the clients can observe the therapist embody not only the physical practice, but also nonverbal disposition. As we have noted elsewhere (Singh et al., 2014), mirror neurons are implicated in learning new skills through observation and imitation (Iacoboni, 2008). Simply observing the therapist meditate might provide the setting event for mirror neurons to fire in the brains of the individuals, thereby enhancing their meditation practice.

Clients often have questions that arise during the early stages of learning to meditate. While it is relatively easy to respond to their questions that arise from their lack of understanding of concepts and practices, the therapist needs to display authenticity and authority in answering questions that arise from the practice itself (McCown, Reibel, & Micozzi, 2017). These come about only with a personal meditation practice and the presence that comes with the practice. The therapist's response arises from deep within rather than from an intellectual understanding of the question and its answer. What arises meets the clients exactly where they are and not where the therapist would assume them to be in the absence of personal practice. The therapist's authenticity and embodiment of the practice enhances the sharing of experiences regardless of whether the experiences were proximal or distal in time, and brings about the oneness of the therapist and client, a mutual trust in the experiences. Having the experience of "been there, done that, and still doing it" enables the therapist to focus on the journey of meditation and not as a goal. These are critical skills that arise with a personal meditation practice.

Meditation Training for the Individuals in Treatment

Although not absolutely necessary for using the SoF meditation, for the reasons stated above, we strongly suggest that if the individual is capable of learning *Samatha* meditation, and wishes to engage in it, the therapist should make every effort to support the individual in this practice. Individuals with intellectual and developmental disabilities are invariably taught to engage in various activities because it is specified as a goal, with attendant objectives and interventions, in their individualized support plans (ISPs). However, meditation should not be specified in the individual's ISP, and hence there should not be a teaching goal, either for the individual or the therapist. The following is a standard instructional outline of a sitting meditation practice that therapists can personalize for individuals with intellectual and developmental disabilities.

Instructions: Sit comfortably on your zafu and zabuton (if you are using them), on a cushion, or on a straight-backed chair. If you have a meditation practice already, assume your posture in a full-lotus, half-lotus, Burmese, or kneeling (seiza) position. In Samatha meditation, you practice focusing just on your breath, which is the object of your meditation, to the exclusion of everything else:

1. Sit comfortably with a straight spine, without slouching or stretching your shoulders.
2. Tilt your head slightly forward, with the chin tucked in slightly toward the throat.
3. Have your eyes slightly open, if this is comfortable, or close them lightly if you have to.
4. Have the tip of your tongue lightly touch the upper palate, near the front teeth.
5. Have the right hand over the left hand at the height of your navel, with thumbs just touching each other (in the Zen mudra), or your hands resting lightly on your thighs.
6. Breathe evenly and try not to either shorten or lengthen each breath.
7. When invited by the meditation bell, focus your attention on the flow of your breath as it moves in through your nostrils into your body, back up, and out through your nostrils. That is, focus your attention on the sensation of breath-

ing—from the beginning to the end of inhalation, the pause before exhalation, from the beginning to the end of exhalation, the pause before inhalation, and so on.

8. If you are novice at meditating and need an aid to keep your attention on your breath, silently count each inhalation and exhalation. Count "1" when you inhale and count "2" when you exhale, and so on until you reach 10. Repeat this process until your meditation deepens and you can meditate without counting. If you are an adept, follow your usual routine.

9. When you realize that your mind has wandered away, gently bring it back to focus on your breathing and begin a new round of counting.

10. When invited by the bell, gently bring yourself back out of meditation.

Therapists should not assume anything about the individual and approach each training session with a beginner's mind (Suzuki, 1970). It is best to spend some time with the individual prior to the formal meditation training so that you can determine how to most effectively communicate with the person, understand what the person is giving you, and identify which aspects you can skillfully use to support the person in the meditation training. As the training progresses, be mindful of the person's progress and be fully present with him (or her) during each session.

Therapists usually begin the preparation by discussing what meditation is, why we do it, its benefits, the time it takes, and, if the individual chooses to learn how to meditate, how you will provide the training and support. Although we may be enamored by meditation and think it is good for everyone, do not present it as a choiceless choice so that the person feels pressured or obligated to participate. If the individual makes a choice to participate, begin the training with a discussion of where (e.g., floor or chair; quiet environment) and how (i.e., posture) to sit during meditation. Begin with the basic instructions for sitting, either on a chair (which may be most convenient for most individuals) or on the floor using a zafu (pillow) and zabuton (flat cushion). If the individual chooses to sit on the floor, the Burmese or kneeling (seiza) postures may be the easiest forms to adopt. Be prepared to model alternative postures and go with what the individual chooses. Demonstrate the entire mediation posture—hands, eyes, jaws, tongue, shoulders, and back.

We have found that some individuals have difficulty understanding "focus on your breath," "observe your breath," or "count your breath," and it is wise to spend some time ascertaining that they understand this concept. We hold a mirror under their nose so that they can "observe" their breath, and we work with them until they understand how they can follow the pattern of breathing in and breathing out, without altering the length or nature of the breath. We also might use concrete objects, such as a balloon to illustrate that when one inhales, the belly is filled with air and when one exhales, the belly empties.

In their enthusiasm, novice meditators sometimes want to meditate for long periods from the first day of training. Therapists should emphasize that the meditation might be kept short at first to enable the mind and body to adjust to the meditation posture and the focus on the breath. We usually begin with 2- to 5-minutes sittings and very gradually build it up to 20 minutes. In our experience, individuals with intellectual and developmental disabilities, especially those with autism spectrum disorder, sometimes get pretty rigid about their routines and may in fact regularly sit for 20-minutes meditation sessions once they have mastered the practice.

Begin the Samatha meditation practice with the individual by sitting with the individual until you are meditating together for 20 minutes a day. Then, gradually fade yourself out of the sitting and support the individual to sit in mediation alone as a personal practice. Experience suggests that individuals with intellectual and developmental disabilities can learn to be mindful of their behavior, but that instructions need to be individualized, the training process customized to their style of learning, and they need lots of practice to be able to be mindful in the rhythm of their life. While it is time-consuming, the outcomes for the individuals are immeasurable in terms of downstream effects in the quality of their life.

Mindful Engagement Support Model for Caregivers

Over the last decade, we have developed a mindful engagement support (MES) model that therapists can use to enhance mindfulness in their clients who are involved in human service delivery systems. Our interest here is to briefly explicate the model and then outline how therapists can utilize this model to train caregivers of individuals with intellectual and developmental disabilities, regardless of whether these individuals live independently in supported living arrangements, community group homes, or in family homes with their parents and siblings. Caregivers include parents, paid staff, school teachers, clinical staff, and anyone else that enable individuals with intellectual and developmental disabilities to have a better quality of life. Therapists can provide this training in either individual or group format and in either clinic or on-site consultation. The central issue is that therapists should be well versed in the component parts of the MES model and embody the mindfulness teachings in a seamless manner.

Mindful engagement involves the active investment of one's self in daily activities. It is the "moment-by-moment awareness and nonjudgmental engagement in an activity, without expectation of specific outcomes" (Jackman, 2014, p. 243). Engagement differs from doing or participation in that it requires the person to be fully immersed in the present, without expectation of a desired result or anticipated outcome. Doing and participation are commonly tied to an external obligation or contingency and can become automatic in nature, resulting in one "going through the motions" in a mindless manner to complete a task. Mindful engagement is a state of being that offers a richness of experience that might be missed when action is guided by a predefined goal or requirement, and/or awareness is diminished. It is a way of living and interacting with one's physical and social environment that one can learn through meditation and mindfulness practice. By cultivating mindfulness practice in daily life, one can experience engagement and the enhanced quality of life that accompanies this state of being.

Some individuals with intellectual and developmental disabilities might lack the requisite skills to practice mindfulness meditation and may not be able to experience engagement without the support of their caregivers. Many individuals with intellectual and developmental disabilities live in community group homes, where daily schedule and activities are often driven by consideration of staffing needs and external agency regulations. The press to adhere to regulatory procedures can result in a culture of rule-governed behavior of both caregivers and the individuals they serve. Individuals can become passive recipients of services dictated by predetermined schedules, while caregivers provide assistance mandated by plans and individual objectives that are developed by the individual's treatment team and shaped by service reimbursement policies and/or regulatory requirements. These requirements can lead to a culture in which clients and caregivers regress to a mindless adherence to participation in daily activities to meet progress or risk management objectives. Interventions designed to meet quantitative measureable objectives can result in limited awareness and insight as to the quality of the individual's daily experiences, even in the most compassionate of caregivers.

Training of Caregivers in MES

Therapists can train caregivers to mindfully support individuals with intellectual and developmental disabilities, regardless of where these individuals live or their level of functioning, by being present, open, and receptive to each individual in each unfolding moment. As therapists, we have found training to be most engaging when we use diverse methods and a flexible structure to teach concepts and practices. To teach just at the right level that makes sense to the caregivers requires skillful presentation of the core concepts of the model.

This method of teaching is aligned with the concept of *upaya*, or skillful means, that may include Socratic methods for eliciting principles of practice, contextual storytelling, humor, pointed examples, references to current research and practice, and open dynamic interactions with the caregivers. For example, while we start with *Samatha* meditation, we may add a body scan meditation (a guided meditation that instructs practitioners to notice the various areas of the body) if caregivers are having some difficulty with aches and pains in their bodies. We also observe caregivers during meditation and adjust the duration of the practice according to how they are responding with their posture, facial expressions, and movements. As *Samatha* is a meditation for calm and tranquility and focus on the breath that may be difficult if the mind is scattered (Sumedho, 2007), we teach them to bring their attention to discomfort, emotions, and thoughts that are present and accept them as "it's the way it is" (Sumedho, 2007, p. 113). If a caregiver is from a specific religious faith, such as Christianity, we may encourage that person to meditate on a meaningful prayer or verse of scripture rather than on the breath as the chosen object of meditation. Meditation is conducted throughout two days of formal training, typically for 5–20 minutes every 1–2 hours, with formal and informal meditations each day thereafter.

Mindful Engagement Training: Part 1

Part 1 of caregiver and clinical staff training includes *Samatha* meditation and an introduction to the principles of mindful engagement with group development of an initial mindful engagement support plan (MESP), followed by immersion training in the MES model. Therapists begin by teaching caregivers and clinical staff the practice of *Samatha* meditation, with a focus not only on form and meditation instructions but also attitude and intention. The emphasis is not on the personal benefits that meditation can provide but on the potential impact of meditation practice for loved ones, co-workers, and clients. They then use errorless learning (Carr, 2012) to assist the caregivers to develop an initial MESP by prompting them to contemplate one simple question, which is "If you could do one thing to make this person's life better, what would it be?" Therapists ask the caregivers to practice *Samatha* daily for 20 minutes, a day and implement the initial MESPs.

Mindful Engagement Training: Part 2

Part 2 of formal training is a full day of training that occurs about three months after the Part 1 introduction, enabling the caregivers to have built up their formal *Samatha* meditation practice to at least 20 minutes a day in the first 4 weeks and to engage in the practice for the remaining 8 weeks. In the interim, between Parts 1 and 2, therapists provide monthly teaching and mentoring to caregivers and clinical staff via direct observation, review of videos, and updating of MESPs using continued errorless learning methodology. Once the caregivers have been able to experience the practice of mindful engagement support via the execution of the MESPs and have stabilized their practice of ongoing formal mindfulness meditation, the therapist provides a formal full-day training. The purpose of Part 2 training is to teach the core concepts (detailed below) of the MES model and the framework for providing mindful engagement support. Therapists have found that once caregivers have an experiential context for the core concepts in practice, they are more likely to begin to understand them in terms of application when presented in a didactic manner. In addition, they are able to appreciate the difference between a medical model of treatment that is typically focused on disease, disorder or disability, and "doing to" an individual and the MES model, which prioritizes quality of life and the importance of "being with" and supporting an individual.

After introduction of the mindful engagement support core concepts, therapists provide training on the practice of mindful listening and mindful communication using games, exercises, and didactic teaching to illustrate these practices. Given that many individuals with intellectual and developmental disabilities have limited communication skills and caregivers are required to frequently work with other caregivers and clinicians, mindful, open, and nonjudgmental awareness is vital to meaningful and accurate information exchange. Experience has taught us that informal *sati* practice during listening and communication is most beneficial at this stage of training, and so these are the focus of our general standards of practice training for Part 2.

Core Concepts of the MES Model

The core concepts provide understanding of differentiation between more traditional Individual Support Plan (ISP) treatment planning, which is typically aligned with a medical and mechanistic model of care and the MES model. While the ISP model is often referred to as person centered, it typically results in planning for daily activities that are selected by the treatment team and/or rendering provider based on goals related to medical care, amelioration of risk, and/or skill building. In contrast, the MES model is rooted in bringing clinical and compassionate awareness to support actualization of individualized quality of life outcomes. The paradigm shift involves moving from a model of care grounded in periodic analysis and practice in a predetermined and structured time-bound format to that of a model that stems from open and intuitive awareness of and response to each individual's needs in each emerging moment. Caregivers use skillful means to support individuals to engage in quality of life activities, as needed, instead of teaching them team or provider-prescribed skills at scheduled times.

Individualized Routines Versus Fixed Schedule

ISP goals and interventions are often implemented in a clinical or convenient environment and performed in accordance with staff, group home, or family schedules. The MES model requires consideration of each individual's rhythm of life and the patterns and routines that are natural to each person's internal time perception. For example, some individuals function better and are happier when they wake up early, but others require more sleep to prepare them for the day. Some schedules typically require all individuals to wake up, receive grooming and dressing care, and eat at around the same time for the convenience of staff or families. Individualized routines follow each individual's preferred pace and sequence for engagement in daily activities and include a physical context that is meaningful to the individual (e.g., performing range of motion exercises during dressing and bathing, rather than in the therapy clinic).

Response Versus Reaction

The ISP and medical model approach often result in a reactive approach to caregiving and risk management. For example, some individuals with intellectual and developmental disabilities might exhibit challenging behaviors due to limited communication, poorly developed flexibility and coping skills, and/or difficulty managing frustration. When an individual exhibits a challenging behavior, such as aggression or self-injury, this elicits a reaction by caregivers and creates the need for a behavior plan to manage the challenging behavior that has already occurred. The MES model emphasizes the importance of response over reaction. While reaction is guided by habit and is often mindless and quick, response is guided by ongoing intuitive awareness of often-subtle cues and precursors of difficult situations. For example, one reacts to a traffic light changing to green by accelerating without regard to surroundings having perceived the signal to "go," whereas one responds by looking to ensure that the intersection is free of errant cars and pedestrians before carefully driving on. We use the term "regret prevention" to describe the use of compassionate awareness to cultivate a practice of responding with regard to the potential consequence of our actions on others.

Support Versus Assisting

Assisting in a community care setting is typically characterized by using predetermined plans to help an individual. Assisting tends to be prescriptive and often follows formulated stages or levels of assistance, one step at a time (e.g., progression from physical assistance to physical prompting). Mindful engagement uses 5-step prompting (no help, nonspecific prompt, verbal prompt, demonstration, assistance) to provide a level of support to enable an individual to engage in an activity. Caregivers provide support that is flexible and allows response to an individual's potentially changing needs within varying temporal, physical, and social contexts, as well as dynamic needs, abilities, and motivation levels. This is where the caregiver's knowledge and use of *upaya* comes into its own.

Activities Versus Prescribed Exercises

Individuals who need support and/or supervision may require specialized therapy programs and protocols to help them to engage in activities that are important to their health, well-being, and quality of life. Under a medical or ISP model, this may involve exercises for skills such as standing, ambulation, balance, strengthening, range of motion, problem solving, and using augmentative communication. An example of an exercise may be pulling on a therapy band to increase arm strength or standing in a standing box to build standing endurance. In contrast, an activity implies a degree of motivation and fun for the individual to achieve the same ends as an exercise. For example, an individual who enjoys games and social interaction that would benefit from arm strengthening and standing endurance to increase and enhance quality of life may be supported to engage in assisted standing to use a lightly weighted tennis racket to hit a balloon back and forth to a peer. For individuals who require care, especially 24-hour care, the majority of social encounters are typically medical and clinical in nature. We train staff to understand that fun and learning are not mutually exclusive and that quality of life can be greatly enhanced by integrating activities that are fun into therapy and learning programs.

Autonomy Versus Independence

Many individuals with intellectual and developmental disabilities are unable to perform daily tasks independently and require support, modification of task, and/or specialized equipment to maximize performance and independence. However, while working toward independence can be beneficial if the individual has increased independence as a goal, it does not necessarily contribute to enhanced engagement or quality of life. Autonomy speaks to the individual's ability to have control and choice over daily activities, which may or may not involve independence. For example, an individual may be physically able to gain skills in ambulating independently, but he may choose to use a walker or power chair to conserve his energy so that he may engage in other activities that he enjoys, such as playing and moving to music. The difference can be subtle, but caregivers are able to discern and understand a client's level of autonomy and how it impacts engagement through the practice of ongoing intuitive awareness and observation.

Engagement Versus Participation

Mindful engagement is a state of being, which requires active presence. Participation can be passive and is typically focused on a goal directed task. There is a qualitative difference during observation of an individual who is participating or doing without awareness, or with a goal directed focus, and an individual who is mindfully engaged. With the former, the expectation of outcome may induce stress if there is a press for time or if the outcome is not meaningful to the individual. Boredom or frustration could occur if there is a mismatch between task demands and skill or arousal level. In the process of mindful engagement, there is enjoyment and reinforcement in the act of being while invested in an activity, i.e., the reward is inherent in the engagement and is not dependent on the outcome of the activity or achievement of an objective.

The CREATE Framework for Mindful Engagement Support Plans

The acronym CREATE represents the framework of elements that therapists can use to enable caregivers to understand how to support each individual to experience an engagement opportunity. These elements are the foundation of client assessment and observation and are used to build MESPs. Though we discuss these elements in the process of developing the initial engagement support plans in Part 1 of the training, we do not introduce the concepts explicitly until Part 2, so that caregivers have experienced some practical exposure to the concepts during the first interim immersion stage. Thus, when we provide definitions of these factors, caregivers have a reference point to support understanding over cognitive knowing.

C: Choice, Control, and Curiosity

Choice is central to an engagement experience, particularly in individuals with difficulties in accessing preferred items and communicating wants and needs. In some settings, choice and control can be limited, as schedule is often predetermined, and interventions and activities might be rigid in design and plan. Therapists can train staff to conduct ongoing preference assessment to ensure that the individual is intrinsically motivated to engage in, rather than passively participate in an activity. In addition, novel items or activities that are interesting to an individual can promote curiosity, which has been shown to promote learning (Gruber, Gelman, & Ranganath, 2014).

R: Response, Regret Prevention, and Reinforcement

The practice of *sati*, or mindful present moment remembrance of the needs of others, requires cultivation of response over reaction. Therapists teach caregivers to be present in the space between stimulus and response to ensure the use of the most compassionate and skillful means of responding for each individual or peer, depending on the time and situation. Thus, the second "R" for this element is what we term "regret prevention." The third aspect is the provision of positive reinforcement throughout interaction and support of each individual, which requires ongoing awareness and attention to individual cues and behaviors.

E: Environment

This factor involves an understanding of how one's environment can support engagement. This may include the physical environment (e.g., temperature, sensory properties), the social environment (e.g., preferred staff), and the temporal context (e.g., time of day). Awareness of the impact of environment on each individual requires not only context-specific present moment awareness but also a broader awareness of individual patterns, habits and trends.

A: Awareness, Attention, and Attitude

This is the most involved factor in terms of training, and therapists teach the practice of both internal and external caregiver awareness using games and exercises. The therapists introduce the concepts and role of perception and fabrication in response to one's thoughts, feelings, and bodily sensations. They discuss attitude as it relates to going with the flow, following the individual and not just the treatment plan or daily planned activities, seeing the person as a new person each time with a beginner's mind, and "giving each moment a chance." Finally, the therapists address the influence of individual attention and awareness on engagement in individuals with intellectual and developmental disabilities.

T: Task Demands

According to flow theory, a flow state is more likely to occur when challenge and skill levels are above average and are in balance—too much challenge can induce anxiety and too little challenge can result in boredom (Csikszentmihalyi & Nakamura, 2011). Similarly, supporting engagement may require careful task analysis and task modification to match individual to meaningful task. At this point in training, the therapists may expand upon the 5-step prompting method of support.

E: Energy

Analysis and discernment of energy level is important in creating an engagement experience. If an individual is too tired or too excited for a planned activity, engagement in that activity may not occur. Once again, therapists emphasize the use of skillful means to modify the activity or engagement plan to fit the individual and/or support the individual to become more alert or relaxed to match the activity and allow for engagement to unfold.

Mindful Engagement Training: Part 3

Between Part 2 and Part 3 of training, caregivers engage in a 1-month immersion period in which they continue to implement MESPs. Part 3 of the training is the second full day of training for caregivers. Therapists continue with *Samatha* meditation throughout the training day for formal practice and use multiple methodologies (didactic, activities, games, video analysis) for teaching informal practice of general guidelines and the implementation of the CREATE engagement framework.

Mindful Pause, Mindful Pace, Mindful Eating, Attitude, and Embodiment

Part 3 of training begins with presentation of the remaining standards of practice for provision of mindful engagement support. Mindful pause and mindful pace are essential to preventing the "hurry up and wait" mentality that is consistent with the

Western culture at large, especially when working with individuals who might have delayed processing ability. Slowing the pace of caregiving can require development of patience, which is a critical component of acceptance and present moment awareness. Sumedho (2007, p. 113) taught, "Patience is an essential ingredient. It means that we are willing to let something be what it is." Therapists emphasize that the practice of *Samatha* meditation can help caregivers to strengthen their ability to stay in the moment and that this mindfulness practice cultivates the art of staying.

Therapists guide caregivers and clinical staff through an exercise to help them to understand the difference between simultaneous multitasking and mindful serial monotasking. This particular exercise provides an experiential understanding of how doing too much at once can compromise the quality of engagement and illustrates how simultaneous multitasking can negatively influence intuitive awareness and presence. Therapists utilize mindful eating and mindful client handling activities in conjunction with sensitivity training exercises to teach caregivers these standards of mindful practice.

Throughout Part 3 of training, therapists continue to emphasize mindful attitude, which is vital to the practice of compassionate care and the use of skillful means to best support each individual. Embodiment of right mindfulness practice can result in positive benefits for individuals directly as evidenced by research on caregiver mindfulness and resultant behavioral changes in individuals with intellectual disabilities and behavioral difficulties (Myers et al., 2014). In addition, caregiver and clinical staff embodiment of *sati-sampajañña* can benefit individuals indirectly by increasing the caregivers' capacity to use *upaya*. That is, when caregivers are able to embody *sati-sampajañña*, they intuitively recognize the needs of each individual in their care and spontaneously use and adapt appropriate supports aligned with the changing needs and wants of the individuals.

Documentation and Creative Response

Therapists conclude Part 3 training with review and analysis of video segments of caregivers working with individuals to implement MESPs. They use errorless learning methodology to guide caregivers and clinical staff to identify aspects of the CREATE framework to provide insightful documentation that informs subsequent support planning.

Experience has taught us that creativity and insight are both vital to the practice of mindful engagement support. When discussing the practice of *upaya* in the workplace, Gallagher and Metcalf (2012, p. 118) suggested that "…begin where you are, work with what you have, and create from there." Therapists use exercises to promote creativity and lateral thinking and to erode habitual and static thinking tendencies—the most basic of which is to ask the question, "What would be the best support or solution if there were no rules?" When discussing mindful creativity, Langer (2005, p. 103) stated that "rules are, by their very nature, mindless limitations on our attention to the context in which we do things." By hypothetically suspending rules that govern practice, daily schedules, and care provision, caregivers are able to think beyond mechanistic and medical model modes of treatment planning and gain new insight into service delivery.

Individuals who practice mindfulness are more likely to exhibit enhanced creativity as measured by divergent and convergent thinking (Capurso, Fabbro, & Crescentini, 2014). Divergent thinking is necessary when brainstorming during mindful engagement support planning. Convergent thinking can assist caregivers in selecting the most appropriate solution to the identified problem or barrier.

Throughout Part 3 of training, therapists emphasize the importance of seeing the individual as a new person in each moment and in being open to all suggestions from all caregivers and clinical team members. With mindful caregivers and clinical team members, frank discussions are not only common but also encouraged. The team members' ability to argue with each other about the quality of life of the individuals they serve and how to provide services that will actualize such quality is one of their greatest assets, individually and as a team. It is the therapist's role to listen to, participate in, and stoke these arguments in the best interests of the individual. The setting for interdisciplinary collaboration is seen as a safe environment where staff can agree or disagree, without fear of having their voice drowned out, belittled, or mocked. The team meeting is a place where people feel safe enough to discuss every aspect of the individual's life in the hope of bringing new dimensions to the MESPs, which ultimately will enable the individual to enjoy, experience, and live life fully even in the face of severe and debilitating disabilities.

Conclusion

Therapists can teach mindfulness practices to individuals with intellectual and developmental disabilities and their caregivers. Indeed, individuals with intellectual and developmental disabilities can learn to successfully use such meditations as *Samatha* for personal development and soles of the feet for specific behavioral reasons, such as to manage anger and aggression. Furthermore, the individuals can also teach their peers to use soles of the feet to successfully control their anger and aggression (Singh et al., 2011). With training in meditation, caregivers of individuals with intellectual and developmental disabilities can provide services in a mindful manner. The MES model provides an alternative to the traditional ISP and medical models of care that have become ossified in their policies and practices to such an extent that the services appear to be mechanistically delivered based on prescriptive goals, objectives, and interventions. With the MES model, caregivers are freed to focus on the quality of life of the individuals they care for. In turn, they experience unexpected and swift positive changes in the individuals that stand out in stark relief to the outcomes of mechanical compliance common with staid programmed interventions of the past.

References

Capurso, V., Fabbro, F., & Crescentini, C. (2014). Mindful creativity: The influence of mindfulness meditation on creative thinking. *Frontiers in Psychology, 4*, 1020.

Carr, J. E. (2012). Training novice instructors to implement errorless discrete-trial teaching: A sequential analysis. *Behavior Analysis in Practice, 5*(2), 13–23.

Csikszentmihalyi, M., & Nakamura, J. (2011). Positive psychology: Where did it come from, where is it going? In K. M. Sheldon, T. B. Kashdan, & M. F. Steger (Eds.), *Designing positive psychology* (pp. 2–9). New York, NY: Oxford University Press.

Felver, J. C., Frank, J. L., & McEachern, A. D. (2014). Effectiveness, acceptability, and feasibility of the soles of the feet mindfulness-based intervention with elementary school students. *Mindfulness, 5*, 589–597.

Foerde, K., Knowlton, B. J., & Poldrack, R. A. (2006). Modulation of competing memory systems by distraction. *Proceedings of the National Academy of Sciences, 103*, 11778–11783.

Gallagher, B. J., & Metcalf, F. (2012). *Being Buddha at work: 108 ancient truths on change, stress, money, and success*. San Francisco, CA: Berrett-Koehler.

Gruber, M. J., Gelman, B. D., & Ranganath, C. (2014). States of curiosity modulate hippocampus-dependent learning via the dopaminergic circuit. *Neuron, 84*(2), 486–496.

Harper, S. K., Webb, T. L., & Rayner, K. (2013). The effectiveness of mindfulness-based interventions for supporting people with intellectual disabilities: A narrative review. *Behavior Modification, 37*, 431–453.

Hastings, R. P. (2002). Parental stress and behaviour problems in children with developmental disability. *Journal of Intellectual and Developmental Disability, 27*, 149–160.

Hwang, Y.-S., & Kearney, P. (2013). A systematic review of mindfulness intervention for individuals with developmental disabilities: Long-term practice and long lasting effects. *Research in Developmental Disabilities, 34*, 314–326.

Hwang, Y.-S., & Kearney, P. (2014). Mindful and mutual care for individuals with developmental disabilities: A systematic literature review. *Journal of Child and Family Studies, 34*, 314–326.

Iacoboni, M. (2008). *Mirroring people: The new science of how we connect with others*. New York, NY: Farrar, Straus and Giroux.

Jackman, M. M. (2014). Mindful occupational engagement. In N. N. Singh (Ed.), *Psychology of meditation* (pp. 241–277). New York, NY: Nova Science.

Lama, D. (2002). *How to practice: The way to a meaningful life*. New York, NY: Atria Books.

Langer, E. (2005). *On becoming an artist: Reinventing yourself through mindful creativity*. New York, NY: Ballantine Books.

McCown, D., Reibel, D., & Micozzi, M. S. (2017). *Teaching mindfulness: A practical guide for clinicians and educators*. New York, NY: Springer.

Myers, R. E., Winton, A. S. W., Lancioni, G. E., & Singh, N. N. (2014). Mindfulness in developmental disabilities. In N. N. Singh (Ed.), *Psychology of meditation* (pp. 209–240). New York, NY: Nova Science.

Shababi-Shad, S. (2014). *Use of a mindfulness practice to decrease problem behavior and increase engaged time of three students in an elementary school setting*. Vancouver, BC: University of British Columbia. Retrieved May 28, 2015, from https://circle.ubc.ca/bitstream/handle/2429/46379/ubc_2014_spring_shababishad_sara.pdf?sequence=4.

Singh, N. N., Lancioni, G. E., Karazsia, B. T., Winton, A. S. W., Myers, R. E., Singh, A. N. A., … Singh, J. (2013). Mindfulness-based treatment of aggression in individuals with intellectual disabilities: A waiting-list control study. *Mindfulness, 4*, 158–167.

Singh, N. N., Lancioni, G. E., Winton, A. S. W., Adkins, A. D., Singh, J., & Singh, A. (2007). Mindfulness training assists individuals with moderate mental retardation to maintain their community placements. *Behavior Modification, 31*, 800–814.

Singh, N. N., Lancioni, G. E., Winton, A. S. W., Singh, J., Singh, A. N. A., & Singh, A. D. A. (2011). Peer with intellectual disabilities as a mindfulness-based anger and aggression management therapist. *Research in Developmental Disabilities, 32*, 2690–2696.

Singh, N. N., Lancioni, G. E., Winton, A. S. W., Singh, J., Singh, A. N. A., & Singh, A. D. A. (2014). Mindful caregiving and support. In J. K. Luiselli (Ed.), *Children and youth with autism-spectrum disorders (ASD): Recent advances and innovations in assessment, education and intervention* (pp. 208–221). New York, NY: Oxford University Press.

Singh, N. N., Lancioni, G. E., Winton, A. S. W., & Singh, J. (2011). Aggression, tantrums, and other externally driven challenging behaviors. In J. L. Matson & P. Sturmey (Eds.), *International handbook of autism and pervasive developmental disorders* (pp. 413–435). New York, NY: Springer.

Singh, N. N., Singh, J., Singh, A. D. A., Singh, A. N. A., & Winton, A. S. W. (2011). *Meditation on the soles of the feet for anger management: A trainer's manual*. Raleigh, NC: Fernleaf (www.fernleafpub.com).

Singh, N. N., Wahler, R. G., Adkins, A. D., & Myers, R. E. (2003). Soles of the feet: A mindfulness-based self-control intervention for aggression by an individual with mild mental retardation and mental illness. *Research in Developmental Disabilities, 24*, 158–169.

Sumedho, A. (2007). *The sound of silence: The selected teachings of Ajahn Sumedho*. Boston, MA: Wisdom.

Suzuki, S. (1970). *Zen mind, beginner's mind*. Boston, MA: Weatherhill.

Whittingham, K. (2014). Parents of children with disabilities, mindfulness and acceptance: a review and a call for research. *Mindfulness, 5*, 704–709.

Wilson, A. N., Kasson, E. M., Gratz, O., & Guercio, J. M. (2015). Exploring the clinical utility of a stimulus avoidance assessment to enhance a relaxation training model. *Behavior Analysis in Practice, 8*, 57–61.

Chapter 16
Teaching Individuals in Chronic Pain

Lone Overby Fjorback and Else-Marie D. Elmholdt Jegindø

> There is no
> greater joy than
> when a person is
> suddenly freed
> from pain.
>
> —Unknown

Pain as a Biopsychosocial Phenomenon

Pain is a complex phenomenon. The International Association for the Study of Pain (IASP) defines pain as "an unpleasant sensory and emotional experience associated with actual or potential tissue damage, or described in terms of such damage" (IASP, 1994). This definition has been accepted worldwide as the standard pain definition not only by most clinics, but also by pain researchers, and indicates that pain is always a subjective experience including both sensory and affective dimensions. On the one hand, tactual tissue or nerve damage is not a necessary condition for pain experience, so pain can be present without actual nociceptive processing. The individual's experience of pain, on the other hand, does in fact serve as both a necessary and sufficient condition for the presence of pain. In other words, when patients express that they are in pain, we need to acknowledge the experience, regardless of other information (e.g., lack of "physical" evidence).

L.O. Fjorback, M.D., Ph.D. (✉)
Danish Center for Mindfulness, Aarhus University Hospital, Aarhus University,
Barthsgarde 5, Aarhus 8200, Denmark
e-mail: lonefjor@rm.dk

E.-M.D. Elmholdt Jegindø, Ph.D.
Research Clinic for Functional Disorders and Psychosomatics, Aarhus University Hospital,
Barthsgade 5, 3rd floor, Aarhus DK-8200, Denmark
e-mail: else-marie@cfin.au.dk

© Springer International Publishing Switzerland 2016
D. McCown et al., *Resources for Teaching Mindfulness*,
DOI 10.1007/978-3-319-30100-6_16

Another important aspect to keep in mind is that the *context* in which the afflicted individual experiences pain is highly influential. Various psychological, social, and cultural factors interact with the underlying brain mechanisms involved in pain processing. Hence, the mental state of the individual and the circumstances in which pain is experienced are known to contribute significantly to neurobiological aspects of pain. Accordingly, defining pain as a biopsychosocial phenomenon is the most heuristic approach, both in pain treatment and in pain research. In order to engage fully with our patients, it is important to understand and keep in mind the various factors that interact with and contribute to pain conditions. The following sections deal with the neurobiological, psychological, sociocultural, and cognitive aspects of pain separately, but one should bear in mind that these dimensions are integrated, reciprocal, and dialectical parts of the individual's complete pain experience. These descriptions will then be followed with sections detailing the application of mindfulness techniques when working with this population.

The Cerebral Signature for Pain: A Salience Detection System

The complexity of pain is demonstrated on the anatomical level by the complex and highly distributed neural components involved in pain processing. René Descartes is famous for his notion of pain as a hardwired system passively transmitting the noxious stimulus through sensory channels to the pineal gland, which he considered "le siège de l'âme" (eng. "the seat of the soul", Descartes & Timmermans, 1649/2010). Thanks to new and noninvasive brain imaging technologies, we now know that the conscious experience of pain is the result of cortical activity and that there are two main pathways: ascending and descending pain processing. Ascending input originating in the peripheral nerves projects to the dorsal horn of the spinal cord and via the brainstem to a large and distributed network of brain regions. In contrast, descending pain processing can either facilitate or inhibit the noxious information processing via this network.

The pain research community now characterizes pain as being part of a "salience detection system": "a system involved in detecting, orienting attention towards, and reacting to the occurrence of salient sensory events" (Legrain, Iannetti, Plaghki, & Mouraux, 2011, p. 111). Thus, the fundamental role of the nociceptive system is to detect salient changes and facilitate appropriate responses in accordance with the homeostatic principle. This perspective stresses the importance of context, and on a larger scale, it is broadly recognized that various psychological and social mechanisms may therefore influence the experience of pain.

Psychological Factors

When we experience pain, a number of psychological factors may mediate and modulate the condition. The psychosocial context surrounding the pain patient is often a major contributor to the subjective experience of pain and to neurobiological pain mechanisms. In previous studies, *expectations* about pain have been shown to account for between 25 and 81 % of the variance in pain intensity scores (see e.g., Price, Finniss, & Benedetti, 2008; Benedetti, 2009; Meissner et al., 2011). Desire for pain relief has also been demonstrated as a critical motivational factor. Desire is related to wanting, in the sense that you either want something to happen (e.g., pain relief) or want to avoid something from happening (e.g., augmentation or persistence of pain).

The role of anxiety in pain experience and pain processing is palpable yet complex. It is unknown exactly how anxiety and pain interact, but it is well established that the two factors mutually affect one another. As a core example of negative affect, anxiety is a pro-nociceptive mechanism, which increases pain sensitivity at a neurophysiological level. Patients who have a high degree of anxiety will thus be more sensitive to pain signals. It may be the case that anxiety enhances pain, but in some circumstances, pain may also generate or exacerbate anxiety. The reciprocal link between pain and anxiety can lead to further negative emotional affect and pain catastrophizing thoughts, which may fuel a vicious cycle, particularly for chronic pain patients. The Pain Catastrophizing Scale (PCS) by Sullivan (1995) is often used in the clinic and in pain research to investigate the possible presence and influence of patients' exaggerated negative mental activity during pain perception or anticipation of pain (Keefe, Brown, Wallston, & Caldwell, 1989; Sullivan, Stanish, Waite, Sullivan, & Tripp, 1998). Studies have established comparable links for depression (e.g., Gormsen, Rosenberg, Bach, & Jensen, 2010) and stress (e.g., Logan et al., 2001). Coping efficacy, sense of control, and personality have also been shown to influence pain processing (Folkman & Lazarus, 1988). Indeed, it seems impossible to isolate a single determining factor, which further illustrates the importance of context.

Sociocultural Factors

From an historical perspective, both conceptualization and treatment of pain have developed over time and across geographical regions. Indeed, cultural and social factors are the foundation for our expression and treatment of pain. That is, cultural contexts shape our perceptions and experiences of pain, pain behavior, and pain treatment strategies (Jegindø, 2012). The social and cultural context that surrounds the person in pain will therefore affect pain expressions, the words (or sounds) used to express pain, and the assessment of pain. It has also been demonstrated that the immediate social environment, especially family history, plays an important role for future pain experiences. The prevalence of pain disorders is significantly higher in patients whose parents have a history of pain disorder and affective disorders such as depression and anxiety (Hudson, Goldenberg, Pope, Keck, & Schlesinger, 1992), and parent behavior and other mental factors may influence pain in children and adolescents.

Similarly, the interactions between pain patients and their spouses often contribute to the "dynamics" of the actual pain experience and of verbal and nonverbal pain communication (Gauthier, Thibault, & Sullivan, 2011). Another critical aspect of the patient's context is the set of cultural beliefs and norms that shape both pain response and pain treatment. For instance, cultural and religious beliefs may produce certain expectations and assumptions about the causes of pain and of diseases in general. In some contexts, illness is interpreted in terms of sin, black magic, bad karma, or impurity. Likewise, treatment strategies and outcomes are likely to be affected by such beliefs (Jegindø, 2012).

Cognition and Pain Modulation

The descending pain modulatory system is considered to be a bidirectional central control of nociception that can either inhibit or facilitate nociceptive processing. In terms of adaptive survival, the former can be advantageous in "fight or flight" situations, while the latter can be useful in situations where attention and care to afflicted tissue is needed. The problem occurs when either hypoalgesia or hyperalgesia (for pain terminology, see IASP, 1994) becomes a chronic state. Some hypoalgesic patients risk serious tissue damage due to reduced cortical processing of noxious input. Conversely, one of the biggest challenges in pain management is to help patients whose hyperalgesic states remain "switched on" long after normal and expected healing time, as is often the case in chronic pain conditions.

Like pain itself, pain modulation is a multidimensional process. The descending pain modulatory system is believed to project from cortical regions, the anterior cingulate cortex (ACC) and via the periaqueductal gray matter (PAG) in the midbrain through the rostral ventromedial medulla (RVM) to the spinal cord. Other areas such as the amygdala, thalamus, and the hypothalamus may also be involved, but evidence seems to suggest that the prefrontal regions serve as the main regulators of top-down pain modulation, especially the ventrolateral and the dorsolateral prefrontal cortices (VLPFC/DLPFC). A variety of cognitive processes are known to influence pain. The main categories are related to attention, coping, and expectations, which are discussed in turn.

Attention: Distraction is one of the most effective and well-documented pain modulators. Several behavioral and neuroimaging studies have confirmed that distraction from the painful stimulus by attention to a non-painful sensory stimulus or a cognitively demanding task can help to relieve pain by reducing attention to the nociceptive input (e.g., Buhle & Wager, 2010). This modulation again relates to the salience detection mechanisms. As mentioned, this system helps to orient attention, and in some situations, the appropriate response may require a shift in attention from one sensory stimulus to another, i.e., the more salient stimulus in terms of adaptive survival.

Coping: The effect of emotional pain regulation is a modulation that occurs when affective states influence pain processing. Emotional stress, negative affect, and especially anxiety increase pain sensitivity, whereas positive affect and positive arousal decrease pain sensitivity. The context of the painful event and the subject's conscious or unconscious interpretations of this context have a major influence in pain regulation. Sense of control and acceptance both decrease pain sensitivity and serve as adaptive coping strategies. Similarly, a coping strategy known as reappraisal helps to reduce pain as input, which would usually be interpreted as (tissue) threatening and detected as such by the relevant brain regions. Pain can be reevaluated through reappraisal mechanisms guided by the prefrontal regions (Ochsner & Gross, 2005). Adding meaning and positive beliefs will also generate positive reappraisal effects. The most familiar example of this reappraisal effect is childbirth. Most women consider it to be an exceedingly painful affair, but in the context of delivering a child, the painful event is often reinterpreted due to the highly meaningful and (now usually) non-life-threatening context, which is driven mainly by positive affect and positive expectations.

Expectations and placebo: Expectations about the outcome of a treatment, the progression of an illness, or experimental conditions are known to contribute to major parts of the variances in outcome measures (see above). They are part of the psychosocial context of (pain) studies and (pain) treatment. They can be induced by suggestions and/or conditioning, and can either be conscious or unconscious to the subject. The psychosocial context of the study or the treatment also depends on more external aspects such as physical properties (e.g., the way a waiting room or an operating room usually looks, the scientific objects that are present, and the profession-specific uniforms worn by the healthcare staff) and context-dependent behaviors/procedures. We expect doctors, nurses, and experimental researchers to do and say certain things—and *what* they choose to do/say, and *how* they do/say it, can have a major impact on the patient's expectations, and therefore on their brains. Renowned placebo and nocebo researcher, Fabrizio Benedetti, is famous for stressing that placebos change the patient's brain, literally speaking (Benedetti, Carlino, & Pollo, 2011). He explains that placebo treatments are based on the administration of inert substances, or sham physical treatments such as sham surgery, but placebos as such are *not* inert. They are made of "words and rituals, symbols, and meanings, and all these elements are active in shaping the patient's brain" (ibid., p. 1). Together with verbal suggestions of clinical benefit and/or conditioning, the inert substances have real and significant neurobiological, behavioral, and subjective effects. The placebo effect is also a learning phenomenon based on different (Bayesian) mechanisms, and the magnitude of placebo analgesia thus depends on previous experience of analgesic effects.

Over the last couple of decades, placebo and nocebo studies have established a highly significant role of positive and negative expectations on neural pain processing and pain modulation. Nocebo effects are the opposite of placebo effects, wherein expectations of a negative outcome lead to worsening of a symptom or a clinical condition. A series of elegant studies by Luana Colloca and colleagues from Benedetti's laboratory have, thus, shown how *words can be painful*, i.e., how negative verbal suggestions can lead to increased anxiety and, thus, to increased pain sensitivity (see Colloca & Finniss, 2012).

Neurochemical underpinnings of doctor–patient relationships: In the late 1970s, Jon Levine and colleagues demonstrated that the opioid antagonist, naloxone, could block both opioid and placebo analgesia (Levine, Gordon, & Fields,

1978). Since then, it has been accepted that at least some types of placebo analgesia are opioidergic. In other words, positive expectations can engage the body's own painkillers. Elegant open/hidden paradigms and protocols have further emphasized the critical role of both positive and negative expectations in neuromodulation. In 1995, Benedetti et al. showed that the analgesic effect of the drug proglumide only occurs in a placebo context when expectations are given and not when the drug is given without the patient's knowledge in a hidden infusion (Benedetti, Mayberg, Wager, Stohler, & Zubieta, 2005). Similarly, morphine and other powerful analgesics have been found to be significantly less effective in hidden trials when patients are completely unaware that a painkiller has been administered. By contrast, an open injection of saline *thought* to be morphine (a placebo trial) can be just as effective as a hidden infusion of 6–8 mg morphine (Levine, Gordon, Smith, & Fields, 1981). Finally, disruption of postsurgical morphine dramatically increases pain levels, except when disconnection of the infusion is unknown to the patient. These perspectives are extremely important for our clinical work as they highlight the fact that our interaction and relationships with our patients fundamentally change the neural basis for their current and future experiences of both symptoms and healthcare. In short, our words and actions can both ease and augment pain.

Mindfulness Therapy

Every year, hundreds of patients who experience multiple, persistent, and disabling symptoms are referred to our hospital clinic. Most suffer from some form of chronic pain condition, and for the most part, these symptoms cannot be explained by well-defined medical or surgical conditions. We term illnesses that are characterized by such symptoms "bodily distress syndrome" (BDS). BDS requires functional somatic symptoms from at least three out of four bodily systems: the cardiopulmonary, gastrointestinal, musculoskeletal, or general symptoms, and moderate to severe impairment in daily living, and at least 6 months of duration. The BDS classification is developed from empirical research and may unite functional somatic syndromes such as fibromyalgia, chronic fatigue syndrome, irritable bowel syndrome, chronic whiplash, and somatization disorder (Fink & Schroder, 2010). These conditions belong to the same family of disorders, and BDS may be a useful, non-stigmatizing designation for the group of closely related conditions that are currently divided into medical and psychiatric disorders. In the following, however, we focus on clinical applications of mindfulness therapy primarily in the context of chronic pain.

   The co-occurrence of negative affect and pain is well recognized, as we have seen, and an impaired ability to evaluate and categorize painful sensations could indicate a deficiency in the cognitive regulation of pain perception in patients suffering from chronic pain. This dysfunction may be due to changes in the parietal and prefrontal cortex, which are the areas that sustained training of mindfulness may improve (e.g., Hölzel et al., 2008). Impairments of sensory processing may also lead to repetitive overloading, which may in turn lead to fear of movement and unhealthy coping strategies.

Patients often describe that they shift between ignoring and being completely overwhelmed by pain and other somatic symptoms. Our patients often describe an inability to detect and react to bodily sensations as a state of stress in the body of which they are not aware. In contrast, mindfulness training may improve stress and emotional regulation, and it may train patients in the ability to notice when bodily sensations, thoughts, and emotions arise and help them embrace these sensations in a friendly, nonjudgmental awareness. Mindfulness training may enable one to notice the selective process or the automatic filters that regulate the flow of energy and information in what may be considered the mind.

No matter what we believe as medical practitioners, the fact remains that the majority of chronic pain patients have experienced an odyssey of treatments through the healthcare system and through alternative treatments. Safety guidelines are therefore highly recommended. When it comes to chronic pain patients, modern medicine and alternative treatments seem to have forgotten Hippocrates' guidance of first doing no harm. The word mindfulness implies to "remember." Remember the body, the mind (intelligence), and the heart (kindness). This triad is so obvious and trivial, but it may, nevertheless, be exactly what is called for in modern medicine. Teaching how to feel whole, physically present, mentally clear, and emotionally balanced may, indeed, be an integral part of modern medicine. Since the patients start out with a problem in the body, learning how to be present in the body, instead of trying to escape from it, is a very practical and useful skill.

Medical assessment is important because it ensures that the patients receive the right diagnosis, which is the basis for the right treatment. Mindfulness is not a cure one can use when nothing else is working, but it may very well be the right treatment if the body is distressed and/or in pain to a level where the person is no longer functioning.

Not a "Fix"

Chronic pain patients are suffering, and mindfulness entails working with the very stress and pain that causes the suffering. According to the Buddha himself, we are all suffering, but, for chronic pain patients, the physical suffering is so present that it cannot be ignored. However, when our patients enter the clinic, they are often looking to have their body "fixed" rather than to look at what it means for them to be suffering and to work with this reality. The tools offered by medicine, including psychiatry, are intended to "fix" or attack the symptoms, not to release suffering or promote flourishing. However, the "real trick" might be to help our patients to recognize that pain is a multidimensional and complex phenomenon. The brain sometimes produces a conscious experience of pain so vivid and intense that we feel certain that "something is seriously wrong with me." However, the fact remains that at times even intense and disabling pain experiences need not be due to physical injuries. At the same time, patients should be reassured that pain is a very common human phenomenon, not an indication or further verification of their own judgements of themselves as a person in whom there is "something wrong."

Instead, many chronic pain patients will need to work with other aspects of their pain experiences, in particular with their *relationship* to the pain, as we shall see below. This step is where mindfulness practice becomes a particularly good ally in their daily battles.

> We habitually declare war on the things that afflict us. The person who lies back and says, 'this is my lot. So be it', is a quitter, a passive, pessimistic, spineless loser who deserves only our contempt. And yet, the very moment I stopped thinking of my condition as 'the enemy', I made a turn and began to get better. I wasn't cured, wasn't forever well, but I was better. Siri Husvedt, Novelist

(Husvedt, 2012)

How to engage individuals with a chronic pain condition in the work of observing and embracing a painful and/or fatigued body, how to inspire them to use what is now known from modern medicine, and how to engage in their everyday lives is an ever evolving process, in which mindfulness can make a real contribution. In the following sections, we elaborate on clinical experiences from the perspective of a physician and practitioner.

How to Work with Chronic Pain

Essentially, this work is all about "relationality"; your relationship to the patients, to what they share/do, to your own practice, and it is ultimately about facilitating a change in your patients' relationship to themselves and the issues with which they are struggling. Your success as a practitioner will also depend on your ability to trust the practice, the patient, and the group. Do not think you know how it is to be in pain, fatigued and anxious all the time, and in case you know, you still do not know what it is like for the particular patients you are teaching. And you do not have to know. What you have to do, however, is to engage with the patients, give safe directions and know what is called for moment by moment.

Thoughts Control Behavior

The way we perceive our problems or pain is an important factor in determining how we react. If you think "this is ruining my life," it most likely will do just that. Many people, including chronic pain patients, speculate about situations or events that have gone wrong. Through psychotherapy, we can examine new and old conflicts and the reasons for why people repeat the same undesirable reaction patterns. In cognitive behavioral therapy, we work with the thoughts that lead to disability, low self-esteem, and disorder-driven behavior. When patients experience a lot of pain and/or other symptoms, it may be difficult to find a cause, particularly in the case of chronic (idiopathic) pain. Even though they learn to change their thought patterns and their behavior, symptoms may persist. This situation is where mindfulness can be particularly helpful, as it can increase acceptance of symptoms that are impossible or difficult to change.

Accepting (life, as it is right now) often involves approaching feelings of denial, anger, and sorrow. Patients may be deluded, thinking how great their lives were before the pain occurred or how they may never get better. There is no need, at this point, to turn the conversation into a debate. Your job as the teacher is to listen and to offer connection. You have to take care of the group, and you may need to schedule an individual meeting at this point. When the connection is strong enough, and the time is right, it may be very useful to start questioning such delusions. Often our participants actually begin to do that by themselves—because insights often come with practice. We spend quite a lot of time on psycho-education in our classes, because many patients have misconceptions about pain and physical symptoms, misconceptions that lead to destructive behavior. We keep asking them about their thoughts, feelings, and behavior related to the symptoms. It helps to take a friendly approach to noticing symptoms and to explicitly view thoughts as just passing thoughts, not permanent truths.

Physical and Psychological are Interrelated

Attempting to divide symptoms into physical and psychological categories is an obsolete approach. As we have seen in the previous sections, the intensity of pain varies over time. Negative thinking makes pain worse, for example, catastrophizing about pain and thinking it will never get better or thinking it will definitely get worse from now on. The mind cannot concentrate for a particularly long period of time, neither can it concentrate on pain all the time. If one really focuses the concentration on the pain, the attention moves, exactly as it does when one tries to keep the concentration focused on the breathing. It may help patients to place a hand where it hurts and have them say to themselves, "I'm taking care of this."

Many MBSR participants say they do not experience any difference in the first weeks. However, by the end of the course, they are surprised to find that they have either completely stopped or use considerably fewer painkillers. By practicing mindfulness daily and learning to focus on, and examining, their pain in a friendly and nonjudgmental way, most find that the sensation of pain tends to move or change in quality and/or intensity over time. This experience is worth directly examining with your patients throughout the course as this perspective may help them to recognize that pain is not "a constant." It allows us to acknowledge and experience that pain is dependent on several factors and thus—at least to some degree and at least in some moments—manageable. As we have seen, the context in which pain occurs changes pain processing and experience. Try, for example, to examine the thoughts and feelings that surround the actual sensation of pain. Your patients may discover that pain is much more than just the physical sensation of pain. Additionally, they can learn to experience pain as "just pain" without its surplus burdens. Potentially, such practices may alter the patient's appraisal of the pain and facilitate more adaptive coping, as discussed above.

Rehabilitation and the Staircase Model

Rehabilitation following stress and chronic pain follows the same principles as rehabilitation after a broken limb or a sports injury. Correct and regular rehabilitation results in fewer complications and fewer relapses. Breaking from the rehabilitation principles (forcing rehabilitation and ignoring warning signs) results in a "jagged" process, with large oscillations in outcome, which often prevent the patients from becoming well.

Life consists of good days and bad days. Many people are not conscious of the fact that when they are facing pain or illness, their mood continues to swing, just at a lower level. Often when our patients are in a good mood, they think, "I better get out and do something." This way, they overstrain themselves and end up feeling even worse. They have started a vicious cycle. The appropriate alternative is for patients to examine how badly they feel on bad days, to accept it, and slowly *practice* their way up from there, one step at a time. This approach is known as the staircase model.

Where We Often Get Lost: Thoughts and Feelings

The mind is inherently critical and judgmental. Negative thinking affects the body. We are all prone to negative thinking when tired, sad, or experiencing pain and other symptoms. If a person has offended us, the mind has prepared a long series of thoughts about how terrible it is. A tone of voice, a movement, and we are caught. It does not take much for the mind to have a whole narrative story or "novel" ready. Becoming conscious of the negative thoughts that are controlling one's life is an important step towards improving one's well-being. In our experience, the most difficult part of mindfulness is the practice of not taking your thoughts seriously. We are used to "existing" in our thoughts, and frequently, we do not discover the other, bigger, and more interesting reality.

When life is difficult, it is almost second nature to think that "something is wrong." We often run into self-blame when we feel lonely, sad, ashamed, or angry. When thinking goes off on such a track and pain or other difficulties are experienced as a personal failure, suffering is amplified. The task is to guide our patients to take responsibility for the original pain, feel it—and let it pass. That is, they need to work on their tendencies to either ignore or to amplify the pain.

Let the feeling pass: During meditation, people may discover emotions, thoughts, or tensions previously unknown to them. Instruct your patients not to try to explain to themselves why a certain feeling overwhelms them. Many people believe they have to find an explanation for their emotions or tensions, but that will frequently trigger even more thoughts. As with all experiences, negative feelings and sensations should be seen, held, and acknowledged. But with mindfulness, we can practice not supressing or holding on and not fueling them with the surplus burdens of fear, anger, and sadness. Instead, we can practice embrazing the feelings and letting them be and pass.

To open and shut the door: At some point, most people feel a need to shut out the world. Reality can be so hard that we cannot confront it. It can be difficult to endure when our loved ones or we face difficulties. The technique of "shutting out" is as old as the technique of opening up. When we meditate, we can practice imagining awareness as a door that can be opened or closed. Instruct your patients to work on their limits. The door should not be held wide open all the time. Each person needs to feel when it is enough, and close the door again. The task is to be awake the whole time and conscious of when you are opening and closing the door. Perhaps this is what the Sufi poet and philosopher Rumi references in the poem, *The Breeze at Dawn*:

> The breeze at dawn has secrets to tell you.
> Don't go back to sleep.
> You must ask for what you really want.
> Don't go back to sleep.
> People are going back and forth across the
> door sill, where the two worlds touch.
> The door is round and open.
> Don't go back to sleep.
> —Rumi

It won't last: As mentioned, chronic pain patients often catastrophize about their condition, for example, by thinking that pain will definitely get worse, that it will never end, or that there is nothing they can do to reduce pain. We therefore suggest that it may be useful to examine and ultimately challenge such thoughts in order to break the vicious cycle. Karen Blixen (author) was once given a letter and was told that she could only open the letter when she was very sad or very happy. She opened the letter when she was very sad, and the letter said, "It won't last."

Yoga and Chronic Pain

Many illnesses, disorders, conditions cause the body to tense unconsciously; stress, depression, sorrow, BDS, etc. This tension causes pain. Some people experience actual weakness or paralysis. Chronic pain patients often refrain from physical activity from fear they might exacerbate pain sensations. Unfortunately, this behavioral pattern fuels a double vicious cycle in chronic pain. Sustained physical inactivity leads to muscle atrophy, decreased flexibility, joint stiffness, and decreased cardiovascular fitness, and, ultimately, more pain and less physical activity. Consequently, patients are more prone to experience sleep disturbance, fatigue, and anhedonia, and they risk further aggravation due to related social withdrawal. Eventually, many patients struggle with both severe pain and depressive states.

I (LF) was extremely excited when I first began teaching yoga to patients suffering from BDS. "Now we are going to do something that will make them feel well," I thought to myself. I had previously taught retired senior citizens and patients suffering from schizophrenia, and my experience was that these people often arrived annoyed and tired, but left happy. Unfortunately, my BDS patients left frustrated and even more tired and sad than when they had arrived. It turned out that many of our patients had a kind of "body phobia." All of their bodily signals told them the exercises were dangerous and they would become ill. Consequently, the patients' reactions tended to represent two extremes. One group would not move, while another group would move too much and, hence, overstrain their bodies.

The technique we use now, and which works well, is to instruct the patients to feel their bodies and to make their own decision about how much they can move. It has become clear that the individual's own way of carrying out the exercise is more important than the instructions. The overall goal here is to help break the vicious cycle of chronic pain by introducing gentle physical exercises while respecting the individuals' unique boundaries.

Guiding yoga: The purpose of yoga poses (*asanas*) is to remove physical tensions, drowsiness, fatigue, and discomfort, in order to ease meditation and concentration, and to awaken energy and live life fully. There are 196 *sutras*, but only two of them cover asanas, and the general guidelines are: (1) they have to be comfortable and stable, (2) future pain should and can be avoided. Many chronic pain patients avoid yoga due to fear of symptom aggravation. The important thing is that they get going at their own pace and come to feel comfortable doing the exercises.

Yoga consists of exercises, where you feel your body by using your breathing and focusing your attention. It is about being as close as possible to your breathing and body, exactly as with body scanning. You learn to respect the body's limits and relax tense muscles. You can do yoga standing up, sitting down, on your back, in a bed, or in a wheelchair. All that is required of yoga is that you breathe and make some kind of voluntary movement.

Yoga should be done in tandem with meditation. This state means you keep focused on the now. Do not try to be somewhere else. Allow yourself to be, as you are. Let go of self-judging thoughts. See your thoughts and feelings and accept them, for example, frustration over what your body cannot do, or the habit of trying to overreach yourself. You are your own expert, so move carefully. If there are exercises, you are not ready to do, lie in a comfortable position, close your eyes, feel your breathing and imagine you are doing the exercises. You need to work with your body, so try to do as many of the exercise as possible, so that you will feel something happening.

You are encouraged to examine your body's limits and to respect them, so that you do not overreach. You are the only one who can feel where your limit is. You can use your breathing as a pathfinder. If you hold your breath and tense your face, you have pushed yourself too far. Go back a little, breathe freely, and concentrate on feeling the exercise. You can also notice if you have begun to compete with yourself or others. The most important yoga exercise is called the "Corpse Pose." You lie on your back with your arms by your side, legs straight out, and feet splayed apart. You concentrate on being completely still and feeling your body in this position. You are as still, and completely let yourself go, as if you were dead.

The word yoga can be translated as "to unite or to create harmony between the body and the mind or between physical and mental energy." Yoga, therefore, is not about fitness. It cannot be emphasized enough that the aim of yoga is to *feel* the body. If you are good at yoga, you are good at feeling your body. Frequently, we conclude a yoga session by asking participants to feel the contact they have with their bodies. Feeling the body, just the way they are feeling it. It can be a very pleasant experience, regardless of the condition of the body.

Teacher Perspectives

As teachers, we may think we know who is "getting it" and who is not. We may place the wisdom, the desire, and the trouble within different participants in the group. It is crucially important to remind oneself that actually, we do not know. In the beginning, I (LF) would be thinking all week between classes how I could formulate my points so that the participants would "get it." I seldom used my points, but very often, some of the participants that I had judged as "untouchable" would come to class and say, "I don't know, I don't believe in any of this, but the meditation is great. I feel like getting started with my life again." Sometimes, however, people that we think are easy to move seem stuck. We never know.

During the first class or two, participants sometimes consider the teaching unclear, and as a teacher you may, therefore, spend a lot of effort trying to refine your points. As discussed above, words can be extremely influential in modulating pain within clinical settings. They are part of the psychosocial context surrounding the treatment and hence constitute a key factor in doctor–patient relationships. Naturally, doctor–patient communication includes nonverbal cues, such as body language, eye contact, and tone. Indeed, all of these "nonspecific" factors are likely to contribute to clinical outcomes. Therefore, future studies of the role of language and psychosocial factors in mindfulness therapy are highly warranted. Yet, in our experience, the essential ingredient, so to say, is that you are able to *engage* people. The only way to attain this engagement is by being genuine, to yourself and to patients. Being in a group is a huge privilege and pleasure. Do not push, do not pretend, do not be afraid. Be still, listen, learn, and trust that something much larger than you will take care of the process. Take good care of your own practice too, learn from life, and admit when you, yourself, are stuck.

A New Beginning

Mindfulness practice can offer a greater insight into how we are feeling and the way we are living our lives. Perhaps you have undesirable patterns of behavior that are difficult to change. Will we continue along the same lines or will we try something new? Every single moment can be a new beginning.

Some years ago on an MBSR retreat, I (LF) decided finally to meet the knot in my stomach. For a whole year, in my daily meditation, I had been crying. At the retreat I decided that I was ready to take on whatever might come. During meditation, I saw an image of myself: I was in a deep and fast flowing river. I was clinging to a stone so that I would not lose control and drown. I realized that the stone symbolized my pain, and that it somehow made me feel safe. I was clinging to my pain because it felt as if my life depended on it. More and more often, I realize that the daily problems I encounter are due to the fact that I am clinging (as warned by the Buddha). This "holding on to pain" is a common experience for many of my patients. Perhaps this image may be of help to your patients, too.

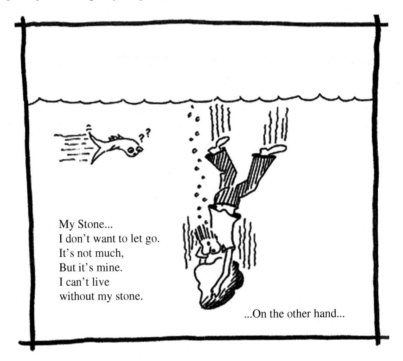

References

Benedetti, F. (2009). *Placebo effects: Understanding the mechanisms in health and disease.* Oxford, NY: Oxford University Press.

Benedetti, F., Carlino, E., & Pollo, A. (2011). How placebos change the patient's brain. *Neuropsychopharmacology, 36*, 339–354.

Benedetti, F., Mayberg, H. S., Wager, T. D., Stohler, C. S., & Zubieta, J. K. (2005). Neurobiological mechanisms of the placebo effect. *The Journal of neuroscience, 25*, 10390–10402.

Buhle, J., & Wager, T. D. (2010). Performance-dependent inhibition of pain by an executive working memory task. *Pain, 149*, 19–26.

Colloca, L., & Finniss, D. (2012). Nocebo effects, patient-clinician communication, and therapeutic outcomes. *JAMA, 307*, 567–568.

Descartes, R., & Timmermans, B. (1649/2010). Les passions de l'âme (Réimpressionth ed.). Paris, France: LGF.

Fink, P., & Schroder, A. (2010). One single diagnosis, Bodily distress syndrome, succeeded to capture ten diagnostic categories of functional somatic syndromes and somatoform disorders. *Journal of Psychosomatic Research, 68*, 415–426.

Fjorback, L. O. (2012). *Mindfulness and bodily distress*. Aarhus: Aarhus University.

Folkman, S., & Lazarus, R. S. (1988). The relationship between coping and emotion: Implications for theory and research. *Social Science & Medicine, 26*, 309–317.

Gauthier, N., Thibault, P., & Sullivan, M. J. (2011). Catastrophizers with chronic pain display more pain behaviour when in a relationship with a low catastrophizing spouse. *Pain Research & Management, 16*, 293–299.

Gormsen, L., Rosenberg, R., Bach, F. W., & Jensen, T. S. (2010). Depression, anxiety, health-related quality of life and pain in patients with chronic fibromyalgia and neuropathic pain. *European Journal of Pain, 14*(127), e121–e128.

Hölzel, B.K., Ott, U., Gard, T., Hempel, H., Weygandt, M., Morgen, K., & Vaitl, D. (2008). Investigation of mindfulness meditation practitioners with voxel-based morphometry. *Social Cognitive and Affective Neuroscience, 3*, 55–61.

Hudson, J. I., Goldenberg, D. L., Pope, H. G., Jr., Keck, P. E., Jr., & Schlesinger, L. (1992). Comorbidity of fibromyalgia with medical and psychiatric disorders. *The American Journal of Medicine, 92*, 363–367.

IASP. (1994). *Classification of chronic pain. Descriptions of chronic pain syndromes and definitions of pain terms (taskforce)* (2nd ed.). Seattle, WA: IASP Press.

Jegindø, E. E. (2012). *Pain and coping in the religious mind*. Aarhus: Aarhus University.

Keefe, F. J., Brown, G. K., Wallston, K. A., & Caldwell, D. S. (1989). Coping with rheumatoid arthritis pain: Catastrophizing as a maladaptive strategy. *Pain, 37*, 51–56.

Legrain, V., Iannetti, G. D., Plaghki, L., & Mouraux, A. (2011). The pain matrix reloaded: A salience detection system for the body. *Progress in Neurobiology, 93*, 111–124.

Levine, J. D., Gordon, N. C., Smith, R., & Fields, H. L. (1981). Analgesic responses to morphine and placebo in individuals with postoperative pain. *Pain, 10*, 379–389.

Levine, J. D., Gordon, N. C., & Fields, H. L. (1978). The mechanism of placebo analgesia. *Lancet, 2*, 654–657.

Husvedt, S. (2012). *Living, thinking, looking*. London, England: Sceptre.

Logan, H., Lutgendorf, S., Rainville, P., Sheffield, D., Iverson, K., & Lubaroff, D. (2001). Effects of stress and relaxation on capsaicin-induced pain. *The Journal of Pain, 2*, 160–170.

Meissner, K., Bingel, U., Colloca, L., Wager, T. D., Watson, A., & Flaten, M. A. (2011). The placebo effect: Advances from different methodological approaches. *The Journal of neuroscience, 31*, 16117–16124.

Ochsner, K. N., & Gross, J. J. (2005). The cognitive control of emotion. *Trends in Cognitive Sciences, 9*, 242–249.

Price, D. D., Finniss, D. G., & Benedetti, F. (2008). A comprehensive review of the placebo effect: Recent advances and current thought. *Annual Review of Psychology, 59*, 565–590.

Sullivan, M., Bishop, S., & Pivik, J. (1995). The pain catastrophizing scale: Development and validation. *Psychological Assessment, 7*, 524–532.

Sullivan, M. J., Stanish, W., Waite, H., Sullivan, M., & Tripp, D. A. (1998). Catastrophizing, pain, and disability in patients with soft-tissue injuries. *Pain, 77*, 253–260.

Chapter 17
Teaching Individuals with Anxiety and Depression

Susan L. Woods

Introduction: Taking One's Seat, Embodying Mindful Practice

A room full of people. I know a little of their personal histories, as I have had the chance to meet with them individually. They are looking for ways to feel better and to discover whether a program offering mindfulness-based skills can help them be less susceptible to feeling depressed and anxious. Many of them have tried a variety of treatments.

Mindfulness meditation practice can be an agent of change transforming how we experience ourselves and as a result how we choose to interact in daily life. But change is not easy and reshaping how we view and relate to the mind and mood states associated with depression and anxiety requires patience, courage, and kindness.

The practice of mindfulness meditation can be seen as essentially a training in waking up. This awakening requires an intention to be present for each moment and to observe the intricate nature of sensations that make up all of our experiences. Supporting and developing this consciousness is an attentional focus on the breath. By attending to the sensations of breathing, we anchor an experiential understanding about the nature of each unfolding moment.

We are frequently not in touch with what we are experiencing. This condition means we might be physically present, but our minds are often elsewhere. This is where the breath becomes helpful as it provides a reminder to return to being a participant observing the actual moment, rather than reliving what has just happened or

S.L. Woods, M.S.W., L.I.C.S.W. (✉)
Mindfulness-Based Stress Reduction and Mindfulness-Based Cognitive Therapy, P.O. Box 3565, Stowe, VT 05672, USA
e-mail: www.slwoods.com

© Springer International Publishing Switzerland 2016
D. McCown et al., *Resources for Teaching Mindfulness*,
DOI 10.1007/978-3-319-30100-6_17

ruminating over what has yet to occur. This attention to breath and the present moment is particularly helpful in depression and anxiety where the tendency is to get caught up in a cycle of negative thinking and low, anxious moods.

Researchers have become interested in investigating outcomes from 8-week mindfulness-based interventions (MBIs), and have also begun to understand what happens in the brain when people participate in mindfulness practice (Hölzel et al., 2011).

In this chapter, we focus on discussing the presence of the teacher in the room and take a look at some characteristics important to consider when thinking about the embodiment of mindfulness. We will also review how these characteristics are important for mood disorders. Of course, what an MBI instructor is essentially embodying are qualities of mind and heart that are founded on the principles and philosophy of mindfulness meditation practices. Along with these practices, the design of the MBI, group interaction and process, the MBI Instructor is also a catalyst for change.

A Contemplative Pedagogy

A contemplative pedagogy based on the practice of mindfulness requires an MBI instructor to find ways to support his or her own mindfulness practice because an instructor *embodies* rather than *explains* the merits of mindfulness. Therefore, any teaching of mindfulness relies on an instructor's personal experience of the practice.

At its heart, teaching an MBI will embrace the following; a present moment focus, mindful awareness, curiosity, loving kindness, and self-compassion. These characteristics epitomize fundamental qualities rooted in the practice of mindfulness. When embodied and articulated by a mindfulness-based instructor, they offer the possibility of engaging in a different relationship to persistent negative thoughts and depressed and anxious mood states. Importantly, these qualities are supporting something else, an explicit path for engaging in everyday life and for long-term general well-being.

In Fig. 17.1 below, the qualities of a contemplative pedagogy are depicted diagrammatically. Inevitably, these will overlap, interconnect, and interrelate; each one informing the other so that the practice of teaching is constantly changing and evolving. This process is not static nor indeed should these qualities be considered a methodology for teaching. Rather, it is a way to consider thoughtfully how you have come to understand and relate to them.

A brief word about self-compassion. In Buddhist literature, the word "self" is not attached to compassion but for our purposes here it is helpful. We are often extremely critical of ourselves when we perceive we have failed to measure up in some way, or are unable to make ourselves feel better or solve an emotional problem. It turns out that the ability to pay attention on purpose to these critical thoughts when they arise, to actually "be" with them, to explore them with friendliness and with kindness

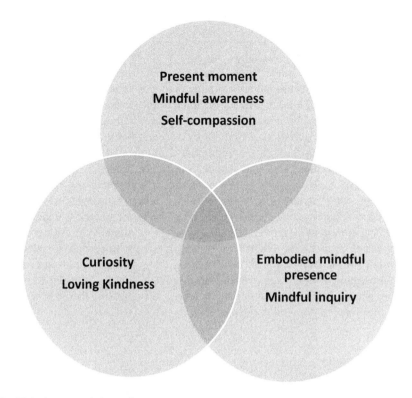

Fig. 17.1 A contemplative pedagogy

creates a very different empathic understanding about the nature of suffering, whether it be depression, anxiety, or indeed anything else we might be struggling with.

The Present Moment

Remembering to stay present requires much practice in patience, intention, curiosity, and friendliness. A mindfulness-based instructor recognizes that each moment is transitory. This understanding is one of the mainstays of an instructor's ability to be present for, and inquire into, challenging and often fear-based negative thoughts and emotions. Realizing this is possible generates a sensitivity and discernment towards what is being experienced.

As steadiness increases in meeting these moments, insight and compassion arise, giving birth to a very different relationship to what has previously been perceived as anxiety provoking or overwhelming. When a gentle, kind, and steady inquiry is brought to these moments by the teacher, it transforms the moments of fear, sadness, and/or anxiety. Compassion provides a key mind and mood state for understanding how we can relate to challenging emotions and anxious thoughts. Mindful awareness supports a consciousness that is not avoidant or fear based.

Mindful Awareness

When we are faced with difficulties, we tend to get distracted and self-absorbed, often on an "automatic pilot" mode of thinking, unaware of what is really taking place in the present. Mindfulness meditation practices help us to "see" this reality, and to understand that it takes time for the mind to settle. Once the mind has settled just enough, we can then notice the way we connect with and relate to thoughts, emotions, and body sensations. It supports us seeing that thoughts are a series of mental events passing through the mind, that emotions and moods are transitory, and that body sensations shift and change. Sowing the seeds for discerning impermanence is especially helpful when encountering difficult mind and mood states.

Once we allow ourselves to witness the vast array of thoughts and emotions associated with depression or anxiety, the "story" becomes much less important and the cyclical power of negative self-talk (rumination) diminishes. Awareness and insight develop about the contributory part played by story and rumination in depression and anxiety. As the ability to witness these moments gently strengthens, self-compassion, insight, and wisdom arise quite naturally. Mindful awareness becomes a key component shedding light on how self-defeating thoughts and rumination contribute to depression relapse.

Self-Compassion

The paradox of mindfulness is that an invitation to rest awareness in the present moment will, of course, include being present for the recognition of difficult emotions and/or thoughts, rather than denying or avoiding them. It is only by staying present (over and over again) and compassionately attending to these challenging moments that, ultimately, reactive mind and mood states are calmed and responsiveness is born. In due course, new and fresh ways of observing challenging sensations are experienced and the possibility of different choices and changed behaviors are shaped. While helpful for all participants, it is particularly useful for those who have a history of a mood disorder because a present moment orientation is an opening to, and an experiencing of, a "being" mode of mind rather than the more common "doing" modes of thinking.

"Being" modes of mind encompass, an experiential and reflective awareness that involves a compassionate engagement towards oneself and others. The "doing" modes of mind tend to include rational and problem-solving skills based on previous experiences of learning. We, of course, need a balance of both, but typically it is more common to have been educated to think using logical and solution-orientated skills. When this problem-solving approach is applied to trying to feel better or escape the negative thinking and feeling states present with a mood disorder, it produces more problems in the form of ruminative thinking and feelings of increased fear and anxiety. This endless cycle of trying to think our way out of feeling sad, anxious, and helpless is especially problematic.

Curiosity and Loving Kindness

An MBI instructor is guided by the philosophy of the dharma and from an understanding of the ethical and practice-based principles that are embedded in this wisdom tradition. These practiced-based principles support a particular form of wakeful consciousness that is naturally curious and caring. By employing all of the six senses (mind being one of them in Buddhist psychology), the ability to observe what is actually present in any given moment is strengthened. This perceptual attunement develops over time and with consistent practice, supports an exquisite experiential understanding of how we respond to internal and external cues. This sensorial information informs the teaching of a contemplative pedagogy which is then expressed through an instructor's embodied mindful presence, through the teaching of mindfulness meditation practices and in facilitating mindful inquiry.

Embodied Mindful Presence and Mindful Inquiry

A friendly, inviting, and kindhearted presence will infuse an instructor's teaching of the body scan, the sitting meditation practices, walking meditation practice, and mindful movement. These qualities inform an instructor's skill for witnessing and inquiring into, while at the same time affirming, a participant's and the group's discovery of the impact of mindfulness practices on their moods, thought processes, and general experiences. Additionally, and significantly, an instructor knows that mindfulness practices are constantly pointing to what it feels like to be inherently whole and not broken.

From his or her own mindfulness practice, an instructor will have experienced many mind and mood states, and be able to see how easy it can be to get caught up in thinking that is often unrelated to the experience of the moment. The MBI instructor appreciates the role of gentle curiosity accompanied by a kindly friendliness in exploring not only the present moment, but past memories and future worries. Through observing this movement of mind and mood, an instructor learns what is helpful and what is not useful in meeting those moments, and teaches from this experiential platform.

MBI instructors who have embraced their own mindfulness meditation practice come to embody a sense of meeting the difficult and unwanted without needing to change, avoid, chase after, or struggle with whatever is showing up. This orientation is not passive but requires mindfully responding to what is arising—bringing clarity, compassion, and a skillful discernment to the moment.

In a world where we often feel pressure to be an instant expert, it is important to acknowledge that an embodied mindful presence and the articulation of mindfulness do not develop overnight. It is a journey for a lifetime. And even if our mindfulness practice fluctuates (as it will), the recommitment to practice is important, not the fact there has been a gap when, for whatever reason, one has been unable to "find the time." Teaching competencies and good practice skills evolve over time as an instructor's personal practice deepens and matures. There is no hurry to this process. Teaching mindfulness takes time to develop.

Depression and Anxiety

Depression and Anxiety are common in our culture. The National Institute of Mental Health (NIMH) reports that Major Depressive Disorder is the leading cause of disability in the USA for adults between the ages of 15–44 years (The World Health Organization, 2008). Once you have experienced one episode of depression, you are far more likely to experience another (50 %) (Kessler, Demler, et al., 2005). If you experience additional episodes of depression, (two or more) your chances of experiencing a major depressive episode are even greater (70–80 %) (Keller et al., 1992). Therefore, depression can have a relapsing and remitting trajectory over a lifetime. And for many people suffering from depression, anxiety is often a significant additional factor.

Anxiety disorders are debilitating disorders that prevent people from feeling free to enjoy their lives. Anxiety disorders include such diagnoses as Panic Disorder, Obsessive-Compulsive Disorder, Post-Traumatic Disorder, Agoraphobia, a Specific Phobia, and Generalized Anxiety Disorder (GAD). Approximately 6.8 million American adults (3.1 % of people aged 18 and older) will experience GAD in a given year (Kessler, Chiu, Demler, & Walters, 2005; U.S. Census Bureau Population Estimates by Demographic Characteristics, 2005).

We all encounter moments of worry, anxiety, and fear. Equally we experience moments of sadness, and even prolonged unhappiness. We cannot escape this part of being alive. However, for those participants who come to us with a history of depression and/or anxiety, these states of mind and mood may have eventually become a way of being, an identity ultimately laying down the roots for negative core beliefs about themselves.

A once-adaptive system is hardwired into our brains designed to alert us to danger. It sets off an alarm system that has enabled us to survive and thrive as a species, allowing us to appraise the situation and quickly decide what we need to do about it, if anything. This adaptation has been called the "flight, fight, or freeze" reaction to a perceived threat. We no longer face the proverbial sabre tooth tigers, but we can find ourselves frequently confronting situations that will activate this flight, fight, or freeze reaction.

Stress can also be subjective, and some level of stress is good when perceived as just enough to motivate us. This kind of stress (called by some "eustress") can help us set goals, stimulate us in all the right ways and allow us to meet challenges with a sense of growing competence and mastery.

However, any stress that causes us to feel undue mental/emotional strain and threatens to overwhelm our ability to cope successfully produces a variety of reactive responses. These responses may actually be rather reasonable attempts to deal with the short-term situation. Unfortunately, they don't help over the long term as they engage the mind in trying to "problem solve" a way out of feeling anxious or depressed. These strategies end up not being successful, and we are left feeling incompetent and unresourceful about managing the situation regardless of whether the stressors are internal (thoughts, emotions, body sensations) or external.

The struggle to escape feelings of anxiety, or protracted periods of sadness, only strengthens the various psychological mechanisms (e.g., denial, avoidance, distraction, rumination) that can actually make the problem worse. In addition, internal critical judgments form about one's failure to avoid feeling depressed or anxious which actually add to increased vulnerability to depression and/or anxiety. Over time the failure to ease this negative landscape leads to more stress and increased attempts to avoid negative thinking and/or feelings of sadness and anxiety. Unattended, this cycle leads to poor coping strategies and maladaptive behavioral patterns.

An orientation to the present moment, and mindful attentiveness create the foundation for seeing thoughts as "mental events," even those attached to a sense of "self." Thoughts are attended to in much the same way as one would notice body sensations or sounds. They arise, are observed, examined for when there is a repeating pattern, and eventually fall away. This process, practiced over time, leads to the profound understanding that we are more than just our thoughts and promotes a process of decentering or defusing from the belief of being less than adequate or inadequate.

The distinctive nature of the conditioned thoughts and emotions related to being a depressed or anxious person can be helpfully attenuated by coming together with others who have had similar experiences. This kind of connecting can be especially helpful in understanding the role of self-identification about "being a depressed or anxious person."

Being with others who have felt and thought the same and employed similar coping strategies lessens the sense of shame, loneliness, isolation, and personal failure. Participants come to understand that there are shared and common ways of reacting to aversive states of thinking that are actually reasonable attempts to deal with feeling depressed and/or anxious.

It is therefore very helpful for participants suffering with a history of depression and/or anxiety to attend an MBI specifically adapted for their needs. The Mindfulness-Based Cognitive Therapy (MBCT) program was created to specifically target the relapsing nature of depression (Segal, Williams, & Teasdale, 2013, Teasdale et al., 2000). In addition, the MBCT protocol has been found to be useful for people suffering from anxiety as well (Evans et al., 2008; Kim et al., 2009).

A word of caution. Someone who is experiencing a major depressive episode, or who has high current states of anxiety, is not a good candidate for taking an MBI 8-week course. There are other methods of acute treatment that would serve them better. Once the acute episode has passed, through the interventions of psychotherapy and/or medication, then it becomes possible to consider mindfulness. One needs to have a certain level of energy to be able to practice mindfulness. If the mind is being affected by profound states of depression or anxiety, there is not enough intentional energy to practice.

Psychological Mechanisms and the Role of Mindfulness

We all employ a variety of psychological mechanisms to ameliorate feelings of discomfort, unease, or a state of feeling that things are generally unsatisfactory. These reactions are quite ordinary to wanting to feel better and more comfortable. For those who have a history of anxiety and depression, the psychological mechanisms of aversion, avoidance, distraction, denial, rumination, reactivity, and attachment are of particular importance since they become primary methods for dealing with unwanted thoughts and feelings (Table 17.1). Understanding how these psychological mechanisms contribute to a vulnerability for depression and anxiety is important for an MBI instructor to be aware of, especially as it relates to teaching mindfulness based practices.

We observe a variety of these psychological mechanisms operating in our participants at different times over the course of the 8 weeks of an MBI as they engage in practicing mindfulness meditation skills. However, you don't need to have had a history of depression and/or anxiety to make use of these psychological mechanisms. But for people who have a history of mood disorders, they are primary strategies for warding off feelings of anxiety, low mood, and hopelessness. Unfortunately, the more they are employed, the less energy is available to be adaptively present for the experiences of life.

Trying to avoid, deny, or push away negative thoughts and low mood fails over time. This failure becomes interpreted as a personal failure, producing additional

Table 17.1 Psychological processes and mindfulness-based skills

Psychological processes	Mindfulness-based practices
Aversion—pushing away the unwanted, the wish to have a different experience	Staying present; being with; investigating; turning towards; approaching; safely enduring
Avoidance—escaping from things perceived as difficult	Staying present; being curious; investigating; approaching
Distraction—a way to escape from something perceived as problematic, challenging	Staying present; patience; kindness; compassion
Denial—pushing away and preventing painful thoughts and emotions	Being present and noticing; being curious; creating space for; investigating
Rumination—cycle of rethinking that tries to "think a way out" of negative thinking, along with feelings of anxiety and chronic sadness	Staying present; noticing; seeing thoughts as no different from any other sensation, just mental events
Reactivity—a knee jerk reaction to the unpleasant	Staying present; slowing down; pausing; being curious about; being with; patience; investigating
Attachment to the pleasant; holding on to the pleasant; not wanting to let go of something being experienced as pleasant because of fear of feeling otherwise	Staying present; appreciating moments of pleasantness and joy; allowing; letting be; letting go
Attachment to negative fixed thoughts about self	Staying present; curiosity; patience; loving kindness; compassion

layers of thinking centered on personally identifying oneself as a depressed or anxious person. The self-referencing stories generated from these negative thoughts and the resulting low mood becomes an important driver for depression and/or anxiety. Such narratives collect around the core concept of "me" that reinforce a largely negative belief about the self which then becomes a main contributor to the remitting and relapsing cycle of these conditions.

Mindfulness-based practices focus on a present moment awareness which is the opposite of avoidance or distraction. This first step is key for developing "bare attention" as a practice of maintaining a relaxed focus on an object, simply observing what may be arising without partiality, as well as noting any concurrent reactions that may be present.

Attending to the present moment, and recognizing how often we are not in the present moment, strengthens patience (an often unacknowledged benefit of mindfulness). It also supports kindness and equanimity. When we become aware of our distractibility, instead of berating ourselves, we can remember to return to the present, steadying purpose and equanimity.

Interestingly, "bare attention" also provides preparation for gradually increasing exposure to what has been avoided. This attention is helpful for both depression and anxiety, but particularly for anxiety. Mental health professionals use various exposure techniques in order to break the pattern of anxiety. These techniques teach a person to stay with the unwanted anxiety in increasingly specified increments while waiting for it to pass, which it eventually does. Mindfulness provides an additional potent ingredient, revealing that our relationship to worry, anxiety, or sadness is determined by how it is perceived and experienced.

Present Moment Focus for Mood Disorders

It is a paradox that we encounter so much internal noise when we first try to sit in silence. It is a paradox that experiencing pain releases pain. It is a paradox that keeping still can lead us so fully into life and being.

—Gunilla Norris

Recognizing when aversive states are around, being present and learning to stay with these states, is particularly helpful for our participants struggling with mood disorders. Whenever we experience something we perceive as unpleasant, our normal reaction is to not like it. This response may be mild and quickly forgotten, or it can be very unpleasant lingering and becoming imbedded in memory. When strong emotional feelings are attached to negative past experiences, we understandably make every attempt to avoid feeling that way again.

Reinforcing a mindful attunement to the present moment helps us recognize the strong pull to move away from negative thinking and/or unwanted feelings. Attending to the present moment, noticing the arrival, ongoing nature, and departure of thoughts, emotions and body sensations provides the platform for becoming a participant-observer of one's own experiences without getting quite so caught up in

being the central character of the story or what it all means. These techniques lessen
the belief around "my story." We learn that narratives can simply be the movement
of thoughts, moods, and body sensations.

The two scenarios below describe a dialogue between an MBI instructor and two
of her participants. The first participant is struggling with negative thoughts and
anxiety and is identifying himself as "an anxious person." The second participant is
sad and stressed by a sense of being a failure brought on by remembering previous
periods of disappointment. Note the instructor's ability to expand on what is being
noticed, reflecting back on the participants' experiences and staying with the present
moment experience and discovery process.

First Scenario: Recognizing Aversion and Learning to Stay Present

Participant: It's hopeless. I've been trying to do the sitting meditation practice and
I start off fine. I can be with my breath and then move on to being with the sensations of the body. I'm pretty okay with being with sounds but when it comes to
noticing thinking, I get all caught up with really anxious thoughts. And off I go
again. I'm just an anxious person.

Many of us will have encountered these kinds of remarks in our teaching of an
MBI especially in the second half of an 8-week course, when our participants have
been practicing mindfulness meditation for a number of weeks and know there is no
quick fix. In fact, it brings up exactly what they have tried to avoid.

In this scenario, we have **aversion** and **attachment** operating. So what will be
useful for the instructor to embody and articulate to help this participant? To some
extent it depends on which session is being taught. For example, let's say we are
half way through the 8 weeks, at session 5. This participant is staying attentive to
the various objects of concentration until he notices thinking and then experiences
being caught up in some unpleasant negative and anxious making thoughts.

Instructor: So you are noticing anxious thoughts?
Participant: Yes. Same old stuff!
Instructor: As you were noticing the thoughts, were you aware of any physical
sensations?
Participant: Um, yes, actually my shoulders felt tight and my breath was faster. I'm
noticing that feeling now. It doesn't feel good.
Instructor: In this moment, there's a physical sense of unpleasantness. I wonder
what might happen if you directed the breath to that area in the body, giving the
unpleasant sensations as much space as they need.
Participant: (Participant spontaneously moves body that he has been holding
stiffly, spine lifts, and shoulders drop. Watching the instructor, he takes some
breaths then closes his eyes. The MBI instructor is naturally modeling a present

moment orientation, kindness, and curiosity. The group is watching. His breath slows down and shoulders relax). My shoulders feel easier ... not so tight. Um, I feel calmer.

Instructor: (Waits a bit before answering). I wonder if this might be helpful when you notice anxious thoughts again. Remember we are not trying to get rid of anything. We're seeing if it is possible to be with those things that are difficult to stay with. So the next time you notice anxious thoughts, allow your attention to include any physical sensations in the body giving them as much space as they need, letting the breath be your guide. And then when you are ready, returning to simply noticing thoughts when that is your primary object of concentration.

Second Scenario: Recognizing Aversion, Rumination, Attachment, Learning to Stay Present

Participant: I get so down on myself. I get this sinking feeling and thoughts about all the ways I have screwed up. Meditation practice is just one more way that I know I'm going to fail because I get sad about all the thoughts I have about things that have happened in the past.

Instructor: A sinking feeling. Do you remember when you noticed this? (Teacher is slowing down the story about what has been observed and not being specific or interpreting what constitutes "this sinking feeling").

Participant: When the instruction was to be with the body, I had this sinking feeling.

Instructor: I'm wondering if you noticed where in the body?

Participant: (Places hands on abdomen.) In this area, I can feel it now. My breath feels tight and I don't want to feel bad.

Instructor: So the breath feels tight? Is it possible to stay with those sensations for a moment or two? Even describe them? (The teacher is staying present with whatever is being revealed; taking the participant step by step through the process rather than having this experience become a run-on story of avoidance accompanied by feelings of failure).

Participant: I feel nauseous, anxious. (The participant has moved off the breath to somatic sensations).

Instructor: There is a feeling of nausea present, anxiety. How about the breath?

Participant: Still tight.

Instructor: I'm curious about what might happen if you brought your full attention to each in- and out-breath?

Participant: (Some time passes. The teacher waits, embodying calmness, curiosity, and genuine interest). The feeling of anxiety has changed. The breath feels a little easier but I feel sad.

Instructor: Right now the breath feels a little easier and there is sadness. (The instructor pauses for a moment or two). So we are staying with the breath moment by moment, as best we can. (The teacher is tracking the movement of sensations, modeling for this participant [and for the group] attentiveness, curiosity, kindness, and steadiness as a key ingredient of learning about staying with difficult thoughts and emotions. She is also following the participant's experience that is demonstrating that sensations do change as we notice them).

Participant: It's interesting. The sadness feels different and my breath is easier. It's sort of changed.

Instructor: So a sense of change, even with these difficult emotions that include thoughts of anxiety and sadness. Noticing the breath, an anchor to the present, grounding a sense of safety for these challenging emotions and thoughts, allowing you to observe them. Letting them be. Watching and noticing the movement of sensations. Nothing to fix or make go away.

Mindful Awareness for Mood Disorders

This is the first, the wildest and the wisest thing I know: that the soul exists and is built entirely out of attentiveness.
                                                                                                    —Mary Oliver

Mindful awareness embraces a way of being present that notices and pays attention to how we respond to ourselves, behave towards others, and how we relate to daily life. The MBI instructor understands that developing mindful awareness calls for two primary mindful-based skills; one that concentrates on focusing on single objects of attention, (such as an awareness of breathing, of body sensations, sounds, or thoughts and emotions), the other choiceless awareness.

By mindfully attending to a particular object of concentration, we become aware of how we relate and respond to what is being noticed. By mindfully attending to whatever object is being observed, we also become aware of any reactions (pleasant, unpleasant, or neutral) that we may have. Mindful awareness is supported and strengthened by bearing witness to these moments. This approach can be fertile ground for any of us and particularly helpful for those suffering from depression and/or anxiety. Thoughts and emotions, no matter how potent or ubiquitous, are no different from body sensations or any other object of attention as all things are eventually subject to movement and change.

Choiceless awareness incorporates a wider lens of attention that is more spacious. It involves noticing whatever arises within the field of attention. Choiceless awareness supports sensitivity to the movements of sensation in our internal and external environments. We learn by opening to all of our senses, revealing an awareness that simply "is," one that requires no prescribing or predicting of any outcome.

This awareness is important for mood disorders as people who suffer from anxiety tend to generate a lot of anxious thinking about future outcomes, leading to more anxiety and worry about outcomes most of which may never even happen. People who have more of a depressed outlook tend to have thoughts about the past, ruminating about what has gone wrong. Tuning into the movements of what is actually present is very different from letting thoughts or mood become the ruler of experience.

An experienced instructor will know when a more expansive approach is needed, and equally, when it will be important to have a finely honed attention for detail. This awareness includes clear seeing (as best as one is able in any given moment) of what is needed in the present when addressing participants. The instructor's decision about how to respond will be based on the maturation of her own mindfulness practice along with a willingness to stay with and investigate a participant's present moment experience with gentle compassion and curiosity.

This determination could be anything from an affirmative nod of the head to a more direct line of questioning, encompassing a finely tuned mindful listening, and paying careful attention to what is being expressed by the participant. An instructor will be attentive to individual and evolving group dynamics, be aware of the thematic structure for each of the individual sessions of the MBI, and be conversant about the progression of the course material and teaching components. And importantly, an instructor must develop a mindful internal attunement to what is being noted in his or her own experiential landscape as part of the process and skill of teaching.

From an experiential understanding born of personal mindfulness practice, an MBI instructor embodies a deep awareness about a mind often on automatic pilot, frequently working from habituated perspectives, ruminating on problem solving and usually seeking distraction. The embodiment of this awareness encompasses unequivocal understanding of the centrality of generosity and compassion. It creates a place of trust where it becomes possible to pause, open to, and investigate gently. This approach is the opposite to reacting, closing down/constricting, denying, and avoiding.

Mindful Self-Compassion in Mood Disorders

Nothing wondrous can come in this world unless it rests on the shoulders of kindness.
— Barbara Kingsolver

When we find ourselves in a situation that produces a strong emotional reactive response, we tend to relive in our minds and emotions what has just happened. It's not long before we are being critical of ourselves in some way, usually about what we said or did, or didn't say or do. No one likes to experience such thoughts, so every attempt is made to ward them off and deny their presence. We become self-absorbed in a process that finds us going over what has happened in an effort to solve the problem and feel better, or we can equally spend time worrying about what might happen next. This cycle becomes an endless series of negative thoughts and anxiety that is unproductive and ultimately ends in physical, emotional, and spiritual exhaustion.

Mindfulness epitomizes something very different. It teaches the possibility of being aware of these moments without getting completely caught up in them, observing them instead. Anxiety lessens when we consistently pay attention in this way, allowing the breath to provide an anchor when necessary (to steady this contemplative awareness). When we come to see this process for what it is, sensations shifting and changing, it provides a relief and release. Along with those feelings of release, there is gratitude and the experience of open curiosity. This approach is very different from struggling with, pushing away, or chasing after, what is perceived to be problematic. Over time and with consistent practice, the manner of perceiving what has previously been defended against (because it is experienced as painful and anxiety provoking) becomes lessened by the steadiness of staying present and attending to the present moment.

This steadiness provides moments of tender friendliness when turning towards oneself and facing what is arising. Mindfulness encourages a resolve to notice, be still for a moment or two, and allow for and create space around fearful thoughts or feelings. This mindful resolve sows the seeds for a warm, investigative questioning, "What's this?" that supports insight, wisdom, and compassion.

With practice this inner mindful compassionate attunement becomes the epicenter for behavioral activation, not by forcing anything to change or embarking on a path of self-improvement, but from a sense of embracing new possibilities by allowing things to be just as they are.

An MBI instructor who has personally encountered such landscapes in her or his own mindfulness practice will offer participants a feeling of security when they too encounter them. In these moments, it is not only the insights, or the relief that is felt, but a deep sense of self-compassion that alters the way these moments are met.

Closing (Mindful) Thoughts

Teaching MBIs requires an instructor to honestly reflect his or her current understanding of the practice of mindfulness. The instructor must be able to demonstrate an understanding that nothing needs to be added to this moment, or taken away from it. We never know what is actually present until we turn towards each moment and pay attention. When an instructor embraces this practice with participants, he or she embodies an openness to welcoming the movement of life that releases joy to be in the flow of each changing moment of sensation.

An MBI instructor allows such moments to arise without directing them. There is no sense of being a manager, but rather a deep connection to the experiences born of a body moving, thoughts coming and going, emotions rising and falling, and the breath moving freely. How would it be to teach expressing this truth and meet participants in this place? A tender permission to be unfettered—meeting each moment as it is, and then letting go, knowing grasping onto anything tightly causes suffering.

An MBI instructor embodies an openness of character that offers an invitation to answer the call of something deeply rooted and natural. A call to meet oneself and others in a place of profound communication; an invitation to drop the mask of uncertainty and the wish to please. To be quiet, listening to the threads of being, a reminder to be grateful. And recognizing the deep well of compassion born from all the moments of meeting this moment, with no beginning and no end.

An MBI instructor knows that compassion can be present for pain. In those places of encountering and acknowledging suffering, he or she sees it as part of the universal condition of being human. It is true that we fear anger, anxiety, and sadness. We see how it can tear down our walls of defense, leaving us feeling vulnerable with a desire to run away, to hide, or to try to deny and forget.

An MBI instructor takes a seat amidst all these considerations, tending to the heart's delight in being present. She or he provides a foundation that does not ask, why? For why has no place where heart, soul, and spirit live. Like lovers meeting for the first time. Moments of love—the passion of the meeting for its own sake and the joy of this release that comes from the permission to be. To witness and be absorbed by this moment and the next—thoughts and emotions moving freely. Not owning the moments, but a delicious surrender to the now of all things and an awakening that reveals the uniqueness of this moment. Unique and blessed. Inimitable because this moment will never be the same, and blessed because being awake and alive notices that.

An MBI instructor understands all of the many moments of experience that have coalesced into story. These stories over time can become the source of the deep cyclical nature of depressions and anxieties. Mindfulness offers a profound awakening to the fact that we are all much more than our stories. In letting go of story, we embrace the uniqueness and deep humanity in each of us, along with all of the universal connections we share in our humanness.

References

Evans, S., Ferrando, S., Findler, M., Stowell, C., Smart, C., & Haglin, D. (2008, May). Mindfulness-based cognitive therapy for generalized anxiety disorder. *Journal of Anxiety Disorders, 22*(4): 716–721.

Hölzel, B. K., Carmody, J., Vangel, M., Congleton, C., Yerramsetti, S. M., Gard, T., & Lazar, S. W. (2011). Mindfulness practice leads to increases in regional brain gray matter density. *Psychiatry Research: Neuroimaging, 191*, 36–42.

Keller, M. B., Lavori, P. W., Mueller, T. I., Coryell, W., Hirschfeld, R. M. A., & Shea, M. T. (1992). Time to recovery, chronicity and levels of psychopathology in major depression. *Archives of General Psychiatry, 49*, 809–816.

Kessler, R. C., Chiu, W. T., Demler, O., & Walters, E. E. (2005, June). Prevalence, severity, and comorbidity of twelve-month DSM-IV disorders in the National Comorbidity Survey Replication (NCS-R). *Archives of General Psychiatry, 62*(6):617–627.

Kessler, R. C., Demler, O., Frank, R. G., Olfson, M., Pincus, H. A., Walters, E. E., … Zaslavsky, A. M. (2005). Prevalence and treatment of mental disorders, 1990 to 2003. *New England Journal of Medicine, 352*, 2515–2523.

Kim, Y. W., Lee, S.-H., Choi, T. K., Suh, S. Y., Kim, B., Kim, C. M., … Yook, K.-H. (2009). Effectiveness of mindfulness-based cognitive therapy as an adjuvant to pharmacotherapy in patients with panic disorder or generalized anxiety disorder. *Depression and Anxiety, 26*, 601–606. doi: 10.1002/da.20552.

Segal, Z. V., Williams, J. M. G., & Teasdale, J. D. (2013). *Mindfulness-based cognitive therapy for depression*. New York, NY: Guildford Press.

Teasdale, J. D., Segal, Z. V., Williams, J. M. G., Ridgeway, V., Soulsby, J., & Lau, M. (2000). Prevention of relapse/recurrence in major depression by mindfulness-based cognitive therapy. *Journal of Consulting and Clinical Psychology, 68*, 615–623.

The World Health Organization. (2008). *The global burden of disease: 2004 update, Table A2: Burden of disease in DALYs by cause, sex and income group in WHO regions, estimates for 2004*. Geneva, Switzerland: WHO.

U.S. Census Bureau Population Estimates by Demographic Characteristics. (2005, June 9). *Table 2: Annual estimates of the population by selected age groups and sex for the United States: April 1, 2000 to July 1, 2004 (NC-EST2004-02)*. Washington, DC: Population Division, U.S. Census Bureau Release.

Chapter 18
Teaching Individuals with Traumatic Stress

Trish Magyari

Applying a Trauma-Informed Framework to Teaching MBIs

This chapter (1) aids in the development of a "trauma-informed" competency in mindfulness teachers and therapists working with general population groups which may contain persons with traumatic stress symptoms and histories; and (2) offers additional guidelines for those teacher-therapists who are delivering dedicated trauma-focused mindfulness-based interventions (MBIs). The chapter includes a description of trauma-informed behavioral health intervention guidelines; applies those guidelines with practical suggestions from screening to follow-up; describes a trauma-informed method for beginning mindfulness meditations; offers specific guidelines for the body scan, mindfulness retreats, and additional adaptations for dedicated trauma-focused MBI groups. "Trauma-Informed Mindful Dialogue," (found in Part IV Chapter 24, D) applies many of these guidelines to inquiry following a mindfulness exercise.

Persons with trauma histories, trauma stress symptoms, or a diagnosis of post-traumatic stress disorder (PTSD) are likely to be in virtually all MBI groups. Many of the most common referral criteria include traumatic components such as chronic pain, anxiety, depression, traumatic illness, traumatic grief, and traumatic stress-related symptoms. Merriam-Webster's dictionary defines trauma simply as "*a very difficult or unpleasant experience that causes someone to have mental or emotional problems usually for a long time*." While not everyone who experiences trauma will be diagnosed with PTSD, many will exhibit some of the symptoms of traumatic stress, either acutely after the trauma or to a degree that may or may not meet the full criteria for a PTSD diagnosis.

Trauma survivors experience a number of challenges to developing mindfulness skills, especially regarding those practices that are still (as opposed to moving),

T. Magyari, M.S., L.C.P.C., N.C.C., R.Y.T.-200 (✉)
Mindfulness-based Professional Training Institute, UC San Diego Center for Mindfulness,
5060 Shoreham Place, Suite 330, San Diego, CA 92122-0980, USA
e-mail: trish@trishmagyari.com

© Springer Science+Business Media New York 2016
W. Goodwin (ed.), *Forensic DNA Typing Protocols*, Methods in Molecular
Biology 1420, DOI 10.1007/978-3-319-30100-6_18

eyes-closed practices with long expanses of silence. This limitation stems from the primary effect of trauma on the brain, namely, chronic and easily triggered fight/flight/freeze reactivity. There is also growing research evidence and clinical experience revealing that trauma survivors can master, benefit from, and experience transformative recovery through a trauma-informed, mindfulness-based approach (Kimbrough, Magyari, Langenberg, Chesney, & Berman, 2010; Folette, 2015; Williams et al., 2015); even more importantly, mindfulness is being recommended as an efficacious component of trauma recovery programs (SAMSHA, 2014; van der Kolk, 2014), including healing from the sequelae of adverse childhood events (ACEs) (Jackson Nakazawa, 2015). With these recent recommendations, it is likely that there will be an increase in referrals to MBIs or mindfulness-based therapists, often as an adjunct to individual trauma-focused therapy. The value of mindfulness training in general, and of MBIs in particular, is in the combination of learning to be present in *this moment* of one's life, along with very specific and concrete instructions on how to "be with" one's own experience in a way that is healing rather than retraumatizing, triggering, or otherwise self-injuring.

All MBI program components can be successfully taught to persons with trauma histories when using a trauma-informed approach. This approach to teaching the full MBI curriculum of mindfulness exercises allows for the greatest chance of mastery, healing, and success by anticipating and creating empowering solutions through skilled attention to the known challenges of working with traumatized populations. In general, what makes trauma-informed teaching successful is more in the "how" of it, rather than the "what" of it. This process is accomplished through four main "trauma-informed" teaching components with specific attention for evoking self-compassion as a resource woven throughout:

1. Offering anticipatory guidance both before and during the course regarding supports and resources for staying present, even while those recovering from trauma are participating fully in the curriculum. This includes the resource of the teacher and any resources the participant already has for staying present, grounded, and out of distress—such as techniques that calm the sympathetic nervous system.
2. Giving control to participants through options, choice, invitations, and seeking permission. Such as the choice for eyes open or eyes closed and normalizing, validating, and supporting choice and autonomy.
3. Working skillfully with trauma-related distress when it arises in class and during home practice through modeling nonjudgment, acceptance, and compassion.
4. Titrating periods of mindfulness meditation in order to stay within the therapeutic window, using resources and supports as well as modulating intensity.

General guidelines for trauma-informed behavioral interventions, of which mindfulness is one, include the following components: Preparing the client; Creating collaborative relationships; Creating safe environments; Supporting choice, control, and autonomy; Putting in place resources and supports for staying present; Monitoring and facilitating stability; and Managing trauma-related destabilization. (SAMSHA, 2014). Each of these trauma-informed components is operationalized and explained in this chapter, citing numerous practical applications to MBI curriculum components. The last guideline, Managing Trauma-Related Destabilization, is also addressed in Chap. 37. Please keep in mind that many of these guidelines overlap, so that "Creating a Collaborative Relationship" is also a part of "Preparing the Client" and "Putting in Place Resources and Supports."

Theoretical Considerations Regarding PTSD

The DSM-V (APA, 2013) places PTSD symptoms into four categories:

- Intrusion symptoms including triggers, flashbacks, and nightmares
- Avoidance, including dissociation, avoiding people/places/things as well as both emotional and memory numbing
- Arousal/reactivity where the fight or flight reactivity is overworking coupled with difficulty calming down
- Negative mood and cognition such as rumination over negative events

Mindfulness interventions are a good fit for addressing these symptom domains. Intrusion symptoms are addressed by teaching skills to stay present and work with intrusive memories and triggers like any other phenomenon—by teaching clients not to react to reflexive inner reactivity. Clients are coached to *move toward* what they are experiencing with a friendly attitude, even when they don't like their experience, thus decreasing avoidance symptoms. Arousal/reactivity symptoms decrease through the calming effect that mindfulness practices have on the nervous system, specifically by activating a parasympathetic response. Additionally, mindfulness of current surroundings can be used to notice the presence of safety when it is there. Negative mood and cognition are addressed by disrupting the downward spiral of depressive rumination and self-loathing by learning not to react, but instead simply to identify thoughts simply as just thoughts. Clients can also learn how to respond to self-critical thoughts in a kind way, creating a more positive relationship foundation with self. MBIs also involve training to identify and stay with positive experiences that are often overlooked or rejected in persons with negative mood states.

According to one theoretical framework, trauma potentially affects the domains of identity, relationship problems, and affects regulation (Briere & Rickards, 2007; Briere & Spinazzola, 2009). Each of these domains is described more fully below, including how MBIs address these domains:

1. Identity issues, including reduced access to self and being other-directed, are addressed through increasing inner-directed awareness and developing self-knowledge.
2. Relationship problems, including difficulty separating past from present in interpersonal relationships, are addressed by increasing the ability to identify and stay with present moment experiences, decreasing reflexive reactivity, and teaching specific mindful communication skills such as listening and speaking.
3. Affect Regulation, including a reduced ability to self-regulate moods, thoughts, and feelings, are addressed by increasing self-calming skills, increasing self-

compassion, and learning to respond vs. react, especially to inner reactivity and negative emotional, or cognitive states.

Research Considerations

A number of research studies have described the quantitative value of MBSR, MBCT, and other MBIs for persons with trauma histories on reducing PTSD symptomatology and are summarized in the book "Mindfulness-Oriented Interventions for Trauma Care" (Follette, et al. 2015). The following comments were collected through written questionnaires during one MBSR clinical trial for women with complex trauma from childhood sexual abuse. These comments illustrate MBIs' ability to address PTSD symptomatology and to have personal meaning for the participants (Magyari, 2015). Comments are disguised to preserve study participants' confidentiality without altering meaning:

Participant A's Words

WK4: "At last, I can let go of the shame and anger. Now I can stay with those thoughts without panicking or trying to avoid them."

WK8: "In this group, I've learned that I am not my crazy thoughts and it's OK to feel scared, sad, or angry. It doesn't mean that I am falling apart. The most important part was that (sic) learning not to bury my thoughts. That's at the core of my being able to forgive myself."

Participant B

WK4: "Before this class, I was stuck. This class is on growing and healing. It's really useful to learn not to be so judgmental of myself."

WK8: "To be in this moment, present, and not dwell on the past. I've learned that I have the strength and to heal myself and to be a friend to myself. It's like I've been awakened. I felt good to be reintroduced to myself."

Participant C

WK4: "This class has given me tool that will help me to handle my life better. The most useful tool for me is the body scan."

WK8: "In this group, I've been formally introduced to myself. I feel like I am finding myself after being lost for a very long time, and I am feeling more secure about who I am during this period of my life. I am also more willing to reach out to people rather than withdraw from everyone. The body scan helped me to get in touch with the places where I hold all the pain in addition to all the normal aches and pains. I found myself again."

Participant C was again interviewed 2.75 years after the MBI course as part of a follow-up study. Some of the behavioral changes that she reports since the MBI course include:

- Recognizing how "stressed" she was in former job and finding a new, more fulfilling job that she's been in for the last 2.50 years.
- Stopping smoking after many previous failed attempts; now, smoke free for over 2.00 years.
- Getting married after a lengthy engagement. "Finally, felt safe enough"; feeling happy in marriage.
- Taking up running. She now runs a 5-mile race on a regular basis.

These reported behavior changes illustrate increased self-awareness, increased relationality, decreased reliance on an addictive substance for coping, and increased healthy behaviors. Such changes were echoed in other participants' follow-up reports.

Notable was the lack of distressing events during the silent, eyes-closed mindfulness meditations or laying down body scan or yoga routines, two activities often considered to be too emotionally challenging for those with complex trauma. The MBI had been delivered utilizing both the trauma-informed and trauma-focused guidelines in this chapter.

The most consistent feedback on the course was that participants liked and valued that they did not need to "tell their trauma story" to the group and that the MBSR curriculum focused on their lives now and moving forward.

Applying a Trauma-Informed Approach

The following guidelines come from (1) the clinical experience of leading MBI groups specifically for women with histories of childhood sexual trauma, who met full PTSD criteria at baseline; (2) facilitating over 60 additional MBI groups for a variety of traumatic stress, chronic pain, and/or chronic illness populations; (3) providing individual therapy for those with traumatic stress and PTSD using trauma-informed mindfulness-based and compassion-based approaches; (4) recommendations gleaned from participants during follow-up interviews; and (4) consultation and collaboration with other MBI teacher therapists working with traumatized populations using a trauma-informed approach.

Clinical Challenges to Providing MBIs to Those
with Traumatic-Stress Histories or Symptoms

The clinical challenges of teaching mindfulness/MBIs come primarily from the PTSD symptoms of *avoidance, reexperiencing, and reactivity*. Rather than seeing these challenges as limiting factors, described here are methods of addressing them that features one of the core mindfulness tenants of "responding" rather than "reacting" to a participant's emotional reactivity. When considering these challenges, it is important to evoke a sense of mastery of the MBI material so as not to perpetuate the cycle of failure so familiar to those with traumatic stress. Specific challenges experienced by survivors of traumatic stress include: (a) increased identification with, and attachment to, a negative story line and memories; (b) increased self-judgment and unworthiness, leading to thoughts of not doing it right, not being good enough, or that one is bad; (c) fear that PTSD symptoms will be triggered (i.e., worry, avoidance) if they become present to their own experiences; (d) feeling hopeless and a failure (i.e., self-doubt, unworthiness); (e) not practicing at home due to not feeling safe; (f) having a tendency to start with the most challenging practices rather than the easiest (Wilkins & Magyari, 2009). The trauma-informed approach responds to these clinical challenges while also maintaining the integrity of the MBI curriculum.

Trauma-Informed Guideline: Prepare the Client
Through Screening for Trauma Symptoms or Events
and Providing Anticipatory Guidance

Screening participants in advance for traumatic symptoms or events prior to the course, and offering all participants the option of one-on-one contact with the MBI teacher prior to or early on in the course is recommended. Specifically reaching out to those who answer positive to these screening questions can help build trust between the teacher and participant. The relationship with the MBI teacher can be a potent support to participants with traumatic stress.

General questions are helpful:

1. "What are your current stressors?" "Your sources of stress?" "Are there any past events that are still stressful for you?" If you limit screening to direct questions about trauma/PTSD, many trauma survivors minimize their own distress and might not mention it. In addition, if they don't have full-blown PTSD, they may say "no" to the question regarding PTSD.
2. "What are your current stress symptoms?"
3. "Do you have a history of trauma?"
4. "Who is helping you with any of the above?"

Flag for follow up anyone who (1) has a diagnosis of PTSD or describes PTSD symptoms—those who meet full criteria, and those who do not; (2) divulges a trauma history or history of traumatic events, regardless of chronology; (3) becomes lost in a traumatic "story"; and (4) is having traumatic stress symptoms such as panic attacks, nightmares, flashbacks, and dissociation.

Appropriate Candidates for MBIs/Mindfulness Groups

MBIs are appropriate interventions for many healing from traumatic stress. However, attention to timing is important. Some clients are best served initially by having individual therapeutic work *prior* to entering a group situation, in particular: those in the immediate crisis phase of their trauma healing, those with ongoing physical safety concerns, and those who are not yet stable on any medications which may be indicated for co-occurring conditions. During this preliminary individual work, it is helpful to put in place basic tools for staying present. Potential MBI participants must be able to organize life on a practical level to attend regular weekly sessions. Participants are best served when MBI teachers aid in this discernment process regarding timing so as to ensure maximum chance of a successful outcome.

Contraindications for group MBIs include being actively suicidal, in an active addiction process, or actively psychotic (unless the MBI teacher/therapist has specialized mental health training to address these situations).

Trauma-Informed Guideline: Developing a Collaborative Relationship Prior to the MBI-Helpful Strategies Before the Class Begins

It can be helpful have opportunities for contact between teacher and participant prior to the MBI, whether in person at an orientation session, in an individual screening session, on the phone so that a trusted relationship might take place. In the words of Brach (2015) a first step in mindfulness-based therapeutic work with those with trauma histories is for the participant to be able to "take comfort in my presence—physically, emotionally, and energetically," a process that may take time. The relationship with the teacher is a valuable support and a resource for those entering into an MBI. Therefore, several points of preparation are helpful to ensure that the course begins smoothly for individual participants and for the group as a whole:

- Have a written registration form and review them as above.
- Touch base in person or on the phone traumatic stress histories or symptoms. Give the option to *all* participants to meet or talk by phone in advance of the first class date if at all feasible.
- In this interview/orientation, inform participants that there will not be a need to "retell" their trauma "story" within the MBI and but neither is it a taboo subject.

Give examples of what might be relevant—if memories or trauma symptoms resurface during meditation or if it relates to any of the practices in the class. Even within trauma-focused MBI classes, the focus is on the here and now—how the past trauma might be interfering with their lives, causing stress or illness—not on the retelling of the traumatic event story.

- In any welcome letter, invite participants to make "special requests" or "let you know of special needs." Control is key to healing trauma. A special request might be anything from wanting to sit in a certain place in the circle (near you, facing the door, near the door) to wanting to know in advance what is happening, to simply needing more reassurance that you know what to do if they get upset in class. Thank them for asking for what they need and be clear about what you can or cannot accommodate. Offer information or reassurance regarding your approach (based on the guidelines in this chapter); anticipatory guidance is often helpful for building trust and calming anxiety and/or reactivity.
- In your MBI class notebook or workbook, provide a listing of the general topics to be covered at each class session. Giving a reasonable amount of structure can help trauma survivors to heal and feel safe enough to trust the process and open to new experiences.
- Encourage participants to contact you if they find themselves in the "distress" zone between classes or find themselves struggling with themselves or the material. Very often, this distress is due to an increased awareness of self-critical cognitions.
- Trauma survivors with PTSDs will often ask in advance if they can just leave class if they need to. This fear is common, but it is a very rare occurrence. Explain that they are free to make their own choices, but you'd prefer that they let you know immediately if they feel distress during the class (see Chap. 37, "Dialogue"); get agreement in advance. Ask what symptoms would make them to want to leave. Normalize any that you can, for example, weeping in class. Weeping isn't disruptive per se and can often be a sign that someone is letting feelings flow instead of numbing or avoiding them.
- Put in place resources and supports for staying present (see below for further details). Even teaching one method for activating the parasympathetic, like taking slow, deep belly breaths when starting to feel activated, can be helpful.

Trauma-Informed Guideline: Preparing the Client Through Putting in Place Resources and Supports for Staying Present

The collaborative relationship with the teacher or therapist, and later, the group, is a valuable resource for the participant with traumatic stress. Other equally valuable resources include tips for grounding in the body (such as contact with the chair or soles of the feet on the ground) or mindful movement; orienting to time and place, which may include opening the eyes temporarily if they are closed; calming the nervous system (through deep belly breaths or audible sighs), and self-soothing (through soothing touch or offering words of encouragement). These can be put in place prior to the MBI at an orientation, individual intake, or early in the first session. Handing out lists of these resources as a reminder for use during home practice can increase a sense of safety and help with emotional regulation when practicing both in session and outside of class.

Teacher/Therapist Characteristics

Teaching *dedicated* MBIs to those with PTSD requires an advanced level of mindfulness training, practice, and embodiment as well as a deep understanding of the traumatized psyche. It is possible to assist those in our mixed groups to a successful completion by using the trauma-informed approach described here. The most important characteristic for the MBI teacher is not reacting in an outer way to a participant's inner or outer reactivity. The teacher models the desired response to reactivity by nonjudgmentally naming the cognitive, physical, and emotional experiences that the client reports experiencing (see Dialogue). It is natural for the MBI participant to react in habituated ways to new experiences that may be frightening to them, which primarily stems from negative cognitive patterns being activated by sensory experiences. Participants may encounter predictable challenges (such as noticing that they can't "feel" parts of their body during the body scan or getting anxious when their mind is quiet) in the first few weeks of the MBI. Dropping out might be reactive, reinforcing a pattern of avoidant behavior toward challenging experiences. Most clients are able to work through temporary challenges brought on by mindfulness practice if they stay with the program and utilize their resources and supports for staying present without distress.

Instead of encouraging avoidance, the trauma-informed MBI teacher gently guides the participant through concrete inquiry with questions such as "what is happening right now in your body?" "What are your feelings?" "On a scale of 1–10, how intense is that feeling?" If the participant can't identify the feeling or says they don't know, ask "which of the four pure emotions comes closest to it—sad, angry, afraid/anxious, or happy/content?" "Where and how do you sense this in your body?" And "Can you be with them in a friendly way?" When negative cognitions arise, as they will, it is important to name them as thoughts and go back to staying with the sensory experiences. Other helpful characteristics include exuding confidence both in mindfulness as a modality and in the participant's potential for recovery and ability to learn mindfulness skills. A sense of humor for the way things are is also helpful. Above all, the teacher is a mindfulness practitioner and embodies the practices in class.

It can be invaluable for individual therapy to continue during the group MBI experience so that the material can be integrated with a known and trusted helper. Signing releases so that you can share the MBI approach and your observations with the individual therapist is recommended.

Incorporating Sensitivities to Trauma into Standard MBI and Other Mindfulness Interventions

Many of these suggestions stem from adhering to good teaching practices, from paying special attention to clarity, safety, trust, and boundaries, and from being aware of how to handle known and expected challenges.

1. **Trauma-informed guideline: Creating safe environments safety concerns**: Choose to hold your groups in a private space and cover any public windows during class time. Sit in a chair where you can watch the door; if a latecomer enters during the opening meditation, state this directly, i.e., "Sally is taking off her coat now and joining the circle." Confidentiality is particularly important; while the MBI teacher may know much about participants' trauma history, the level of sharing is left up to group members. Confidentiality guidelines are discussed/decided upon in the first session. MBI teacher insures group members' feeling of safety with a question such as, "Is there anything else you'd like to ask for to feel safe in this group?" Dim or turn lights off only with the explicit assent of all class participants. In early classes, it is preferable to have lights on, especially if the class is in the evening.

2. **Trauma-informed guideline: Supporting control and autonomy to participants through options and choices**: Language your instructions to invoke "invitations"; permission, emphasizing choice, and giving people time to go at their own pace. For example: "When you're ready, I invite you to open your eyes and rejoin the group." Helping participants to maintain a sense of control over the process of the intervention is empowering and helpful to recovery. Using declarative instructions like "Close your eyes" may raise up resistance, story, and distress; better to say, "You may have your eyes open or closed. If open, I invite you to rest them on the floor in front of you. If closing your eyes, let them gently close when you are ready." Areas of choice might be around eyes open/eyes closed; standing, sitting, or laying down for the body scan; having lights on for the meditations; choosing where in the body to be with the breath; to shift position when needed; to "opt out" or pass for an portion of the class, etc. Those with traumatic stress do not often advocate for their own needs, so explicitly giving options and supporting autonomous choice whenever possible, is helpful.

3. **Trauma-informed guideline: Monitoring and facilitating stability introducing mindfulness in a concrete fashion/titrating silent practice**: "Mindfulness" is often equated with a silent meditation on the breath. While persons with trauma histories/PTSD can benefit over time from extended silent periods of breath meditation, they often benefit from other, more concrete and guided mindfulness practices as a first introduction. I introduce participants to any mindfulness meditation using a grounding and orienting sequence:

   (a) Mindful movement, even a brief stand and stretch before any still, silent practice.

   (b) Orienting to time and place: "I invite you to notice that you are here, now, in [this place] on [this day of the week, this date, this year]"; inviting to practice with eyes open or closed.

   (c) Grounding in the support of the chair/cushion and floor, especially the soles of the feet (Pollak, Pedulla, & Siegel, 2014).

   (d) Down-regulating with a few deep diaphragmatic breaths with long audible exhale to activate the parasympathetic nervous system (Hanson, 2009).

   (e) Reminders to bring calming resources, especially self-kindness (Germer & Neff, 2015) into the practice when inner struggle is arising.

This sequence, which takes 1–2 minutes allows for temporary down-regulation and can also be helpful for those with not also traumatic stress, but also anxiety, ADHD, racing mind, or simply those arriving to class with sympathetic activation. Beginning in this way paves the way for an experience that is self-affirming rather than defeating. Speaking too softly or leaving long silences may encourage distress, getting lost in story, or spacing out.

Balance permissions/autonomy/control with structure and guidance. Beginners need concrete instructions for where to place their awareness while navigating silence on their own. Emotional reactivity is often found in the domain of emotions and thoughts, and traumatic experiences are often stored in the body. Therefore, providing a structured way of working with experiences in these domains can be helpful for evoking confidence and the ability to stay present, especially during meditations using bodily sensations, emotions, or thoughts as the anchor; open awareness (choiceless awareness) practices; and any meditation that involves long periods of silence. Neuroscience has a tenant, "if you can name it, you can tame it"; encouraging participants to name experiences while experiencing them is calming to the nervous system. Linehan (1993) developed a 3-step process as part of the mindfulness training in DBT that is particularly stabilizing: (1) observe: notice the experience; (2) describe: choose concrete, descriptive words to name it; and (3) participate: fully experience it.

Especially when you are leading challenging practices or exercises, be clear on the purpose of the exercise. Articulate the reason for the exercise/practice and how it fits into the curriculum.

4. **Addressing reactivity** ("I can't do this," "I'm not doing it right"). Listen carefully for these self-judgments, which are natural responses to beginning mindfulness practice that often cause a great deal of distress. Reframe these cognitions as examples of self-judgment that can be acknowledged and responded to appropriately: becoming aware, naming (i.e., "judging"), noticing how one experiences self-judging on a somatic level, and responding in a kind way to any reactivity that has already occurred following the self-judgment. Use brain science to depersonalize and normalize the "I'm not good enough" story of traumatized/stressed mind.

5. **Normalizing PTSD coping strategies and honoring their role in the past**: It is important to tell the participant "We aren't trying to 'get rid' of anything," especially in regard to past coping mechanisms. Participants may feel shame in regard to maladaptive coping such as avoidant behavior, an inability to control

reactivity to flashbacks or triggering experiences, perfectionism, or dissociation. For participants with childhood trauma histories and adult PTSD symptoms, it is helpful to explicitly state, perhaps in the initial meeting, that the "hurt little girl (or boy) was doing the best he/she could at the time," and is to be honored for keeping the participant alive until adulthood, and that now we are learning another way to respond to past traumas that will allow for a fuller way of living (Wilkins, 2014). Use motivational interviewing techniques to tie the MBI curriculum to participants' personal goals for reducing their trauma symptoms.

6. **Being explicit about how to maintain mindfulness that fosters healing** during class and at home should be done before any meditation practice. Teach participants how to differentiate between the constructive challenge of staying present with unpleasant experiences vs. the unproductive "staying with" once a participant has lost mindfulness and is living within a distressing experience or is in the "distress zone." Suggestions for using supports if participants find themselves in distress at home may include: stop meditation temporality, open eyes, stand, use senses to notice your surrounding, get water, take deep belly breaths, and/or do something self-soothing, along with naming the experience: "distress," "dissociating," "flashback," etc. When the ability to be mindful of present moment experience has returned, it is possible to rejoin the meditation. In later sessions on stress reactivity, discuss how to know whether one is entering the distress zone, seeing clearly the cognitions that take one there, and using present moment experiences to avoid, or exit the distress zone once in it. Give explicit words to track and note inner reactivity ("judging," "adding-on," "telling stories," "spinning"). Since participants are apt to swamp themselves with taking on too much in the beginning, it can be helpful to guide them to "Pick up the 5-lb weight, not the 50-lb weight" (Wilkins, personal communication, 2009); alternatively participants can be reminded "we're practicing meditation, not masochism" (Santanello, 2014). In practical terms, this means not doing extended silent practice without guidance from a CD or teacher until skills to constructively use the meditation are developed, generally after the first two or three weekly sessions.

7. **Balancing awareness and compassion**: Participants may develop focused attention and increased awareness early in the course. It is important to achieve balance in distressed individuals through the addition of compassion. Kindness and friendliness to one's own experience is woven throughout the MBI course from the beginning in implicit and explicit ways. A concrete and structured way to approach self-compassion that is well tolerated by those with traumatic stress is the loving-kindness meditation — especially offering the well wishes to those they love easily or who make them happy.

8. **Giving instructions on how to transcend the cycle of self-loathing** by responding instead of reacting to cognitive self-judgments. Since self-loathing and self-judging cognitive habits are generally very strong in this group, give explicit instructions for working with this habit in order to break the downward spiral that comes from then feeling bad about this habit, i.e., judging our judging as bad or wrong. If mindfulness is strong and there is no inner reaction stemming from "believing" these self-judgments, the participant may note, "judging," and keep

going. However, more often there *is* an inner reaction—some sense of feeling bad or wrong or defective stemming from the self-judgment. In this case, it is helpful for the participant to respond with self-kindness: self-soothing before continuing. Responding in this way sets up a new, more healing habit and sense of inner relationship to self. It can be helpful to check in with clients with trauma histories and ask them which method of self-soothing is working the best for them. If they don't know, exploring in a brief session can help ensure continued productive participation.

9. **Emphasis on naming the "habits of the mind"**: From the first session, the teacher discusses the therapeutic value of getting to know the habits of the mind. Cognitive neuroscience is helpful in this regard; participants may be able to understand the concept of "neural grooves" and the value of noticing and naming cognitive habits as just that—habits or "grooves" that may or may not be relevant to the present moment. I challenge participants to notice and acknowledge their most common mental habits—planning, worry, analyzing, judging, spinning stories, fantasizing, or "spacing out."

Adaptations to Standard MBIs: Applying a Trauma-Focused Approach

Running trauma-focused MBIs—that is, groups in which all members have traumatic stress symptoms or full PTSD—requires considerable skill and trauma training beyond that required to run a trauma-informed MBI. It is recommended that those teaching trauma-sensitive or trauma-focused groups and adaptations have mental health licenses or qualifications, and work in consort with other mental health professionals who may be working with the client. Those offering Trauma-focused MBIs for specific populations will want to incorporate all of the proceeding trauma-informed guidelines in addition to the following additional considerations. These additional considerations are directly related to monitoring and facilitating stability—within each individual member, as well as the group as a whole.

1. **Increase contact before, during, and after the course or extending the length of the MBI**: A trauma-focused group often has additional intensity simply from the fact that everyone in the group has been affected by trauma and a higher degree of emotional destabilization may be present in the group. Spending time upfront creating a collaborative relationship through having an individual session with every participant, as well having an orientation session where participants can meet each other and ask questions before the MBI begins, builds the resource of the teacher and the group to draw on prior to the MBI. Additionally, building in time for beforehand to put in place resources and supports and tapering off rather than having an abrupt ending, is helpful. As an example, the 8-week MBSR course could be extended to 14 weeks, to allow for an intro week 1, a "pre" session putting in place resources and support such as touch points, soles

of the feet, soothing touch in week 2, the 8-week intervention in weeks 3–10; and then 2 additional sessions to integrate, 2 weeks apart in weeks 12 and 14. Extending integration time through monthly dedicated grad classes for up to 12 months is ideal. If not possible, suggest having integrated sessions with a trusted therapist, or joining an ongoing mindfulness practice group to integrate and stabilize.

2. **Predictable class structure**: Participants benefit from having a reliable structure to the class, which can be deliberately, but slowly, made more flexible as needed as the group progresses. I use the following structure within each class: (a) formal meditations learned in the preceding class (to evoke a sense of confidence or orientation within the 8-week structure); (b) inquiry check-in to encourage naming of raw experiences rather than "storytelling" and identify participants in distress; (c) dyad sharing regarding at-home practices, using a mindful listening/speaking format to stay present to one's own experience; (d) inquiry; (e) new material; (f) check-in; (g) review of pertinent notebook pages; (h) assignment of at-home practices; (i) ritualized ending involving holding hands while standing in a circle, emphasizing connection to self (body/breath), group members, and the earth.

3. **Increased processing time**: While there may not be time to do a full inquiry after every meditation, it is possible to check-in with everyone through brief inquiry methods. After every meditation, include at least a go-around mindful inquiry: "one or two words of your current experience: physical, emotional, or mental," with attention paid to the degree of presence. This provides additional opportunity to process experiences and identify participants having trauma-related distress. (See Dialogue, Chap. 24, for how to work with distress once identified).

   Making time in the curriculum for participants to express their experience of being in a dedicated group where everyone shares this history, perhaps in the second or third meeting is helpful. Participants may find the shared history comforting on one hand, and destabilizing on another, as the reality of their history is reinforced by their inclusion in this group. Allowing for noticing, naming, and expressing their experience, and the additional vulnerability this might stir up, is helpful. The teacher normalizes and validates any experiences, including ambivalence for being part of the group.

4. **Additional practice for staying in contact with the self during dyads**: Dyads are helpful to practice mindful listening and mindful speaking on a weekly basis as well as to process at-home experiences. Even with mindfulness in place, participants can be pulled out of themselves through the process of relating to others. Participants can thence practice coming back to themselves through the "three breaths break" between dyad questions While participants stay with their experience of three breath cycles, the teacher reinforces the idea that they are moving from "outer" to "inner," from "doing" to "being," and invites participants to notice what this movement feels like; cue to the support of the chair and the floor, for additional grounding.

5. **Positive psychology enhancements**: Class material is taught in a manner designed to emphasize the positive psychology tenets of mastery, cultivating gratitude, acknowledging one's efforts, savoring positive experiences, connec-

tion, noticing what works, coping effectiveness training, and honoring one's own inner wisdom. It is important to encourage acknowledging one's experience first, only then applying positive psychology. Otherwise "being positive" can engender resistance. Instead, invite curiosity. Rather than saying, "be grateful to yourself for completing the course" (which can sound like a demand ask) say, "notice if there is anything you feel grateful for towards yourself, whether you appreciate anything, and how you might like to express that towards yourself."

6. **Retreats**: If the MBI includes a retreat, offer it in a trauma-informed and trauma-focused manner. See retreat section, below, for specific recommendations.

Example of Trauma-Informed Practice: The Body Scan

Spending unstructured silent time focusing on bodily sensations (or lack of sensations) may stir up uncomfortable sensations, "story," and potentially be retraumatizing, especially if the participant doesn't feel safe in the practice. On the other hand, increasing one's ability to "be with" physical experiences is very helpful for healing from trauma, so much so that some trauma therapists feel this is a critical component of the healing process (van der Kolk, 2014). In addition, some MBI participants feel the body scan to have been the most helpful mindfulness practice for them in their trauma recovery, as noted earlier. The trauma-informed approach relies on giving participants preparatory suggestions for practice, either in a session before the course or in the first class, so there is a better chance of having an affirming experience. The following guidelines are useful in helping participants feel safe, in control, and able to participate to whatever degree they are choosing to participate during the body scan by applying many of the trauma-informed guidelines already delineated. Most may only be necessary during the first or second sessions, while participants are becoming familiar with the space, the process, and the experience.

Create a Safe Space Where You Are in Control of the Room

Please refer to the basic logistics discussed/outlined previously in the chapter, regarding the teacher's location in the room, and the room's lighting (see also Chapter 1, Stewardship).

Let Participants Know They Are in Control of Their Experiences

- Invite them to choose whether to sit or lie down. Normalize either choice.
- It is alright for them to take a break and simply rejoin the scan when ready; there is no point in getting overwhelmed on the first try.

- If they can't locate particular parts of the body, simply note "can't locate," or "no sensation," and rejoin the scan at the next body part. Normalize physical numbing.
- If they become swamped by distress and lose mindful awareness (see below), they should let you know immediately.

Give Participants Tools for Self-Soothing, as Necessary

- Let them know, if they are heading toward distress, that they can open their eyes and take deep abdominal breaths, or place a hand on their heart, and focus on being in the room or practice behavioral compassion—standing up, getting a drink of water; then rejoin the scan when ready.

Guidance and Assurance Through the Body Scan Practice

- If some are sitting and others are lying down, finish with a very brief "downward" scan, always ending with feet. This practice is most grounding for those sitting up.
- Invite them, as beginners, to "see what we are experiencing today," invoking curiosity.
- Give everyday metaphors that garner interest, such as walking through a museum whose exhibit changes everyday often—"some things you might like, others you might not, but we can honor and respect them all."
- "Normalize imperfection": validate physical numbness, validate lack of sensation or inability to locate a part; acknowledge the validity of historical developmental dissociation or avoidance or bodily numbing (Wilkins, 2014).
- Avoid dissociative visualizations in the midst of the scan.
- Scan the room occasionally yourself to check whether anyone is experiencing signs of distress, knowing that those who have dissociated may *not* exhibit any outward signs.

Inquire About Participants' Experience After the Body Scan

Inquiry regarding participant experiences can be especially helpful after the body scan, either through dyads, a brief "go-round" or full group inquiry. Brief go-rounds—hearing 1 or two words about "right now" from each participant can be especially helpful for trauma-focused groups where participants have experienced physical or sexual trauma. Not only does naming experience help to calm the nervous system but it also helps participants to recall the resource of the group and teacher. Assess for signs of dissociation and check in before end of class to see if anyone "hasn't come back yet" (see Dialogue). When responding to inquiry, it is helpful to validate what participants *can* feel and model acceptance of the what can't yet be sensed in the body.

Body Scan Recordings and Instruction for Practicing at Home

Recording two lengths of the body scan provides choice and a point of entry for more participants: a 20 minutes brief body scan focused on finding and sensing relatively large swaths of the body, with many concrete cues and very little silence (1–2 breath cycles per pause); and a 40 minutes body scan including cues to smaller and more subtle sensations (i.e., individual toes or fingers,) with longer silence (up to 3–4 breath cycles per pause). Encourage starting with the shorter scan, and moving to longer scan only if shorter one does not provoke distress. Emphasize making wise choices, including stopping in the middle if "too much."

Ask participants to discover "Where in your body you can rest your awareness most comfortably? It doesn't have to be a comfortable sensation, but it might be. Ie. in your hands or feet for instance [name examples of areas that might be neutral]. Once you've found that place, you can use it as a 'home base' to come back to whenever you want during the body scan or during any of the silent meditation practices if you get lost or need a break from the practice" [this puts in place a powerful resource for them].

Cueing to resources: Opening eyes, stretching your body, offering self-soothing touch or words; taking deep belly breaths." Rejoin the scan when you're ready.

Especially in trauma-focused groups, participants may benefit from additional external support at home, such the picture of a supportive person, pet or spiritual figure; or an object that reminds them of support and/or inner strength. They may wish to do the body scan having it near-by, holding it, or putting it on their chest by their heart.

Cue to down-regulating resources: Suggest exercising, doing some mindful movement, or taking three deep belly breaths before the body scan can be helpful for calming the nervous system.

Mindfulness Retreats: Trauma-Informed and Trauma-Focused

Trauma-Informed Retreats

Trauma-Informed Silent Retreat Days: Retreats offer the opportunity to reap the benefits of extended periods of mindfulness meditation and their completion are often a point of pride and accomplishment. For many in an MBI, this is their first silent retreat and the newness may be anxiety provoking; a new location or additional people attending may be a source of anxiety. The following are helpful trauma-informed considerations: Providing anticipatory guidance regarding any new element such as additional people attending.

Bracketing the day with a structured opening and closing sequence, which includes brief sharing. During the opening sit, include grounding elements and a reminder of resources (including self-soothing and the group itself); follow with dyad sharing around present moment experience and setting an "intention" for the day (a mindful quality); brief "go-round" sharing 1–2 words of "right now" and one's intention; teacher reinforces that all intentions are now in the room as a resource.

Providing a brief orientation, defining silence as a "companionable silence"; silence doesn't mean you can't sneeze or cough or laugh, if those arise naturally; state that questions about "what we are doing" are welcome at any time. State directly when entering silent period. Doing yoga as the first formal practice after entering the silence can help down-regulate. Gathering before unstructured time (ex. meal time), to sense resource of the group and orient briefly to activities during this time; offer to talk with anyone during meal break "if they're in distress"—just knowing someone is available is often all that is needed to increase safety. Cuing to their chosen intention and reminding of resources before any meditation with extended silence.

Ending with structured closing, including opportunity for verbal sharing. Trauma-informed inquiry questions include: "what was most helpful?," "what was most pleasant?," and "what would you most like to remember?" Offer to "be around for a few minutes" if anyone wants to talk and check-in directly those who expressed verbal or non-verbal cues of distress. Sexual trauma can take the form of rape, incest, assault, or other sexual violations.

Trauma-Sensitive and Trauma-Focused Retreats

The considerations in the previous section on trauma-informed silent retreat days (ex. structured beginning, etc.) can be tremendously useful for trauma-focused retreats; trauma-focused groups may also benefit from additional stabilizing adaptations, such as:

Shortening the hours of the silent retreat, to perhaps half-day.
Starting with brief mindful movement before the 30-minutes structured opening described earlier.
Shortening the unstructured time after the meal.
Adding additional "check-ins" with participants, especially right before and after the unstructured meal period, and after any still silent practices.
Reinforcing a shared experience of the mindful eating by sharing potluck or provided food. Standing together experiencing sights and smells of the food prior to eating.

Delaying the retreat until later in the series, especially if there are more than eight sessions; ensure there is at least one more session after the retreat for integration. Having the retreat follow directly after one of the regular weekly sessions, if the class is during the day and the venue is available.

This has the advantage of grounding in the "known" of the class structure, venue, and course participants, and the stress-relieving aspect of the mindfulness practice in the class first before the retreat.

Conclusion

This chapter has reviewed guidelines for applying a trauma-informed approach to teaching MBI's as well as additional suggestions for teacher-therapists who may be offering trauma-focused MBIs. There are a variety of clinical challenges for this population. Those with traumatic stress symptoms and histories benefit from mindfulness interventions, including trauma-informed titrated instruction, thoughtful adaptations, and helpful collaboration between the referring therapist and mindfulness provider. With attention to these factors, MBIs and other mindfulness approaches may allow persons to free themselves from the sequelae of past traumatic life events, and to move forward with renewed mental health, increased resilience, and enhanced coping strategies with which to meet future life events.

Acknowledgement With deep gratitude to all of the men and women who have entrusted their sufferings to our care, and whose lives are blossoming moment by moment. *May they be well. May they be safe. May they be happy and free.*

References

American Psychiatric Association. (2013). *Diagnostic and statistical manual of mental disorders* (5th ed.). Washington, DC: Author.

Brach, T. (2015). Healing traumatic fear: The wings of mindfulness and love. In V. Follette, J. Briere, D. Rozelle, et al. (Eds.), *Mindfulness-oriented approaches to trauma care* (p. 32). New York, NY: Guilford Press.

Briere, J., & Spinazzola, J. (2009). Assessment of the sequelae of complex trauma: Evidence-based measures. In C. A. Courtois & J. D. Ford (Eds.), *Treating complex traumatic stress disorders: An evidence-based guide [e-book]* (pp. 104–123). New York, NY: Guilford Press.

Briere, J., & Rickards, S. (2007). Self-awareness, affect regulation, and relatedness: Differential sequels of childhood versus adult victimization experiences. *Journal of Nervous and Mental Disease, 195*(6): 497–503.

Follette, V. M., Briere, J., Rozelle, D., Hopper, J. W., & Rome, D.I. (eds.) (2015). *Mindfulness-oriented interventions for trauma.* New York, NY: Guilford Press.

Germer, C. K., & Neff, K. D. (2015). Cultivating self-compassion in trauma survivors. In V. Follette, J. Briere, D. Rozelle, J. Hopper, & D. Rome (Eds.), *Mindfulness-oriented interventions for trauma* (pp. 43–58). New York, NY: Guilford Press.

Hanson, R. (2009). *Buddha's brain: The practical neuroscience of happiness, love and wisdom* (p. 81). Oakland, CA: New Harbinger Press.

Jackson Nakazawa, D. (2015). *Childhood disrupted: How your biography becomes your biology and how you can heal* (pp. 161–160). New York, NY: Atria Books.

Kimbrough, E., Magyari, T., Langenberg, C., Chesney, M., & Berman, B. (2010). Mindfulness intervention for child abuse survivors. *Journal of Clinical Psychiatry, 66*(1), 17–33.

Linehan, M. M. (1993). *Cognitive-behavioral treatment of borderline personality disorder.* New York, NY: Guilford Press.

Magyari, T. (2015). Teaching MBIs and mindfulness to women with complex trauma. In V. Follette, J. Briere, D. Rozelle, J. Hopper, & D. Rome (Eds.), *Mindfulness-oriented interventions for trauma* (pp. 140–156). New York, NY: Guilford Press. Retrieved from http://www.merriam-webster.com/dictionary/trauma.

Pollak, S., Pedulla, T., & Siegel, R. (2014). *Sitting together: Essential skills for mindfulness-based psychotherapy.* New York, NY: Guilford Press.

Santanello, A. Personal communication, October 2014.

Substance Abuse and Mental Health Services Administration (SAMHSA). (2014). *Trauma-informed care in behavioral health services* (Treatment improvement protocol (TIP), Vol. 57). Rockville, MD: Author. HHS Publication No. (SMA) 14-4816.

van der Kolk, B. (2014). *The body keeps the score.* New York, NY: Penguin.

Wilkins, C. (2014). Mindfulness, women, and childhood abuse—Turning toward what's difficult. *Social Work Today, 14*(2), 10.

Wilkins, C., & Magyari, T. (2009). *Shelter in the storm: Teaching mindfulness for those with PTSD.* Paper presented at the annual meeting presentation: Mindfulness in medicine, health care and society, University of Massachusetts Medical School, Worcester, MA.

Williams, G., Mark, J., Fennell, M., Barnhofer, T., Crane, R., & Silverton, S. (2015). *Mindfulness and the transformation of despair: Working with people at risk of suicide.* New York, NY: Guilford Press.

Chapter 19
Teaching Individuals Mindful Eating

Jean L. Kristeller and Andrea E. Lieberstein

Teaching Mindful Eating: A Practical Guide

Helping individuals to explore their relation to eating and food can provide a door into all aspects of mindful engagement. As it is in the mindfulness-based stress reduction (MBSR) program, savoring a few raisins is also the first window into mindfulness in the mindfulness-based eating awareness (MB-EAT) program. This simple experience brings a quality of full attention into the moment of tasting and eating a raisin. While eating is usually considered a behavioral process, it also involves the full range of human experiences: the body, thoughts, emotions, self-identity, and social engagement. Our relationship to food can also be a spiritual experience, as beautifully addressed in several books on mindful eating (Altman, 1999; Bays, 2009; Kabatznick, 1998). Helping people bring mindfulness to their relationship with eating food can be powerful in applying and understanding the broader value of mindfulness practice in cultivating self-regulation and wisdom (Kristeller, 2007, 2015; Kristeller & Epel, 2014; Marlatt & Kristeller, 1999).

This chapter explores how teaching MB-EAT overlaps considerably with teaching mindfulness in other contexts. Yet there are unique challenges in its focused application to eating behavior, whether for individuals with relatively balanced eating patterns, or for those with a range of eating disorders and issues (Kristeller, 2016a; Kristeller & Wolever, 2011). We first present some broad underlying concepts that are distinct to MB-EAT, and which are particularly important to keep in mind when teaching the program. Then, we review key points that illustrate teaching the unique content elements.

J.L. Kristeller, Ph.D. (✉)
Department of Psychology, Indiana State University, Terre Haute, IN 47809, USA
e-mail: jkristeller@indstate.edu

A.E. Lieberstein, M.P.H., R.D.N., R.Y.T.
Mindful Eating Training, Novato, CA, USA
e-mail: andrea@mindfuleatingtraining.com

© Springer International Publishing Switzerland 2016
D. McCown et al., *Resources for Teaching Mindfulness*,
DOI 10.1007/978-3-319-30100-6_19

Research over the last 50 years has documented the degree to which eating involves complex processes, only some of which are related to our biological need for food energy and nutrition (Capaldi, 1996). Basic physical needs are complemented by many other uses of food—to celebrate, to socialize, to obtain pleasure, or to soothe and comfort. The first set of physical needs involve maintaining a relatively homeostatic energy balance in the body. The second set involves finding satisfaction and enjoyment with food. Healthy eating arguably encompasses maintaining a flexible balance between homeostatic and hedonic needs for food. Other psychological factors that also affect food intake, in even balanced and healthy eaters, are: eating in response to social pressures; eating "mindlessly" while doing other tasks; eating more whenever larger portions are served; continuing eating patterns and preferences learned in childhood. Maintaining a balance between physical needs for food and the psychological influences on eating often occurs without much awareness for many individuals, while for others, physical needs for food are very much out of balance with meeting other needs. Research evidence to date supports that working towards this balance appears to be facilitated by increasing mindful awareness of these different aspects of our relationship to eating, food, and our bodies (Kristeller & Hallett, 1999; Kristeller, Wolever, & Sheets, 2013).

Background: Connecting the Mind and the Body

We all eat mindlessly at times, and we are all influenced by the interplay between physiological need for food, and all the other influences on eating. Wansink (2007) has identified that individuals with no particular issues with weight or eating make on average 200 decisions per day about food (what to eat, when to eat, when to stop, etc.), many of which are relatively automatic and mindless. This number of decisions increases to about 300 for those with significant weight problems (Wansink & Sobal, 2007). This complexity may be one reason why diets that prescribe particular food choices hold considerable appeal, but restrictive approaches provide little training in how to negotiate the reality of food choices in more flexible, sustainable, and balanced ways.

Cultivating a greater capacity for mindfulness, using a range of general and guided meditation practices, supports the key goal of the MB-EAT program to help individuals make more mindful decisions as they navigate their usual eating environments. Rather than prescribing new patterns from without, individuals are encouraged to first become aware of their current patterns and then to begin to explore how to modify them in ways that will be sustainable, rather than temporary. Group participants are shown how to use mindfulness to observe their own unique challenges, explore options, cultivate awareness of their own inner experiences, make new choices, and weaken dominant patterns.

Much as other MB-programs have grown out of a melding of traditional practices and contemporary psychological theory, MB-EAT has been informed by a combination of theoretical models, cutting edge research on eating behavior and therapeutic intervention, and meditative practices. From the initial development of key elements, beginning in the late 1970s and early 1980s, through to the more recent clinical trial research, MB-EAT has drawn on self-regulation theory (Cuthbert, Kristeller, Simons, Hodes, & Lang, 1981; Davidson, Goleman, & Schwartz, 1976; Kristeller, 1977; Lutz, Slagter, Dunne, & Davidson, 2008; Schwartz, 1975), and theories of eating regulation that acknowledge the interplay of both psychological and physiological processes as modulated by attention and awareness (Rodin, 1978, 1981; Schachter & Rodin, 1974).

The concept of "wisdom" or insight, a core aspect of traditional mindfulness practice, is also central to the MB-EAT program. In the context of this program, wisdom is defined as the ability to recognize solutions to challenging situations as they arise into awareness in the mind, rather than having such solutions defined by someone else. This definition of wisdom is consistent with those that have been proposed within contemporary psychological theory (Baltes & Staudinger, 2000; Sternberg, 1990), but is also intended to resonate with the traditional context of mindfulness meditation as cultivating wisdom or insight (Kristeller, 2003).

The neurocognitive models of meditation that focus on re-regulation, such as Self-Determination Theory (Deci, Ryan, Schultz, & Niemiec, 2015; Ryan & Deci, 2000), explicitly hypothesize that mindfulness practice helps shift the balance from *external regulation* (as imposed by structured diets, for example) to *integrated regulation* in which intrinsic processes meld with external factors for optimal self-regulation. Mindfulness practice also cultivates the capacity to disengage undesirable reactivity, and to engage processes that more "wisely" inform behavior. Even novice meditators have been shown to improve their ability for creative or insight-oriented problem solving (Meeks, Cahn, & Jeste, 2012; Ostafin & Kassman, 2012). Heightening this capacity is particularly relevant to issues related to eating and food choices (Kristeller & Epel, 2014; Kristeller & Wolever, 2011). Throughout the MB-EAT program, mindfulness practices, regardless of their forms, are framed repeatedly as ways to connect with one's own "wise mind."

This model of cultivating wisdom meshes particularly well with the goals and perspectives of MB-EAT. The MB-EAT program places a strong emphasis on cultivating personal "wisdom." There is evidence suggesting considerable variation in regard to underlying patterns even in healthy eating behaviors (Drewnowski, 1996; Kristeller & Rodin, 1989) and there are a remarkable number of decisions regarding eating that are made daily, as noted above. While some models of imbalance focus primarily on biological, genetic, or epigenetic explanations for lack of eating regulation, most individuals can become "disconnected" from internal experiences of hunger and satiety, resulting in "mindless" eating. Furthermore, given evidence supporting the influence of these largely uncontrollable biological/genetic factors, it is all the more reason that individuals deepen their ability to tune into those aspects which are indeed more responsive to personal choice and which may provide a balance to other influences. Therefore, it is important that anyone leading the MB-EAT program, or addressing mindfulness and eating in their program, stay attuned to the complexity involved in eating, and in supporting individuals in the challenges presented, while also respecting the wide variability among individuals in regard to what constitutes relatively healthy patterns of eating.

From the first session, the program is presented to participants as a means for cultivating both greater "inner wisdom" and greater "outer wisdom" to increase balanced eating. "Inner wisdom" involves tuning into immediate physical experiences of hunger, taste, and fullness, and also to related emotions, thoughts, desires, and satisfaction related to eating. "Outer wisdom" involves making use of knowledge of nutrition, healthy choices, portion sizes, and food energy (calorie) information, but in a way that meets both personal health needs and personal food preferences, rather than rigidly following externally set dietary guidelines or rigid rules. We emphasize to participants that such wisdom will emerge from the richness of their own experiences, when engaged with "mindfully," rather than mindlessly. For example, one man with type 2 diabetes had fluctuated between avoiding eating any ice cream, and overeating it compulsively. He realized he could be satisfied by very small amounts of his favorite kind when he fully savored the taste, and while holding an attitude of acceptance rather than guilt. Furthermore, he realized that this amount was still acceptable within his dietary guidelines, whereas the amount he'd previously been eating, mindlessly but guiltily, was needlessly out of balance. He also discovered by mindfully checking his blood sugar, that having the ice cream with a meal had far less impact on his blood sugar than when he had it as a late evening snack. We encourage individuals within the treatment groups to share insights or moments of such wisdom related to making new types of everyday food choices (such as discarding part of a sandwich—not because they "should," but because they realize they are satisfied and don't want more). We regularly emphasize in the program that mindfulness practice assists in accessing such "tacit" wisdom and identifying creative solutions in any situation, including seemingly trivial, but often complex, decisions regarding food choice and eating.

Cultivating Inner Wisdom

With regard to our relationship to eating, the most important aspect of "inner wisdom" is cultivating *interoceptive awareness*. This process brings awareness inward, particularly in relation to physical hunger, taste, and satiety cues, as core elements of balancing internal regulatory processes. Tuning into hunger and satiety signals has, for example, been shown to be effective for promoting weight management in Linda Craighead's Appetite Awareness model (Brown, Smith, & Craighead, 2010; Craighead, 2006). Again, this type of focus is in marked contrast to diet-oriented or prescribed/restrictive approaches to managing eating or losing weight.

The physical signals available to interoceptive awareness include hunger signals, such as the stomach growling and low blood sugar; experiences of physical fullness and body satiety; and experience of taste and taste satiety (Capaldi, 1996; Ogden, 2010). However complex overall patterns of eating may be, involving numerous micro-decisions, the process of reconnecting to internal hunger and satiety signals (interoceptive awareness) is relatively simple and easily experienced for most individuals. Indeed, it begins with eating those first few raisins. As people come to be more aware of these experiences and use them as a counterbalance to all the other pressures to eat and overeat, including emotional distress, they begin to replace the sense of struggle with a sense of choice.

Hunger. Hunger is a complex process, involving multiple biological and psychological elements (Berthoud, 2012; Drewnowski, 1996). Tuning into physical hunger, in contrast to simply craving or desiring a food, involves several elements: (a) becoming more aware of a range of hunger signals, from the absence of hunger, to just a bit hungry, to "starving"; (b) discerning the difference between feelings of physical hunger and the pull of all other types of eating triggers; and (c) responding to hunger signals in more balance, neither denying oneself inappropriately nor overeating to the extreme. By tuning into the experience and range of hunger signals, participants learn to recognize and respond to moderate levels of hunger. For example, some participants, particularly those with a background of food insecurity, may realize they eat whenever they feel the slightest bit of hunger. In contrast, others, who may have been on many restrictive diets, tend to limit their intake to try to be "good," leading to feelings of intense hunger and ultimate overeating. In either case, these individuals benefit from learning to tune in to more moderate hunger signals.

Fullness. Stomach fullness is, of course, another signal that people use to decide when to end a meal. Individuals who regularly eat larger amounts of food at one time tolerate higher levels of stomach fullness because their stomachs are stretched (Geliebter & Hashim, 2001; Geliebter, Hassid, & Hashim, 2001; Sysko, Hildebrandt, Wilson, Wilfley, & Agras, 2010), but they also fail to attend to these signals at lower levels (i.e., moderately full), or they purposefully seek out higher levels of fullness. Whether someone's pattern is to habitually "super-size" their meals, or choosing to eat until they are "too full to eat anymore," we help them tune in mindfully to more moderate levels of fullness. Again, we take a supportive, flexible approach, reminding them that there is no precisely "right" amount to eat, and that even balanced eaters may eat to a point of discomfort on occasion, such as at holiday meals.

Taste. The experience of taste is a core focus of the program. Paradoxically, while individuals with weight problems and/or binge eating disorder (BED) will often describe themselves as "loving" food too much, or being "addicted," we've found that much of the time, they are consuming food mindlessly, and paying little attention to the sensory value of what they are eating. From a Buddhist perspective, they are "attached" to the food they eat, yet in conflict about it, caught in a perennial struggle. At the same time, we find that failing to truly tune into taste extends to most individuals at times, as illustrated by the powerful experience of mindfully eating a few raisins within MBSR. We encourage people to cultivate their "inner gourmet" as a way to balance their eating, choosing foods mindfully, and then fully savoring them. This inner gourmet provides a message that differs dramatically from an abstinence approach. It is also one that most people find surprisingly easy to attain, with many reporting how amazed they are at the differences they experience in foods they'd previously craved or even considered "addictive," often finding that these foods have far less appeal, or that far smaller amounts suffice. They may discover that while eating less, they are enjoying food more.

They also learn that the sensory experience of food is truly fleeting. Decrease in taste intensity is the quickest feedback signal for when to stop eating, helping people to cut down substantially on portion sizes. Sensory-specific satiety (or "taste satiety," as we refer to it) is the process by which food loses its appeal as the taste buds in our mouths habituate to specific flavors (Blundell & Bellisle, 2013; Remick, Polivy, & Pliner, 2009; Sørensen, Møller, Flint, Martens, & Raben, 2003), often after only a few bites. We ask people to assess the pleasure and satisfaction they are gaining from each bite of food, from 1 to 10, considering, after each bite, whether to eat more or not, rather than "chasing the flavor." People are always surprised when they realize that they don't want the fourth raisin, the third piece of cheese and crackers, or the last bite of cookie. They realize they can stop at that point without struggle, truly savoring their eating experience. They can even let themselves gain comfort from food, but now from smaller, rather than larger amounts, quite in contrast to addiction models of excessive food intake (Brownell & Gold, 2012; Grosshans, Loeber, & Kiefer, 2011; Lustig, 2012).

Thoughts and Feelings. Suppressing thoughts about foods and inappropriate metacognitions play a role in compulsive overeating (Barnes, Masheb, White, & Grilo, 2013; Olstad, Solem, Hjemdal, & Hagen, 2015). Therefore, core to "inner wisdom" is learning to tune into both habitual thought patterns about eating, and to the use of food to meet other needs. We also emphasize that such thoughts as "I should always clear my plate," or "Nobody can tell me what to eat—so I'm going to have it all," are habitual patterns that can simply be mindfully observed, rather than responded to (e.g., Bowen, Witkiewitz, Dillworth, & Marlatt, 2007).

Interoceptive awareness can also be applied to the arising of emotions. How does the body feel when anxiety arises? When anger arises? Boredom? Habitually eating "from the middle of emotions" can be interrupted by bringing mindful awareness to the thoughts and feelings that are present when an urge to eat arises by discerning physical hunger from emotional hunger, working with emotions mindfully as in MBSR, and making a mindful choice in that space created, as to whether or not to eat and how much. Being pulled towards eating in response to thoughts or to handle emotions is not in itself unusual, but may be more intense in individuals with disregulated eating patterns and obesity (Appelhans, 2009; Appelhans et al., 2011). Wisdom comes from becoming aware of such tendencies, exercising mindfulness, and bringing them into better balance with physical needs for food.

Stress-related eating. Although meditation offers a powerful tool for relaxation, we are careful to not frame the primary role of meditation practice as "stress-reduction," as that carries the implication that decreasing "stress-related" eating is all that is needed to end the struggle, when it is generally only one of many challenges. While individuals with BED are more likely to use eating to manage stress (Goldfield, Adamo, Rutherford, & Legg, 2008), it may still range from relatively benign use of food for comfort, to overusing eating as a coping strategy or distraction, to more extreme reliance on eating as a way to dissociate from overwhelming and unresolved emotions, such as those linked to a history of trauma (Grave, Oliosi, Todisco, & Vanderlinden, 1997; Grilo & Masheb, 2002; Peterson, Miller, Crow, Thuras, & Mitchell, 2005).

Indeed, as noted earlier, many people with reasonably balanced relationships to food are drawn to using eating for comfort or other non-nutritive reasons. By normalizing this tendency—in moderation—we find that even individuals with BED realize that they can modulate these cravings, letting themselves enjoy and savor smaller amounts of favorite foods, while exploring other ways to cope with negative feelings and thoughts, including individual therapy. Mindfulness helps support individuals with eating problems in moving past the self-blame and sense of struggle that often occurs when they eat something "bad," or eat in response to emotions, desires, or cravings. In truth, such self-blame often triggers further compulsive eating (the "I've blown it" effect), fueling the sense of being addicted and unable to manage the complex food choices that abound. The MB-EAT program normalizes emotion-related eating, when it occurs in smaller amounts in balance with other food choices, while assisting individuals to identify and engage other ways to handle stress.

Within the weight regulation area, this approach is in marked contrast to the "will-power" or abstinence-based models that abound, drawing increasingly on addiction models of obesity (Brownell & Gold, 2012; Lustig, 2012). While some individuals do maintain weight loss by internalizing recommended restrictions, many individuals rebound. Our data shows that individuals in the MB-EAT program, regardless of their previous degree of disordered eating, improve substantially in what could be considered "healthy restraint" and in more positive attitudes towards engaging self-management, making far more discerning choices about their eating. At the same time, they are able to enjoy smaller amounts of the foods that they had previously perceived as "addictive." In Buddhist terms, we are helping people find the "middle way" between addiction and abstinence. We do not explicitly refer to the Buddhist concept of nonattachment. However, the program is very much informed by the value of skillfully releasing oneself through mindfulness practice from strong cravings, a sense of "addiction," and struggling with food. At the same time, responding in a more balanced way to perceive desires and immediate pleasure arguably provides a "middle path" between addiction and abstinence.

Self-Acceptance. The concept of accepting what is arising (thoughts, feelings, and sensations), without judging, is repeatedly emphasized in the MB-EAT program, as it is in other mindfulness-based programs. Self-acceptance is encouraged, over and over, as a general attitude to hold in relation to the self. It is also encouraged in the moment as an alternative to reacting judgmentally to every self-perceived slip in choices made about eating, or to judgmental thought about the body and weight. Critical self-judgment/guilt is a hallmark of eating disorders, but is also present for many individuals simply struggling with weight. For many women, it may start during early teen years, and may continue even into old age (Kristeller, 2016b). Self-acceptance is also an alternative to the sense of simply giving up—eating whatever seems to appeal and suppressing immediate concerns about subsequent weight gain, which we find occurs in many of our heavier binge-eaters. Self-acceptance and self-forgiveness are particularly powerful for interrupting cycles of binging, self-recrimination, and over-restraint. Therefore, self-acceptance and mindfulness form a foundation for bringing a state of open curiosity to overeating episodes in order to cultivate awareness of triggers, and then being open to their own "wisdom" in looking for alternatives.

There is a negative "charge" on eating forbidden foods from food rules that chronic dieters, binge eaters, and those struggling with weight so frequently have. It can lead to overeating when "breached," but is mitigated by developing more flexibility and self-compassion. One woman, with a history of binge eating since young adulthood, developed a kind inner voice for herself as she worked on cultivating self-compassion and nonjudgmental awareness. When she ate what was previously a forbidden food, she found herself eating smaller quantities and not moving into binging. She would say to herself with a nurturing attitude and tone of voice, "that's okay" and move on. She was able to stay with her increasingly healthier way of eating, while occasionally enjoying what used to be binge foods but in small quantities. The frequency and size of her binges decreased to a non-diagnostic level.

The body work we introduce (the body scan, a healing self-touch practice,[1] chair yoga, and mindful walking) are also framed in the context of becoming more aware and self-accepting of the body and the body's capacity. However, in comparison to MBSR, some of the practices are adapted, introduced later, and play a smaller role in the overall program, given the intense anxiety present around body issues. This modification is particularly true for many of our heavier participants, some of who simply cannot get up and down off the floor. Again, in contrast to emphasizing simple solutions (i.e., intensely increasing exercising), MB-EAT encourages an attitude of experimentation, and self-compassion in developing new patterns that feel sustainable, rather than temporary.

Engaging Outer Wisdom

The "inner wisdom" components reviewed above are complemented throughout the program by helping participants also cultivate their "outer wisdom." In the initial development of the program, only a limited amount of attention was given to addressing decisions based on nutritional information or to systematic weight loss (even though that was a goal for most of our participants). We discovered that while some individuals did lose weight, others actually gained weight (Kristeller et al., 2013), perhaps due to misconstruing the message of self-acceptance as "self-indulgence." So we came back to the question: rather than minimally addressing these topics, how could we infuse them with a sense of mindfulness, rather than the self-judgment and guilt that often accompany any mention of calories and nutrition? As is outlined in more detail below, we found that we were able to accomplish this goal in several ways. With respect to food choices, we emphasize healthier foods, but within a "more of this/less of that" context, encouraging people to make more

---

[1] The healing self-touch exercise was developed by Sasha Loring, M.S., M.Ed. at Duke Integrative Medicine.

discerning choices about which foods they really wish to keep in their diets, and which they might remove with little loss or regret. We also encourage more exercise, but from a broader, healthier framework of overall health, rather than with a primary goal of weight management.

We also found that many of our participants, while knowledgeable about "food energy" in low calorie foods (from many years of dieting), had little knowledge of the calories in their favorite, higher calorie foods, usually underestimating what they were actually taking in. As people learned to savor and enjoy far smaller amounts of favorite foods, they discovered that they could incorporate such amounts into a more balanced energy "budget." Again, we emphasize that while the nutritional and calorie/energy value of any food is indeed simply reality, it should be their choice of whether and how much to eat—not someone else's—and that such choices come from cultivating wise awareness. Introducing these elements into the program led participants to have more systematic success with weight loss, using an element we created for this program called the "500 Calorie Challenge" (see below for details) without reducing the value of the program on other indicators of success (Daubenmier et al. 2012, 2016; Kristeller, Jordan & Bolinskey, in preparation).

MB-EAT: The Practice Components

In this second part of the chapter, we provide an overview of some of the clinical and programmatic considerations informing the MB-EAT program. We share examples of some of the practices specific to the program, and some more depth in regard to key conceptual issues reviewed above. We first briefly review the client populations appropriate for the program, and the related expectations for professional background for teachers. Fuller details of the program are provided in the manual (Kristeller & Wolever, in press) and are addressed in depth in the professional training programs (see www.mb-eat.com).

Client Populations

We all eat mindlessly at times, and MB-EAT can be helpful for anyone wanting to have a more balanced relationship to food. Nevertheless, the program was originally designed to assist individuals with relatively severe imbalances, including BED and serious levels of obesity. Clients who are working with mindful eating, regardless of whether they have a diagnosable eating disorder, often are extremely judgmental towards themselves and their eating, and have internalized the culture's judgments towards body size, self-image, and food choices. Clinical trial research has documented the value of the program for individuals with more disordered eating and obesity. It has also shown value for individuals with a wider range of eating and weight issues, including those from mildly overweight to moderately obese, with a range of eating issues, and with type 2 diabetes (Miller, Kristeller, Headings, Nagaraja, & Miser, 2012). Experimental versions, still under development, have been used with overweight children, adolescents in school settings, and for women during pregnancy to reduce excess weight gain. In the current format, the program is not recommended for individuals with anorexia nervosa, nor is it appropriate for individuals invested in following restrictive weight-loss programs (though limited dietary restrictions for health or personal reasons can be accommodated). The program has been developed primarily to be used in group settings, in which the sharing among individuals enriches the experience, but elements can be adapted for use with individual clients.

Leadership and Teaching

The primary foundational training for the MB-EAT (and related programs) is a 5-day residential professional training program. Further training and supervised experience in providing the course is needed for certification. Teachers of mindful eating are expected to be firmly grounded in mindfulness meditation practice, along with experience and training in a professional capacity for working with the population to whom they intend to offer MB-EAT. Professionals who offer the program include psychologists, psychotherapists, registered dietitians, other nutritionists, nurses, and health coaches. In general, leadership background, training, and experience is best matched to the population enrolled; a co-leader with complementary background may be able to provide specific expertise. For example, a group targeted towards individuals with type 2 diabetes (such as the MB-EAT-D program adapted for this population (Miller et al., 2012) should include a leader with related experience. In particular, it is not recommended that individuals with clinical eating issues such as BED be included in a program unless there is a leader with training and experience working with these specific types of presenting issues. Experience pertinent to that population, including general knowledge of evidence-based psychotherapeutic and nutrition practices, psycho-educational group facilitation skills, and behavioral change principles are important.

As noted, teachers of mindful eating should have a solid foundation in mindfulness practice. Such background preferably includes an 8-week MBSR course or equivalent experience, a 7–10 day residential *Vipassana* retreat, and a regular personal mindfulness meditation practice. In addition, the practitioner should be well versed in their own personal understanding of mindful eating in order to be a compassionate and effective guide for their clients. This orientation also entails leaders being mindful about communicating to group participants about their own particular food choices (e.g., being vegan; never drinking sodas or alcohol; or only using locally grown products). Such choices might be brought up within discussion as an element of "outer wisdom," but unless a group is so advertised (i.e., MB-EAT for vegans), such messages run counter to each group participant developing his or her own mindful choices.

Creating a safe container to explore what arises from the many exercises and guided eating practices is essential. As in MBSR, the inquiry process is an important skill for the mindful eating instructor. Group leaders encourage the participants to share about their experiences both inside and outside of the sessions. First, each week there is an invitation to participants to share what they noticed during the previous week. Then, each exercise is followed by inquiry into insights that arise. Inquiry then circles back to exploring how this awareness might help in daily life with relation to food, weight management, or other goal and intention they have set around eating. Because eating patterns have so many elements inherently unique to each person, the challenge is always to balance sharing from as many individuals as possible with reflection on integrative principles and common experiences.

Core Components

The core components of the MB-EAT program cover a range of meditative practices, including both breath awareness and guided meditations. Guided mindfulness practices encourage awareness of a specific targeted experience, and help individuals cultivate awareness of distinct aspects of their eating, viewing them with curiosity instead of judgment. These practices focus on physical vs. emotional hunger, taste experience, fullness/satiety, and making healthier and wiser food choices. Other guided visualizations relate to different aspects of the program from meal-intake to emotional issues, such as working with forgiveness and anger, self-acceptance, eating triggers, cultivation of wisdom, body awareness and acceptance practices, and guidance in how to make nutritionally mindful food choices. These visualizations could be considered parallel to other focused therapeutic applications of mindfulness meditation, such as cultivating awareness of specific aspects of depressive thinking in Mindfulness-Based Cognitive Therapy (Segal, Williams, & Teasdale, 2002), or urges to drink within Mindfulness-Based Relapse Prevention (Bowen, Chawla, & Marlatt, 2011). Throughout the program, participants are encouraged to share their experiences both in dyads and with the full group, exploring mindfulness as related to their eating, body, emotions, thoughts, and food choices. The use of the fluid and flexible interplay of inner and outer wisdom is explored through group practices and daily life examples or challenges, At the end of practice discussions, the question is posed: "*How might the awareness gained or experience of this practice help with* (inserting here the appropriate issue of focus, such as…) '*your relationship to food/losing weight/eating smaller amounts of food*'?"

Meditative Practice

Sitting meditation. Sitting meditation practice is an integral part of cultivating and strengthening mindful awareness of eating, and the associated thoughts, feelings, and behaviors that impact choices, including what, why, and how we eat. In

MB-EAT, participants are introduced to 10 minutes of mindfulness meditation at the first session and asked to practice 10 minutes a day during the first few weeks with a provided recording. This amount of practice is increased to 20 minutes, and then to 30 minutes as the weeks go on, with encouragement for practicing without the audio file as the program progresses. The instructor helps participants understand the practice and explore barriers to regular practice, as in other MBIs. Through inquiry, instructors help participants see parallels between how they can simply observe their experiences, or work with distress, uncomfortable physical sensations, feelings, and thoughts during sitting practice, and apply this same nonjudgmental observation while eating.

Mini-Meditations. Sitting meditation is complemented from the beginning with what we refer to as "mini-meditations," just a few moments of breath awareness that can easily be incorporated into the immediate experience of eating. The mini-meditation can last from a few seconds to a few minutes such as in the 3-minutes breathing space used within the MBCT program and can be used before snacks or meals and/or in moments of stress arousal. Using mini-meditations before eating throughout the day, or during stressful moments, becomes a new way of being and working with food and relationship to stressors. Evidence from the research suggests that engaging mini-meditations regularly is one of the more powerful predictors of improvement in relationship to eating and to weight loss (Kristeller et al., 2013).

Body Scan and Yoga

A body scan unique to MB-EAT is introduced in the third session but plays a less central role than does the practice in MBSR. In addition to bringing awareness throughout the body, participants are asked to choose areas of the body to which to bring nonjudgmental awareness, including both areas that feel problematic and areas that they can feel proud of. This approach is gentler for many of our participants who suffer from extreme judgment and nonacceptance of their bodies. A session later a body-oriented self-compassion practice builds upon the body scan already introduced. Chair yoga and mindful walking are also introduced and taught as practices to increase awareness of the body with mindful motion, with the participants invited to integrate the quality of practice into their lives as they wish.

Kind Awareness: Balancing Goals with Self-Acceptance

Regular sitting practice and kind attention to thoughts and feelings in daily life can help facilitate less judgment, and more self-compassion in moment-to-moment experience. Negative self-judgment is pervasive among individuals struggling with weight and eating issues. However, identifying and setting goals for change is inherent to the intent of creating healthier, more balanced eating patterns within the hundreds of micro-level, often mindless, decisions made daily.

To support flexibility in facing the complexity of eating patterns, the program incorporates a self-monitoring tool, the KEEP IT OFF.[2] This consists of about 30 eating-related items (plus items related to mindfulness practice and physical activity), designed to help diffuse the all-or-nothing mindset about eating that most of our participants carry: that they are either always eating inappropriately, or they have to be eating in some "perfect" way. Instead, they rate each item (such as *"eating because of boredom"*) on its occurrence during a given week from "never" to "several times per day." During the program, they are encouraged to choose a few items each week to be particularly mindful of, and to mindfully do something less often (from "several times per day" to "once per day") or a little more often (e.g., *"I left food on my plate* "several times", rather than "never"). Intentionally cultivating kind awareness helps reduce the judgments that can contribute to disordered eating and the unhelpful beliefs that keep people locked in shame cycles and disordered eating patterns, such as the "I've blown it" effect. Additional guided meditations in MB-EAT, such as forgiveness and self-acceptance meditations, help directly address these issues as well.

Cultivating Interoceptive Awareness

Increasing interoceptive awareness of physical hunger and satiety cues, particularly fullness, is a core part of the program, connecting body and mind. As outlined below, these points are engaged in the first half of the program and reinforced throughout. Taste awareness, a third component, is embedded within mindful eating practices beginning in the first session, and also actively engaged throughout the program in the context of a wide range of mindful eating practices. Participants are encouraged to practice all these aspects on their own, beginning with 1–2 meals or snacks per day, and extending to all eating experiences.

Physical hunger. We introduce the concept of rating level of physical hunger on a 10-point scale, utilizing a basic tool of psychophysics (as has been widely adopted in rating pain in medical settings) that lends itself well to mindful awareness. People are often surprised at how revealing this tool can be. We ask everyone to reflect on the number that comes to mind, and then ask, "How did you know that?"—reinforcing the value of cultivating interoceptive awareness. As noted earlier, learning to discern whether the pull to eat is driven by physical hunger versus other triggers is very powerful. When asking people to check in on physical hunger, we engage a discussion of the types of experiences (stomach growling, weakness) that might be experienced, but emphasize that everyone is different. Participants are then encouraged to check in on physical hunger multiple times per day, and also to

[2] The Kristeller Eating and Exercise Patterns of Food and Fitness (KEEP IT OFF©) self-check list is completed at the beginning, end, and several times during the program. Kristeller, Jordan, et al. (in preparation). "KEEP IT OFF: A measure of mindful eating for weight management."

engage "outer wisdom" by noticing how this experience varies by time of day, what they had eaten most recently, the presence of food, etc.

Stomach fullness. The physical sensations of fullness are differentiated from those of hunger as they involve different physiologic and biological processes, so a separate 1–10 scale is used to rate awareness of fullness. As part of the practice, we have participants drink a 16–20 ounce bottle of water to simulate the experiences of fullness that one would have with food and with liquid. During the following weeks, as with hunger, participants are encouraged to tune into fullness at varying times of the day both during and after eating different types of food to get to know their own unique sensations of fullness at different levels, and to try to identify levels that feel more comfortable for them. For most, even those with BED, they are surprised at how easily this awareness is achieved, and what a strong counterpoint it is to their tendency to often eat as much as they possibly can. The link with outer wisdom is made by pointing out that feelings of fullness vary tremendously by the type of food. For example, 300 cal of popcorn is far more filling than 300 cal of a granola bar, and on some occasions they might prefer the popcorn and on others, the bar.

Mindful Taste Awareness: Quality Versus Quantity

Multiple practices focus on cultivating interoceptive awareness of taste and choice, increasing in their level of challenge from eating raisins to enjoying a buffet meal. The practices build a foundation from which to be able to enjoy food in smaller amounts, to choose which foods are most appealing, and to enjoy quality over quantity. The foods used in the exercises represent standard brands and types of food and can be modified locally taking into account regional and socioeconomic differences in food preferences.

The raisin experience. Similar to the MBSR program, participants engage in eating a few raisins in the first session as their introduction to mindfulness, and more specifically to mindful eating. Four raisins are used instead of three and other elements are added to deepen the experience and bring out additional teaching points. There is a greater emphasis than in the MBSR program on being aware of thoughts and feelings while eating the raisins, with more guided attention to details such as the taste and texture and the satisfaction derived while eating the first two raisins. Participants then lead themselves through eating the third raisin mindfully as in MBSR, thus initiating their first self-guided mindful eating practice. They are then asked to choose whether they want to eat the fourth raisin and are directed to notice how they make their choice. Making mindful choices is a core theme in the program and the subtleties of awareness of choice builds upon this initial experience. Finally during the practice, participants are instructed to contemplate how the raisins were cultivated, harvested, and arrived into their hands, and to experience appreciation for all the people involved.

Participants often are surprised at the taste and satisfaction from eating just a few raisins. They will also notice how the taste and pleasure goes down substantially by the third raisin. Many choose not to eat the fourth raisin. This is particularly surprising to those with a history of binge eating. Participants are queried about their thoughts or feelings, particularly related to choosing whether to eat the fourth raisin. Common thoughts include, "I shouldn't leave food," "Just one won't matter"; feelings may involve shame, excitement, conflict, positive or negative associations with raisins from childhood, and surprise at the complexity of eating just a few raisins.

Cheese and crackers. The second mindful eating exercise uses small crackers, each topped with a thin slice of cheese, a food more substantial than raisins, and one often labeled a "bad" food in diet programs. It may also be a trigger food for overeating at parties or at home. The exercise offers an opportunity to challenge the "bad food/good food" dichotomy and to learn to be more flexible in enjoying this type of food. Still, participants are again often surprised at how quickly the taste and appeal goes down when eating this food mindfully. They may find they enjoy the flavor for a few bites but then elect to stop earlier than they normally would. Others may be surprised to find they don't even like the cheese and crackers when eaten mindfully. This exercise helps to reinforce the experience of quality vs quantity, and enjoying more while eating less.

Considering the energy value of food, as part of outer wisdom, is also introduced here, with participants asked to guess the caloric value of one cracker and cheese. Most overestimate by 2–3-fold the actual value, which is about 20 cal. Exploring this helps participants feel freer to include small amounts of favorite foods in an overall balanced healthy way of eating.

Chocolate snack. A chocolate snack is used to bring mindful taste awareness to a sweet food that may elicit both intense approach and avoidance, aversion, and desire. We use medium quality chocolate cookies. Emotions during this exercise range from excitement to trepidation and fear of overeating. Thoughts may include "I shouldn't eat this," "This is not on my healthy eating plan, it will make me sick," or "Once I start, I won't be able to stop." This practice is also used to introduce the 10-point taste satisfaction meter. Participants are surprised to notice how much the taste can go down after a small amount. And how satisfied they can be with just one or two pieces when they really slow down and attend to the experience of eating it mindfully. Again, the principle of eating less but enjoying more is reinforced.

Other mindful eating experiences. Being mindful when selecting food is introduced by challenging participants to choose between two snack foods, one sweet and one salty. Participants are directed to notice, in the moment, which is drawing them more, and to notice how memories, thoughts, and/or judgments are contributing to their choice. See Chapter 23, J, for the full script of 'Making Mindful Choices: Cookies vs. Chips'. The challenge of making mindful choices is increased as the group participates in a potluck meal. Group members contribute two food items, a healthier one which they would like to eat more often, and a more challenging food that they would like to keep in their regular diet, but perhaps in smaller amounts. Macaroni and cheese almost always shows up. This potluck experience is used to highlight both inner and outer wisdom. Other practices include bringing in a favorite snack food for oneself and to share, and going out for a meal to an all-you-can-eat buffet, a culminating experience often met with trepidation, but one that reinforces for individuals how much they have shifted in their experiences of eating and food.

Outer Wisdom: Quality and Quantity

Mindful nutrition. "Inner wisdom" experience is integrated throughout with the "what" of eating. In MB-EAT, the outer wisdom components focus on developing a wise relationship to evidence-based nutrition and exercise knowledge. The U.S. dietary guidelines and MyPlate diagram are used as examples of healthy nutrition recommendations in the program, but a facilitator may choose to present other evidence-based models as well, such as plant-based models, the Mediterranean diet, other culture-specific dietary guidelines, or guidelines specific to those enrolled, such as for type 2 diabetes. Individuals are encouraged to find their own "wise" relationship with the nutrition information, taking into account personal health issues, food preferences, available food sources as well as their own values around food and health, and what is important to them and their family. For example, in one program, a man initially decided to remove all sodas from his usually daily intake. When he ended up feeling somewhat deprived by doing so, he added back in one soda during a work break, and cut back on something else. But by the end of the 10-week program he was finding any amount of soda overly sweet, and cut that one out also. This message is very different from condemning any intake of a particular food, even one as problematic as sodas.

Mindful weight loss. Some degree of weight loss is virtually always a goal for our participants, whether 10 lb or 100 lb, but we try to provide a healthier and more balanced context for this than do most weight loss programs. "Quality over quantity" is again emphasized, and "eating less but enjoying more" is encouraged. For weight loss, knowledge of calories is framed as an initial tool for awareness of the energy value of different foods. The "500 Calorie Challenge" invites participants to reduce calories by making small dietary changes that add up throughout the day to about 500 calories, and which seem personally sustainable. This level of decrease is consistent with an initial gradual weight loss of 2–4 lb/month, and is designed to encourage each person to take on the responsibility for such choices, to explore what foods (or amounts of food) they are willing to "give up" indefinitely, and to cultivate an attitude of nonjudgmental curiosity about their food choices. Although we ask individuals to use a structured self-monitoring approach for a few weeks to identify appropriate foods to give up or decrease in amount, we encourage them to do so in an exploratory and nonjudgmental manner. The goal is to cultivate self-knowledge of both caloric and nutritional value of foods, particularly in relation to portion size. Therefore, in many respects, this approach is dramatically in contrast to the structured and abstinence-oriented diets that most participants have tried before. Restricted diets can be appealing because they simplify food choices markedly. But as we may note to our clients:

> If you've been eating 3000 cal per day, and drop down to 1200, you will indeed lose weight relatively quickly (perhaps 2–3 lb/week). But you now know how to eat 1200 cal—and you know how to eat 3000 cal, but you know nothing about how to eat a balanced level in between, for example, about 2000 cal, how to eat flexibly, or how to integrate smaller amounts of favorite foods into your regular eating pattern.

Calorie awareness can be a helpful tool leading to balanced and flexible eating but this is not a calorie counting program. Each individual uses this information as it is helpful to him or her, along with the variety of tools, practices, and awareness developed in the program.

Summary and Conclusion

The ability to be present to the pleasure of food as one eats, while staying attuned to levels of hunger, fullness, and overall satisfaction, helps individuals make informed choices that support their health and well-being. Mindfulness helps to moderate the amount, quality, and enjoyment of food. At the same time, regular sitting practice, utilizing mini-meditations, and attention to thoughts and feelings in daily life can help decrease critical self-judgment, and cultivate self-compassion in moment-to-moment experience.

Mindful eating is an art comprising learned foundational practices and mindful awareness that supports the practice moment to moment. Skilled teacher's of mindful eating help model and facilitate flexibility, kindness, and self-compassion in their own relationship to food and eating and for those of their participants. Food as joy and pleasure, food as nourishment, and eating in moderate quantities, all become attainable for those who have long suffered and can now come into balance with this part of their lives. For all those who simply want to discover a new way of eating that promotes these principles, MB-EAT promotes health and well-being, and a way of eating that is sustainable and sensible, meeting each moment with wisdom and flexibility.

References

Altman, D. (1999). *Art of the inner meal: Eating as a spiritual path.* San Francisco, CA: Harper Press.

Appelhans, B. M. (2009). Neurobehavioral inhibition of reward-driven feeding: Implications for dieting and obesity. *Obesity, 17*(4), 640–647.

Appelhans, B. M., Woolf, K., Pagoto, S. L., Schneider, K. L., Whited, M. C., & Liebman, R. (2011). Inhibiting food reward: Delay discounting, food reward sensitivity, and palatable food intake in overweight and obese women. *Obesity, 19*(11), 2175–2182.

Baltes, P. B., & Staudinger, U. M. (2000). Wisdom: A metaheuristic (pragmatic) to orchestrate mind and virtue toward excellence. *American Psychologist, 55*(1), 122–136.

Barnes, R. D., Masheb, R. M., White, M. A., & Grilo, C. M. (2013). Examining the relationship between food thought suppression and binge eating disorder. *Comprehensive Psychiatry, 54*(7), 1077–1081.

Bays, J. (2009). *Mindful eating.* Boston, MA: Shambala Press.

Berthoud, H.-R. (2012). Central regulation of hunger, satiety, and body weight. In K. D. Brownell & M. Gold (Eds.), *Food and addiction: A comprehensive handbook* (pp. 97–102). New York, NY: Oxford University Press.

Blundell, J., & Bellisle, F. (Eds.). (2013). *Satiation, satiety and the control of food intake.* Cambridge, England: Elsevier-Woodhouse.

Bowen, S., Chawla, N., & Marlatt, G. A. (2011). *Mindfulness-based relapse prevention for addictive behaviors: A clinician's guide.* New York, NY: Guilford Press.

Bowen, S., Witkiewitz, K., Dillworth, T. M., & Marlatt, G. A. (2007). The role of thought suppression in the relationship between mindfulness meditation and alcohol use. *Addictive Behaviors, 32*(10), 2324–2328.

Brown, A. J., Smith, L. T., & Craighead, L. W. (2010). Appetite awareness as a mediator in an eating disorders prevention program. *Eating Disorders, 18*(4), 286–301.

Brownell, K. D., & Gold, M. (Eds.). (2012). *Food and addiction: A comprehensive handbook.* New York, NY: Oxford University Press.

Capaldi, E. D. (Ed.). (1996). *Why we eat what we eat: The psychology of eating.* Washington, DC: American Psychological Association.

Craighead, L. W. (2006). *The appetite awareness workbook.* Oakland, CA: New Harbinger.

Cuthbert, B., Kristeller, J., Simons, R., Hodes, R., & Lang, P. J. (1981). Strategies of arousal control: Biofeedback, meditation, and motivation. *Journal of Experimental Psychology: General, 110*(4), 518–546.

Daubenmier, J., Lin, J., Blackburn, E., Hecht, F. M., Kristeller, J., Maninger, N., … Epel E. (2012). Changes in stress, eating, and metabolic factors are related to changes in telomerase activity in a randomized mindfulness intervention pilot study. *Psychoneuroendocrinology, 37*(7), 917–928.

Daubenmier, J., Moran, P.J., Kristeller, J., ….. Hecht, F.M. (2016/in press). Effects of a mindfulness-based weight loss intervention in adults with obesity: A randomized clinical trial.

Davidson, R. J., Goleman, D. J., & Schwartz, G. E. (1976). Attentional and affective concomitants of meditation: A cross-sectional study. *Journal of Abnormal Psychology, 85*(2), 235–238.

Deci, E. L., Ryan, R. M., Schultz, P. P., & Niemiec, C. P. (2015). Being aware and functioning fully: Mindfulness and interest taking within self-determination theory. In K. W. Brown, J. D. Creswell, & R. M. Ryan (Eds.), *Handbook of mindfulness: Theory, research, and practice* (pp. 112–129). New York, NY: Guilford Press.

Drewnowski, A. (1996). The behavioral phenotype in human obesity. In E. D. Capaldi (Ed.), *Why we eat what we eat: The psychology of eating.* Washington, DC: American Psychological Association.

Geliebter, A., & Hashim, S. A. (2001). Gastric capacity in normal, obese, and bulimic women. *Physiology & Behavior, 74*(4–5), 743–746.

Geliebter, A., Hassid, G., & Hashim, S. A. (2001). Test meal intake in obese binge eaters in relation to mood and gender. *International Journal of Eating Disorders, 29*(4), 488–494.

Goldfield, G. S., Adamo, K. B., Rutherford, J., & Legg, C. (2008). Stress and the relative reinforcing value of food in female binge eaters. *Physiology & Behavior, 93*(3), 579–587.

Grave, R. D., Oliosi, M., Todisco, P., & Vanderlinden, J. (1997). Self-reported traumatic experiences and dissociative symptoms in obese women with and without binge-eating disorder. *Eating Disorders, 5*(2), 105–109.

Grilo, C. M., & Masheb, R. M. (2002). Childhood maltreatment and personality disorders in adult patients with binge eating disorder. *Acta Psychiatrica Scandinavica, 106*(3), 183–188.

Grosshans, M., Loeber, S., & Kiefer, F. (2011). Implications from addiction research towards the understanding and treatment of obesity. *Addiction Biology, 16*(2), 189–198.

Kabatznick, R. (1998). *The Zen of eating*. New York, NY: Penguin Putnam.

Kristeller, J. (1977). Meditation and biofeedback in the regulation of internal states. In S. Ajaya (Ed.), *Meditational therapy*. Glenview, IL: Himalayan International Institute Press.

Kristeller, J. L. (2003). Mindfulness, wisdom, and eating: Applying a multi-domain model of meditation effects. *Constructivism in the Human Sciences, 8*(2), 107–118.

Kristeller, J. L. (2007). Mindfulness meditation. In P. Lehrer, R. Wookfolk, & W. E. Simes (Eds.), *Principles and practices of stress management* (pp. 393–427). New York, NY: Guilford Press.

Kristeller, J. (2015). Mindfulness, eating disorders and self-regulation. In B. D. Ostafin, M. D. Robinson, & B. P. Meier (Eds.), *Handbook of mindfulness and self-regulation*. New York, NY: Springer.

Kristeller, J. (2016a). *The joy of half a cookie. Using mindfulness to lose weight and end the struggle with food*. New York, NY: Penguin Books.

Kristeller, J. (2016b). The struggle continues: Addressing concerns about eating and weight for older women's well-being. *The Journal of Women and Therapy, 39*, 1–11. DOI:10.1080/02703 149.2016.1116855.

Kristeller, J., Jordan, K., & Bolinskey, K. (in preparation). *A mindful eating intervention in moderately to morbidly obese individuals*.

Kristeller, J. & Jordan, K. (in preparation). *The KEEP IT OFF: A measure of mindful eating for weight management*.

Kristeller, J. L., and Wolever, R. Q. (in press). Mindfulness-Based Eating Awareness Training. New York: Guilford Pres.

Kristeller, J., & Epel, E. (2014). Mindful eating and mindless eating. In A. Ie, C. T. Ngnoumen, & E. J. Langer (Eds.), *The Wiley Blackwell handbook of mindfulness* (Vol. 2, pp. 913–933). Chichester, England: Wiley.

Kristeller, J. L., & Hallett, C. B. (1999). An exploratory study of a meditation-based intervention for binge eating disorder. *Journal of Health Psychology, 4*(3), 357–363.

Kristeller, J. L., & Rodin, J. (1989). Identifying eating patterns in male and female undergraduates using cluster analysis. *Addictive Behaviors, 14*(6), 631–642.

Kristeller, J. L., & Wolever, R. Q. (2011). Mindfulness-based eating awareness training for treating binge eating disorder: The conceptual foundation. *Eating Disorders, 19*(1), 49–61.

Kristeller, J., Wolever, R. Q., & Sheets, V. (2013). Mindfulness-based eating awareness training (MB-EAT) for binge eating: A randomized clinical trial. *Mindfulness, 5*(3), 282–297.

Lustig, R. H. (2012). *Fat chance*. New York, NY: Penguin Group.

Lutz, A., Slagter, H. A., Dunne, J. D., & Davidson, R. J. (2008). Attention regulation and monitoring in meditation. *Trends in Cognitive Sciences, 12*(4), 163–169.

Marlatt, G. A., & Kristeller, J. L. (1999). Mindfulness and meditation. In W. R. Miller (Ed.), *Integrating spirituality into treatment: Resources for practitioners* (pp. 67–84). Washington, DC: American Psychological Association.

Meeks, T. W., Cahn, B. R., & Jeste, D. V. (2012). Neurobiological foundations of wisdom. In C. K. Germer & R. D. Siegel (Eds.), *Wisdom and compassion in psychotherapy: Deepening mindfulness in clinical practice* (pp. 189–201). New York, NY: Guilford Press.

Miller, C. K., Kristeller, J. L., Headings, A., Nagaraja, H., & Miser, W. F. (2012). Comparative effectiveness of a mindful eating intervention to a diabetes self-management intervention among adults with type 2 diabetes: A pilot study. *Journal of the Academy of Nutrition and Dietetics, 112*(11), 1835–1842.

Ogden, J. (2010). *The psychology of eating*. Chichester, England: Wiley-Blackwell.

Olstad, S., Solem, S., Hjemdal, O., & Hagen, R. (2015). Metacognition in eating disorders: Comparison of women with eating disorders, self-reported history of eating disorders or psychiatric problems, and healthy controls. *Eating Behaviors, 16*, 17–22.

Ostafin, B. D., & Kassman, K. T. (2012). Stepping out of history: Mindfulness improves insight problem solving. *Consciousness and Cognition, 21*(2), 1031–1036.

Peterson, C. B., Miller, K. B., Crow, S. J., Thuras, P., & Mitchell, J. E. (2005). Subtypes of binge eating disorder based on psychiatric history. *International Journal of Eating Disorders, 38*(3), 273–276.

Remick, A. K., Polivy, J., & Pliner, P. (2009). Internal and external moderators of the effect of variety on food intake. *Psychological Bulletin, 135*(3), 434–451.

Rodin, J. (1978). Stimulus-bound behavior and biological self-regulation: Feeding, obesity, and external control. In G. E. Schwartz & D. Shapiro (Eds.), *Consciousness and self-regulation* (Vol. 2, pp. 215–239). New York, NY: Plenum.

Rodin, J. (1981). Current status of the internal–external hypothesis for obesity: What went wrong? *American Psychologist, 36*(4), 361–372.

Ryan, R. M., & Deci, E. L. (2000). Self-determination theory and the facilitation of intrinsic motivation, social development, and well-being. *American Psychologist, 55*(1), 68–78.

Schachter, S., & Rodin, J. (Eds.). (1974). *Obese humans and rats.* New York, NY: Wiley.

Schwartz, G. E. (1975). Biofeedback, self-regulation, and the patterning of physiological processes. *American Scientist, 63*(3), 314–324.

Segal, Z. V., Williams, J. M. G., & Teasdale, J. D. (2002). *Mindfulness-based cognitive therapy for depression: A new approach to preventing relapse.* New York, NY: Guilford Press.

Sørensen, L. B., Møller, P., Flint, A., Martens, M., & Raben, A. (2003). Effect of sensory perception of foods on appetite and food intake: A review of studies on humans. *International Journal of Obesity, 27*(10), 1152–1166.

Sternberg, R. J. (1990). *Wisdom: Its nature, origins, and development.* Cambridge, England: Cambridge University Press.

Sysko, R., Hildebrandt, T., Wilson, G. T., Wilfley, D. E., & Agras, W. S. (2010). Heterogeneity moderates treatment response among patients with binge eating disorder. *Journal of Consulting and Clinical Psychology, 78*(5), 681–690.

Wansink, B. (2007). *Mindless eating: Why we eat more than we think.* New York, NY: Bantam Books.

Wansink, B., & Sobal, J. (2007). Mindless eating: The 200 daily food decisions we overlook. *Environment and Behavior, 39*(1), 106–123.

Chapter 20
Teaching Individuals with Life-Limiting Illness

Susan Bauer-Wu

> **Case Report**
> Gary, a successful businessman with a self-described type A personality, was fifty-eight years old when he learned that the cancer he'd had for many years had progressed and the available treatment options offered little hope of achieving long-term remission. He knew that his days were indeed limited. His mind raced as he worried about how much time he had left, whether he will be able to complete things left undone, what will happen to his family and his business, how will his body feel as the disease progresses, and how he will die. He grew frustrated by increasing physical limitations. Anger, irritation, sadness, and anxiety infused his waking moments, and he felt disconnected from the world around him and those he loved most.
>
> (Bauer-Wu, 2011a, p. 1).

Introduction

Life-limiting illness refers to a serious and progressive medical condition that has high likelihood to limit both longevity and quality of life. With this type of illness, for which there is no definitive cure, there are usually significant physical symptoms and functional debilitation over time. People living with such diagnoses, like

S. Bauer-Wu, Ph.D., R.N., F.A.A.N. (✉)
Mind & Life Institute, 210 Ridge McIntyre Road, Suite 325, Charlottesville, VA 22903, USA
e-mail: susan@mindandlife.org

© Springer International Publishing Switzerland 2016
D. McCown et al., *Resources for Teaching Mindfulness*,
DOI 10.1007/978-3-319-30100-6_20

379

advanced stage cancer or neurodegenerative disease, for example, amyotrophic lateral sclerosis (ALS), face enormous life changes and challenges. They also recognize that they will likely die as a result of the disease and that death will occur in the foreseeable future.

All of the usual issues that come up in the Mindfulness-Based Stress Reduction (MBSR) class are magnified in those with life-limiting illness. It's like a "perfect storm" of unpleasantness—a barrage of physical and mental suffering greater than during other life experiences. The mere word of a "terminal" disease—that life will end sooner than you anticipated—can put people into a tailspin and quickly conjure up images and stories of pain and misery. Indeed, physical discomforts and limitations abound with everyday activities requiring more effort and even needing assistance from others. Mentally, it is a struggle to not be feeling well most of the time, and needing to ask for and accept help while coming to terms with the grim prognosis. A flood of overwhelming thoughts and related negative emotions can easily consume one's precious moments: fear (e.g., of dying in pain, not being able to make amends before one dies, the unknowns of after death experience), anxiety (e.g., running out of time, a sense of losing control, when to stop aggressive medical intervention, concern of what will happen to loved ones), sadness and anger about the many changes and losses (e.g., not fulfilling personal and professional roles and goals, not being able to do usual recreational activities or get around independently, dramatic differences in the way the body looks and feels), and regrets about past mistakes or things not done. Existentially, one may be drawn to more deeply explore the meaning of life, to ponder what happens after death, and to try to make sense of what is happening. Finally, personal relationships often shift at this time, sometimes distancing and sometimes becoming closer, while navigating difficult conversations and figuring out new ways to enjoy one another and be intimate.

There are other unique issues in the context of life-limiting illness to be considered and skillfully addressed in teaching Mindfulness-Based Interventions (MBI). For some, especially as the disease progresses, *breathing* can become challenging, so that breath awareness practice typically taught may not be appropriate. Physical limitations may make some individuals homebound (or bound to a hospital or hospice) and sometimes even confined to bed. Therefore, attending and participating in an in-person MBI group format may not be feasible. Innovative and flexible teaching formats, such as one-to-one instruction conducted wherever the participant is located, either in-person or online, will be necessary. In addition, these kinds of medical conditions and associated treatments often leave one feeling drowsy, making it difficult to stay awake or focused for more than a few minutes at a time. For these reasons, it is often necessary to shorten the guided meditation recordings and teaching sessions. Living with serious, life-limiting illness poses particular concerns and opportunities for both the person experiencing the illness and the mindfulness teacher.

Essential Teaching Skills: Considerations and Adaptations for Life-Limiting Illness

In *Teaching Mindfulness* (McCown, Reibel, & Micozzi, 2010), four essential teaching skills are described: engaging the group, presenting didactic material, inquiring into participants' experience, and guiding meditations. This chapter provides a discussion of how to effectively teach mindfulness to those living with serious illness using these four essential teaching skills as a frame. Table 20.1 provides a snapshot of the five core teaching intentions of MBSR (McCown et al., 2010) and how they are exemplified in the context of life-limiting illness.

Engaging the Individual or Group

To effectively engage those living with life-limiting illness, it's essential that the mindfulness teacher be comfortable in being with individuals who are facing overt physical suffering and debilitation. If the teacher has unresolved or unexplored issues related to observing someone with serious illness, and who may be dying, perhaps based on past experiences or not having witnessing such circumstances before, she/he may have trouble engaging such participants. I once worked with (supervised) a teacher who was clearly unsettled in the presence of very sick patients. Her anxiety was palpable. In later discussion about her with one of the patients who requested to withdraw from the MBI, he reflected that the teacher's anxiety and very solemn manner made him feel uneasy and actually worse than before the mindfulness sessions. It's critical that the mindfulness teacher feels comfortable working with such individuals and doesn't carry angst or heaviness.

Being comfortable and relaxed in such contexts provides fertile ground to cultivate a caring and healing space. Teachers who embody calm, and unconditional receptivity, especially in moments of silence, can simply and kindly hold the reservoir of being present together. Such true "compassionate silence" is comforting, safe, and affirming and offers the possibility of mutual understanding and trust to emerge (Back, Bauer-Wu, Rushton, & Halifax, 2009).

It's also prudent for the mindfulness teacher to proactively address pragmatic issues that can affect engagement. Consider, for example, the most conducive format to teach people with life-limiting illness. A traditional MBSR group that meets in person, either exclusively for people living with serious illness or in a mixed group, may be very difficult for some to attend. Therefore, it's important to be flexible and creative in finding a format that meets the unique needs of those with whom you are working. With technology's increasing capability, ubiquity, and improving ease of use, doing a Web-based, interactive MBI tailored for this clinical population makes good sense, although it hasn't been adequately studied yet. Another possible format is dyadic (one-to-one) sessions with the teacher going to where the participant is located, such as home or the hospital or hospice. However, this latter format has many logistical challenges like feasibility, cost, time, and legal and credential-

Table 20.1 Five core teaching intentions in the context of life-limiting illness

Teaching intention	Example in life-limiting illness
Experiencing new possibilities	• It's possible to live fully and experience moments of delight and meaning even while facing imminent death
	• Simple pleasures abound, if you wake up to them
	• It's possible to laugh, listen, and love, even if you don't feel well
	• It's possible to reframe roles: de-identifying with the role of "sick/dying person" to re-identifying with significant roles of spouse/partner, parent, child, and friend
	• It's not just about receiving help, but it can be reciprocal: helping and giving to others, too (perhaps in new ways)
	• There can be great satisfaction in considering and working toward leaving one's legacy
Discovering corporeality	• Tuning in and exploring direct sensory experiences is initially scary as the body has been a source of discomfort and disappointment
	• Thoughts (images and self-narratives) are associated with physical sensations in the body
	• Physical sensations in the body change from moment to moment
	• Stories and narratives around pain can lead to a worsening of pain (see Fig. 20.1)
	• Parts of the body are not in pain
	• There's a difference between pain and suffering
	• There's incessant energy and aliveness in the body
Cultivating observation	• Mental narratives of worry, fear, doubt, and expectations are just stories, not what's actually happening in the present moment
	• Getting lost in such stories wastes precious, limited time
	• It's possible to simply notice one's experience (thoughts, emotions, sensations, and behaviors) without getting caught up in it
	• Simply watching one's experience can foster a sense of spaciousness
Moving toward acceptance	• Resisting what's happening and being indignant, angry, and upset can interfere connecting with others and with what matters most
	• Turning toward and befriending changes and challenges don't mean you have to like them
	• Genuine acceptance in the face of loss brings a sense of ease and an opportunity to feel whole after feeling broken
Growing compassion	• Equanimity, love, and joy have ripple effects
	• Receiving and sharing kindness and loving care are mutually nourishing, both to the caregiver and the care recipient
	• Gratitude and forgiveness provide the entry to healing and authentic connection
	• Moments of connection—especially without words through open-hearted presence, a gentle touch or looking into each other's eyes—are reciprocally rewarding
	• Having a generous spirit pays unquantifiable dividends and has the potential to leave a beautiful legacy

ing issues. Moreover, the value of dyadic MBI compared to group classes is highly questionable (Bauer-Wu, 2011b). Tremendous insights in MBSR often come from the group experience. Sense of belonging and resonance in hearing others' stories and questions, and recognizing common elements in each other's experiences, can lead to major insights.

Another practical issue that impacts engagement is choosing a time of day when participants are most alert, since fatigue and drowsiness are common with serious illness. Late morning is often a good time as people have more energy than after lunch and later in the day, while daily pain medication has taken effect. Early morning is not ideal as it usually takes longer to take care of personal care needs when living with serious illnesses. Also, given low energy levels and difficulty con-centrating, shorter class times may be necessary: an hour or less may be as long as can be tolerated. It is important to think through and address such pragmatic issues. Not doing so can greatly impair the mindfulness teacher's ability to effectively engage the individuals or group and negatively impact what the participants will gain from the mindfulness training.

Presenting Didactic Material

When presenting didactic material, it should be made real and relevant to the par-ticipants in the context of living with a life-limiting illness. For example, a key teaching point with these individuals is the vicious cycle of pain whereby how one reacts to pain can lead to worsening pain (see Fig. 20.1). Here, an explanation and exploration of the distinction between *pain* and *suffering* is often a pivotal learning opportunity for those living with serious illness. Furthermore, discussion on *acute* versus *chronic* pain (and other symptoms) is especially relevant. Take time to explain differences in symptom experiences—acute and chronic; mild to moderate to severe; intractable, excruciating and tolerable; new and lingering; and how pain and other symptoms are valuable messengers of important information about the body. The person with serious illness may be more open to tuning into and investi-gating her/his body and unpleasant symptoms. Such thoughtful explanation by the teacher open a "crack in the door" that can provide entry into authentic inquiry into participants' direct experiences.

Inquiring into Participants' Experiences

Sparking curiosity into the experience of living with a serious illness (often infused with tremendous discomfort and loss, and ultimately leading to demise) sounds like a monumental task for the mindfulness teacher. How can the teacher most skillfully navigate turning toward such unpleasantness? The two most important qualities to bring to this process are gentleness and patience. Skillful inquiry is not forced. Gentle invitations are followed by time and space to respond and express emotions.

Consider again the experience of pain or other significant physical symptoms, so common with life-limiting illness. The notion of turning toward discomfort seems

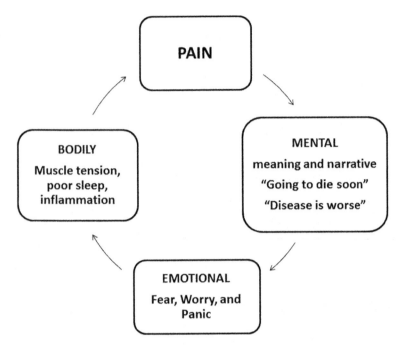

Fig. 20.1 Typical response to pain (or other unpleasant symptom) with life-limiting illness

counterintuitive. A natural reaction is to resist, push away, or flee from it. In our MBI teaching, we foster a fresh perspective and contemplative response (see Fig. 20.2) by gently asking questions about the direct experience. We invite participants to curiously attend to their experiences of pain (or other unpleasant symptoms) and allow them time to tune in and thoughtfully respond to our questions:

What are the qualities and subtle sensations that you're feeling right now?
Perhaps dullness, burning, pulsing, radiating, or something else?
Does the feeling change from moment to moment or is it constant?
What does this sensation mean to you?
Are there narratives or stories that you're telling yourself about this sensation?
What emotions arise as you consider these stories?
Are there parts of your body that aren't in pain right now?
Describe the parts of your body that feel well now.

Throughout this exploration, we also encourage participants to be compassionate, kind, and gentle (toward self and perhaps others who may be trying to help them) and notice any resistance in doing so.

The process of inquiry helps to dissect and more fully understand direct experience. Participants come to realize that pain is not just one big overwhelming "thing," but rather a constellation of many, sometimes subtle, bodily sensations can change from moment to moment. They may also notice breaks in the sensations and

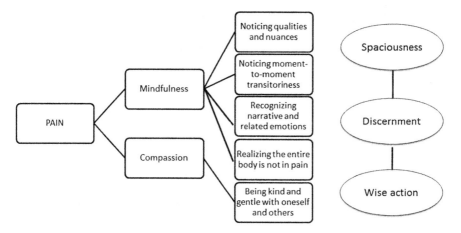

Fig. 20.2 Contemplative response to pain or other unpleasant symptom with life-limiting illness

moments of not feeling anything. Seeing sensations as merely sensations and noticing their nuanced qualities and fluctuations can be liberating and empowering.
Inquiry also helps them to recognize self-created stories or narratives (often worst-
case scenarios or self-blame) that are often not grounded in fact or what is known
for sure in the present moment. Participants can then realize the distinction between
suffering and pain, and that they are *not the pain* (or any other discomfort), not *just
a patient, not a disease*—and that the entire body isn't in pain. As noted in Fig. 20.2,
this process brings spaciousness to a previously constricted experience. In that spaciousness lies an ability to see more clearly what is happening and what the choices
are. Through clear seeing they can then move forward with wise action for how to
best take care of themselves.

Guiding Meditations

In teaching MBIs to people experiencing serious illness, one-size does not fit all,
and modification to guiding meditations is necessary. Some general issues to consider: (1) drowsiness and fatigue are common; (2) finding a comfortable position
can be challenging (lying down is generally better tolerated than sitting); (3) mobil-
ity and flexibility may be quite limited; (4) eating and/or swallowing may be difficult; (5) breathing may be labored. Therefore, it's important to tailor the meditations
in ways that make sense to the participants and are most tolerable, palatable, and
doable. Overall, relatively short-guided meditations (no longer than 20 minutes)
will allow participants to more fully engage with the practice as they are more likely
to stay awake and be comfortable throughout.

Adaptations to the standard MBSR practices that I have co-developed and
studied(Bauer-Wu, 2011a; Bauer-Wu et al., 2008) include: ice chips in lieu of raisins,

very gentle mindful range-of-motion movement (even done lying in bed) in lieu of mindful yoga, and alternatives to awareness of breathing. Some people with breathing challenges can be skillfully guided to have a sense of ease in awareness of breath practice (Benzo, 2013). For others it can be problematic and lead to anxiety and more trouble breathing. Alternatives to breath awareness (as a neutral point of focus to stabilize the mind) can be explored. In addition, a new practice was created in response to working with patients who were essentially limited to staying inside. It's called "Listening and Looking" and emphasizes awareness of sounds and sights. This practice can shift feelings away from being confined and hostage to bodily limitations and circumstances; instead to begin to notice the infinite possibilities of experiences accessible in the present moment. Examples of these adapted practices can be found in the Learning Resources section of this book.

Ice Chips Practice: Variation on Raisin Exercise

When experiencing a serious illness, there may be a period of time when the person isn't able to, or interested in eating or drinking anything except ice chips. Ice chips are soothing to a sore, dry mouth and they quench thirst. This exercise sets the foundation to incorporate mindfulness into routine, everyday activities. In guiding the participants, each begins with having a cup of crushed ice and a spoon; then, everyone can go through the practice together:

> *Intentionally picking up the cup of ice chips and spoon, noticing your body as you move to pick up the cup and spoon. Sensing the temperature as you hold the cup. What does it feel like?*
>
> *Slowly scooping up one ice chip. Paying attention to the movement of picking up the ice chip. Noticing how you choose one ice chip over the other. Noticing if the chip gets stuck when putting it on the spoon or if it slides right onto the spoon. What do you notice?*
>
> *When you have the ice chip on the spoon, stop and look at it. Looking at the size and shape of it. Noticing how the light shines on or through the chip. You might want to move the chip toward the light and notice how it glistens. As you continue to look at it, what do you notice? (maybe it is starting to melt and the shape is changing or there is a small pool of water on the spoon)*
>
> *Next, bring the spoon to your mouth. Don't put the ice chip in your mouth yet. Simply allowing the ice chip and spoon to touch your lips. What does it feel like on your lips? You may close your eyes and notice what that is like.*
>
> *Then, putting the ice chip in your mouth. What do you notice? What does it feel like? Where do you feel it in your mouth? Again, you may close your eyes if you care to.*
>
> *Then, slowly swallow it. Where do you sense it? What does it feel like?*
>
> *You may also take this moment to be aware of your ability to see, feel sensations, and to swallow. You may experience gratitude in your ability to do this.*

Repeat this with several ice chips. Do not rush. Stop whenever you care to or when you have finished with all of the ice chips in the cup.
What have you noticed from doing this? Feel free to share any insights that you've gained from this experience.

Mindful Range-of-Motion Practice: Variation on Mindful Yoga

This practice can be done by those who are frail and may not be able to get out of bed. It involves simple lifting of arms and legs and rotation of joints in fingers, wrists or ankles, while paying attention to the subtleties of the experience. It may be done with the eyes open or closed.

For each of the following, the person is guided to gently and slowly move, and to bring awareness to the experience and sensations of moving as well as holding a position. They are also guided to notice their breathing, during and between the movements (if breathing is not an issue). About thirty seconds to a minute is spent doing each movement:

Turn head to one side; look over the shoulder (repeat on other side)
Roll shoulders forward and backward
Curl each individual finger in, and then each finger roll out
Extend arms to sides, shoulder height and stretch hands out
Bend then extend knees, one leg at a time
Roll ankles, turning feet in one direction then the other, one foot at a time

Alternative to Breath Awareness: When Breathing Is Challenging

Focusing one's attention on a neutral point of awareness can help get centered and stabilize the mind. *Neutral* here means that it doesn't evoke a strong emotion or physical reaction. The breath is a common neutral point of focus because it generally does not involve conscious effort and is always with us. However, for some people, breathing poses considerable challenges due to underlying health problems. In such cases, awareness of breathing practices should be carefully and skillfully explored.

If breath awareness is too troubling, it's important to identify another neutral point of focus that could be used as an anchor to help the participant return to the present moment, time and time again. This anchor should be a body part or specific bodily experience rather than something external because participants need to be able to use that point of focus as a resource regardless of where they are—it must be with them at all times. The hand is an option that generally works well.

Guidance Considerations:

Settle into a comfortable position, which may be sitting, lying down, or standing.

Mentally scan your body and identify a neutral part of your body. This is somewhere that doesn't trigger strong emotions, memories, or discomfort.

You know best what areas feel neutral to you.

Choose to focus on a single body part on one side of your body.

Bring awareness to that body part. Notice internal sensations associated with it, such as tingling or pulsing. Notice any external sensations, like cool air or the feeling of clothes or linens.

For a few minutes, imagine that you are breathing in and breathing out from this area of the body.

Postscript

For the case presented at the beginning of the chapter, the gentleman, Gary, proceeded to participate in an MBI. While at first reluctant, he decided to do so at his wife's urging and because he was uncomfortable and concerned about how he was coping with his situation. A few months later, he shared the following reflection about the mindfulness training:

It has changed the whole quality of my life and the (meditation) practices have become a daily ritual. It has been one of the most important parts of my healing. It lowered my anxiety and increased my sense of control. When I meditate, I feel relaxed and refreshed. The more I practice, the more calm I become. Before I was always someone who fretted about things. Now I'm focused on the pleasure of the moment, and the days are not agonizing—even if I'm feeling really ill.

(Bauer-Wu, 2011a, p. 2)

References

Back, A. L., Bauer-Wu, S. M., Rushton, C. H., & Halifax, J. (2009). Compassionate silence in the patient-clinician encounter: A contemplative approach. *Journal of Palliative Medicine, 12*(2), 1113–1117.

Bauer-Wu, S. (2011a). *Leaves falling gently: Living with serious & life-limiting illness through mindfulness, compassion & connectedness.* Oakland, CA: New Harbinger.

Bauer-Wu, S. (2011b). Insights gained from a decade of research: Mindfulness based practices for cancer patients undergoing stem cell transplant. In *9th Annual International Scientific Conference for Clinicians, Researchers and Educators: Investigating and Integrating Mindfulness in Medicine, Health Care, and Society, Norwood, MA, March 31, 2011.*

Bauer-Wu, S., Sullivan, A., Rosenbaum, E., Ott, M. J., Powell, M., McLoughlin, M., & Healey, M. W. (2008). Facing the challenges of hematopoietic stem cell transplantation with mindfulness meditation: A pilot study. *Integrative Cancer Therapies, 7*(2), 62–69.

Benzo, R. P. (2013). Mindfulness and motivational interviewing: Two candidate methods for promoting self-management. *Chronic Respiratory Disease, 10*(3), 175–182.

McCown, D. Reibel, D. & Micozzi, M. S. (2010). *Teaching Mindfulness: A Practical Guide for Clinicians and Educators*. Springer: New York.

Chapter 21
Teaching Health Care Professionals

Michael S. Krasner

Mindful Practice: An Overview

Mindful Practice, a mindfulness-based intervention developed by a team of physicians at the University of Rochester School of Medicine and Dentistry (Rochester, New York, USA) was designed to enhance medical students', residents', and physicians' resilience and well-being, improve the physician–patient relationship, and advance the quality of medical care they provide. This educational intervention was built on a strong biopsychosocial foundation and contains three major components—mindfulness meditation, narrative medicine, and appreciative inquiry—each integrated with the others into a seamless approach.

Mindful practice refers to qualities of exemplary clinicians that transcend clinical specialty and clinical experience (Epstein, 1999). These qualities include the ability to be present, attentive, curious, and to adopt a "beginner's mind," and have the goal of greater awareness and insight into one's own work. Mindful practice contributes to clinician well-being and reduces burnout (Krasner et al., 2009) . Additionally, it improves quality of care by helping practitioners to become more aware of their own clinical reasoning processes and to be more vigilant. Mindful practitioners tend not to oversimplify, ignore the obvious, cover up deficiencies, or engage in premature closure.

Our current health care environment makes mindful practice very challenging for health professionals. *Mindful Practice* addresses these external barriers as well as learners' own internal barriers to self-awareness such as unexamined emotions, over-concreteness, and emotional exhaustion—which then manifest as feeling overwhelmed by suffering, ignoring the obvious, being reactive rather than responsive,

M.S. Krasner, M.D. (✉)
University of Rochester School of Medicine and Dentistry,
42 Lilac Drive #8, Rochester, NY 14620, USA
e-mail: michael_krasner@urmc.rochester.edu

© Springer International Publishing Switzerland 2016
D. McCown et al., *Resources for Teaching Mindfulness*,
DOI 10.1007/978-3-319-30100-6_21

withdrawing from unpleasant or anxiety-provoking discussions, having difficulty tolerating ambiguity and uncertainty, and making hasty decisions.

Our model of mindful practice describes four qualities of exemplary physicians—attentive observation, critical curiosity, beginner's mind and presence (Epstein, 1999). Attentiveness refers to being able to observe without making judgments that would otherwise distort or diminish one's capacity to understand. This quality involves monitoring one's own biases, thoughts, and emotions: observing the observer, observing the observed. Critical curiosity refers to opening up to possibilities, rather than falling into the cognitive traps of premature closure and the discarding of disconfirming data. Beginner's mind refers to addressing the mind's tendency to take only one perspective—the most familiar one—on a problem; by allowing a fresh perspective and taking more than one perspective simultaneously, more diagnostic and therapeutic options become available. Presence involves being there physically, mentally, and emotionally for patients, accurately communicating an understanding of the patient's concerns and feelings back to the patient (empathic connection through reflective interaction) and enacting compassion. Physicians have written powerful narratives of these experiences. Yet, "being there" is challenging in demanding, noisy, high-paced, and stressful medical environments. This program elicits from participants their own strategies that already exist, helping them become more present, and sharing these strategies with each other in ways that they can be made more generalizable.

Mindful practice depends on developing a capacity for *mindfulness*. Mindfulness includes: (1) the capacity for lowering one's own reactivity (e.g., paying attention to experiences without having to react to them); (2) the ability to notice and observe sensations, thoughts, and feelings even though they might be unpleasant; (3) the ability to act with awareness and intention (not being on "automatic pilot"); and (4) the ability to focus on experience, not the labels or judgments one applies to them (e.g., feeling an emotion rather than wondering if it is okay to feel that emotion). While mindfulness has been used in connection with "mindfulness meditation" or "mindfulness-based stress-reduction" and "mindfulness-based cognitive therapy," for example, mindfulness is a naturally occurring human capacity, and can be cultivated in many ways, including with a wide variety of meditation traditions, physical activities, educational methods, and music.

Mindful practice focuses on contemplative practices as a "container" for holding several other approaches (technologies) that promote the capacity for bringing mindfulness to bear on the clinical experience. The mindful practice curriculum is specifically focused on cultivating mindfulness in clinical work settings with two goals: to improve the quality of care and to improve physician and other health professional well-being. Clearly, these two goals are linked. It may seem as if becoming a "mindful" clinician requires yet another set of techniques and behaviors for the busy health professional to master. However, both the intention for cultivating mindful practice and the integration of mindful practice into the lived experience of health professionals, and hence into the relationships they have with their patients, reflect a return to the foundational qualities of the healing relationship as developed throughout history in the Hippocratic tradition.

Burnout

The problem with health professional burnout has been discussed for several decades, with the first published reports appearing in the United States in the mid-1970s (Freudenberger, 1975; Maslach, 1976). The factors influencing physician burnout are many (Cole & Carlin, 2009), the issue of burnout arises early in the medical education process (Dyrbye et al., 2008; Shanafelt, 2003), and burnout affects not only physician well-being but also the quality of care delivered (Doherty & Burge, 1989; O'Connor & Spickard, 1997; Spickard, Gabbe, & Christensen, 2002). There is a paucity of well-studied interventions for addressing burnout (Dunn, Arnetz, Christensen, & Homer, 2007).

A recent report of practicing physicians demonstrated that nearly one-half of US medical doctors met criteria for burnout, a rate that exceeds that of other US workers (Shanafelt et al., 2012). The specialties most at risk for burnout are those on the "front lines" such as family medicine, general medicine, and emergency medicine. Previous investigations have shown that burnout is quite common among medical students and residents training in a variety of specialties, with rates ranging from 20 to 80 % (Dyrbye et al., 2010; Prins et al., 2007). In one large survey of over 4000 medical students, approximately 50 % of students experience burnout, and burnout was associated with an alarmingly increased likelihood of subsequent suicidal ideation while in medical school, with over 10 % of this sample reporting suicidal ideation within the prior year (Dyrbye et al., 2010).

Physician burnout has been linked to poorer quality of care, including patient dissatisfaction, increased medical errors, and lawsuits, and decreased ability to express empathy (Shanafelt, 2003). The consequences of burnout among practicing physicians include not only poorer quality of life and lower quality of care but also a decline in the stability of the physician workforce (Williams et al., 2001). Evidence exists that the effects of burnout coupled with the natural attrition among currently practicing physicians have already had a significant effect on patient access to primary care services (Bodenheimer, 2006; Buchbinder, Wilson, Melick, & Powe, 1999; Treadway, 2008; Williams et al., 2001).

Although the causes of burnout are many, several deserve highlighting in that they seem to be particularly sensitive to the effects of a lack of mindfulness, and that the capacity to be present within these difficulties may turn these problems into challenges that are workable. Historically, the current unease within the medical profession today is unlikely to be a historical aberration, where the history of medicine is one of a troubled profession, wherein the practitioners often felt mortified by the inadequacy of their clinical tools (Zuger, 2004).

Managed care is often cited as one major reason for physician dissatisfaction, with administrative burdens, limited choice of referrals, limitations on drug prescribing, and financial incentives to curb medical workups suggested as contributing to physician discontent (Grumbach, Osmond, Vranizan, Jaffe, & Bindman, 2003). Additionally, disparate expectations between patients and the physicians, and a lack of enough time to accomplish necessary tasks in the clinical encounter further burden the busy medical practitioner. This occurs within a context of rapid scientific knowledge growth, patient's access to this knowledge, and limited translation of this knowledge into promised outcomes (Zuger, 2004). Finally, burnout may be related to a sense of loss of control and meaning (Dunn et al., 2007).

One answer to address this problem involves promoting activities among physicians and other health professionals that encourage self-care, reflection, and personal development, where these at-risk professionals not only develop their capacity to be present but also benefit from interacting with compassionate and nonjudgmental listeners (Cole & Carlin, 2009).

Resilience and Self-Care

Resilience has been identified as a central element of physician well-being. Findings from a recent study of strategies experienced physicians employ to promote health and resilience suggest that diverse social resources and fields of interest, together with realistic expectancies and good self-knowledge, support sustainable coping which, in turn, create experiences of efficacy that confirm health-promoting attitudes and practices and build resilience (Zwack & Schweitzer, 2013). But what is resilience? And how might self-care practices in general and in particular mindfulness-based practices enhance resilience?

Resilience refers to the ability of an individual to respond to stress in a healthy, adaptive way such that personal goals are achieved at minimal psychological and physical cost; resilient individuals "bounce back" after challenges while also growing stronger (Epstein & Krasner, 2013). Put slightly differently, resilience refers to a dynamic capacity that allows people to thrive on challenges and includes the capacities for self-efficacy, self-control, self-monitoring, adaptability, ability to engage help and support, learning from difficulties, and persistence despite blocks to progress (Howe, Smajdor, & Stockl, 2012).

Personal or self-awareness lies at the center of these definitions. The ancient maxim "know thyself" is inscribed at the Temple of Apollo at Delphi, referring to long established wisdom. It was employed by Plato through his use of the character of Socrates to motivate his dialogues. Evidence suggests that experiences with activities that enhance personal awareness can improve physicians' clinical care and increase satisfaction with work, relationships, and with themselves (Novack et al., 1997). Emotional self-awareness and self-regulation can be consciously cultivated as habits for physicians to better function in clinical situations, with attention to cognitive and emotional factors that, when left unexamined, may lead to medical errors (Borrell-Cario & Epstein, 2004).

According to Michael Kearney and colleagues in discussion of self-care for physicians who work in end-of-life medicine, self-awareness involves both a combination of self-knowledge and the development of dual-awareness that allows the clinician to simultaneously attend to and monitor the needs of the patient, the work environment, and his or her own subjective experience (Kearney,

Weininger, Vachon, Harrison, & Mount, 2009). Methods of self-care that do not enhance self-awareness have limitations, and he cites evidence that it can result in clinicians who are less emotionally available and experience work as less rewarding (Kearney et al., 2009; Spickard et al., 2002). Greater self-awareness of clinicians may enhance self-care, improve patient care and satisfaction, and allow the work itself to be regenerative and fulfilling (Kearney et al., 2009; Meier, Back, & Morrison, 2001; Novack, Epstein, & Paulesn, 1999; Novack et al., 1997).

However, little research exists on what self-care and self-awareness promoting practices are available and which are effective. There are also questions of personal motivation and institutional and organizational support. In summary, members of the health care workforce and health care institutions together can support evidence-based efforts to enhance physician and health professional resilience. These efforts have the potential to increase the quality of care while reducing burnout and attrition (Epstein & Krasner, 2013).

Mindful Practice

The physician–patient relationship can contain both technical and human aspects, sometimes referred to as "Hippocratic" and "Asklepian," for the kinds of attention that physicians use in their work. They can also be either detached and humanly connected, to self and to others (Downie, 2012). Flexner's Carnegie Foundation report had a substantial impact on the shape of medical education in the twentieth century and beyond. Not only was competency in the basic sciences emphasized, but also the importance of a liberal education (Flexner, 1910). One of the objectives of medical professional formation is to integrate these competencies, thereby addressing both the art and science facets of quality medical care. Elements of medical education that include experiential and reflective processes, the use of personal narratives, integration of self and expertise, and candid discussion among learners are all approaches that are suggested to meet these objectives (Rabow, Remen, Parmalee, & Inui, 2010).

Situated at the center of these elements, mindfulness can be considered a universal human capacity to foster clear thinking and open-heartedness. It assists in developing a greater sense of emotional balance and well-being. The original purpose of mindfulness in Buddhism is to alleviate suffering and cultivate compassion. This purpose strongly suggests a rational role for mindfulness in medicine (Santorelli, 1998). Ludwig and Kabat-Zinn point out that mindfulness facilitates the physician's compassionate engagement with the patient (Ludwig & Kabat-Zinn, 2008). It has also been suggested that mindfulness represents a central competency for effective clinical decision-making (Epstein, 1999). This competency may be promoted through practicing attentiveness, curiosity, and the presence as part of a medical educational approach for developing useful "habits of mind" (Epstein, 2003). Indeed, mindfulness can be seen as a core competency that can be cultivated, and can be considered as a potential antidote to the depersonalizing effects of the current medical environment (Stange, Piegorsh, & Miller, 2003).

Mindfulness training has been shown to be both acceptable and effective in medical student, nursing, and health professional training. Medical and premedical students participating in an 8-week mindfulness-based stress reduction (MBSR) program demonstrated reductions in anxiety and overall psychological distress and increases in empathy (Shapiro, Schwartz, & Bonner, 1998). Similar results with anxiety, empathy, and reducing stress were shown among nursing students enrolled in an MBSR program (Beddoe & Murphy, 2004). And among a mixed group of health professionals, an MBSR program showed improvements in stress, quality of life, and self-compassion (Shapiro, Astin, Bishop, & Cordova, 2005).

In addition to the personal benefits of mindfulness for health professionals in training, clinician mindfulness may play a role in promotion of greater patient safety and reduction of medical errors (Epstein, 1999; Ludwig & Kabat-Zinn, 2008). Prominent among strategies delineated for reducing cognitive biases from which diagnostic errors stem is metacognition—the self-awareness of one's own thinking process (Croskerry, 2003). Metacognition and mindfulness are related phenomena, with increased mindfulness associated with greater awareness of intrapersonal experiences, including thoughts, emotions, and body sensations. Therefore, mindfulness training, which has been demonstrated to increase mindfulness (Carmody & Baer, 2008) may help clinicians practice with more awareness of their cognitive biases. Sibinga and Wu effectively illustrate the inverse relation between mindfulness and errors through mapping accepted qualities of mindfulness (e.g., beginner's mind, non-judging, acceptance) with cognitive dispositions that lead to errors (e.g., attribution error, affective heuristic, anchoring, confirmation bias) (Sibinga & Wu, 2010).

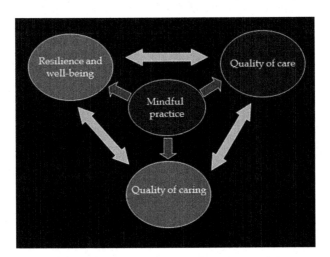

(Epstein & Krasner, 2014; Shanafelt et al., 2005; Shanafelt, Bradley, Wipf, & Back, 2002)

Mindful Practice Curriculum

The Mindful Practice curriculum was designed in 2005–2007 as a mindfulness-based intervention for medical students entering their clinical years to address professional formation, and simultaneously, for practicing physicians interested in addressing burnout and resilience through a contemplative, self-care-oriented strategy. (This intervention was supported by several sources of funding including the Arthur Vining Davis Foundation, the Arnold Gold Foundation, the Mannix Foundation, and the Physicians Foundation for Health Systems Excellence.)

The curriculum is designed to be modular, with each separate module intended to address a theme of professional relevance to the participant. Within each module, there are contemplative exercises, didactic content, and interpersonal dialogues. These components are not considered separate. They are integrated into a seamless experience whereby the participants apply mindfulness practices in the service of reflecting on clinical experiences and discovering interpersonal and intrapersonal qualities already present that can enhance meaning, quality of care, and quality of the caring offered.

Many of the themes can be considered reflective of challenges experienced by clinicians and students, and thus focus on the "problems" they experience. The nature of the reflections and dialogues that develop from those reflections are designed for participants to focus on already present qualities and capacities within the clinician, health care teams, and systems. This "appreciative" approach does not discount the toll that these challenges exert on physician well-being. Rather, it shifts the orientation of the participant to an empowered position. Practical responses to difficulties already present are recognized and the potential for carrying those responses forward are discussed.

Components of Mindful Practice

Components of the program can be viewed as *techniques*, and the intervention viewed as the acquisition of a set of skills for application in the practice of medicine. The program also has a more fundamental aim: transforming one's *way of being* as a physician or physician in training. Expressed in another way, *Mindful Practice is* designed to change the way that physicians relate not only to their patients, but also to their colleagues and to themselves. This expanded view includes recognition that through care and attention to oneself the physician can become a better clinician, more attentive and aware of the needs of patients.

The acquisition of medical knowledge, assimilation of clinical information, and continued honing of manual skills are vital to medical competence. Likewise, the continual honing of interpersonal skills, the steady development of increased intrapersonal and interpersonal awareness, and the capacity to attend to patients with presence are also central tasks toward achieving the goal of practicing high quality and relationship-centered medical care. A desirable outcome of *Mindful Practice* is for these skills to become integrated into the practitioner's clinical understanding and individual expression as a clinician in much the same way as the understanding of organ systems and their physiology and pathology become integrated into an approach to problem solving in the clinical encounter.

With these goals and understandings in mind, the following components are included in an integrated fashion into the *Mindful Practice* curriculum:

Mindfulness Meditation in many ways forms the foundation as well as container for the other two components. It is the medium through which Narrative and Appreciative dialogues operate. The quality of mindfulness, cultivated through the meditative practices, functions as an ever present lens through which personal stories are contemplated, written, shared, and discussed.

In this training, the cultivation of the qualities of mindfulness involves the regular practice of formal meditations which include those with which the reader may already be familiar:

Body Scan — in which participants practice an awareness of the state of the body just as it is from moment to moment through slow guidance through the body, with attention directed toward the body sensations experienced as well as thoughts and feelings arising during the exercise.

Mindful Movement — also known as mindful *hatha yoga* in which participants are guided through a series of gentle movements, postures, and stretching exercises, nonjudgmentally attending to feelings, thoughts, and sensations that arise.

Sitting Meditation — quietly sitting while observing the flow of thoughts, feelings, and sensations.

Walking Meditation — involves bringing meditative awareness with the same nonjudgmental attention to thoughts, feelings, and sensations to the experience of walking.

All these formal practices are designed to enhance the participant's awareness of the stream of thoughts, the flow of feelings, and the presence of sensations that are very often not noticed, yet inform action and behavior from moment to moment. Through the enhancement of the awareness that develops from the regular practice of these mindfulness exercises, it becomes possible at times to step out of the *automatic pilot* mode of living, and instead experience and act with greater awareness.

In order to assist the participant in applying the lessons learned through formal practice to their daily lives, participants are encouraged to bring the same quality of awareness to other activities, both in the classroom (during discussion, while developing and sharing narratives, when engaged in appreciative inquiry exercises) and also outside of the classroom (while engaged in life's activities at work and at home). The cultivation of mindfulness is best supported by regular practice and is the foundation underlying the techniques of narrative medicine and appreciative inquiry. Participants are encouraged to engage in daily home exercises. Supportive materials such as audio recordings of formal mindfulness meditation practices are provided to guide these daily home exercises.

Narrative Medicine provides a way of understanding the personal connections between physicians and patients and the meaning of medical practice and experiences for individual physicians. It also reflects the physicians' values and beliefs, and how they become manifest in the physician–patient relationship, and how that connection relates to the society in which it develops. According to Charon, narrative medicine helps imbue the facts and objects of health and illness with their consequences and meanings for individual patients and physicians (Charon, 2001a, 2001b). The use of narratives in medicine grants access to knowledge about the patient and about the practitioner himself/herself that would have otherwise remained out of reach. Narrative medicine in the Mindful Practice program includes the sharing of stories that arise from the participants' clinical experiences and takes the form of reflection, dialogue, and discussion in large and small groups, specific writing exercises, and journaling. Narratives are chosen by the participants about their own personal experiences of caring for patients. Thus, the narratives are grounded in the real, lived, experiences of the physicians, not in philosophical or rhetorical "what-ifs" that impact on cognitive and emotional challenges.

Appreciative inquiry (AI) strives to foster growth and change by focusing participants' attention on their existing capacities and prior successes in relationship building and problem solving (as opposed to an exclusive focus on problems and challenges). Much of medical training focuses on what is wrong rather than what is right. Patients are described in terms of problem lists, but there are no defined places to describe their strengths and resources. Morbidity and mortality rounds focus on analyzing bad outcomes, but there are few opportunities to explore effective teamwork and joint decision-making. The theory behind AI is that reinforcement and analysis of positive experiences with patients and families are more likely to change behavior in desired directions than the exclusive critique of negative experiences or failures (Cooperider & Whitney, 2005). Appreciative inquiry involves the art and practice of asking unconditionally positive questions that strengthen the capacities to apprehend, anticipate, and heighten positive potential. It is an inquiry tool that fosters imagination and innovation. The AI approach makes six assumptions: (1) for every person or group there is something that is working; (2) looking for what works well and doing more of it is more motivating than looking for what doesn't work well and doing less of it; (3) what we focus on becomes our reality and individuals and groups move toward what they focus on; (4) the language we use to describe reality helps to create that reality; (5) people have more confidence to journey to the future if they carry forward parts of the past; (6) we should carry forward the best parts of the past.

Traditionally, the steps of AI involve the following: (1) *definition*-what we wish to see or grow in ourselves and our groups; (2) *discovery*-what gives life; (3) *dream*-what might be; (4) *design*-what should be; and (5) *delivery*-what will be. AI's impact on fostering change includes a strengthening of the confidence and positive dialogue about the future, increased feelings of connection and participation, and an appreciative mindset and culture.

In the Mindful Practice curriculum, the first two steps of AI, *definition* and *discovery*, are integrated into the structure of interpersonal dialogues in the sharing of participants' narratives. Participants are guided in using AI techniques when engaged in appreciative dialogues, discussion, and reflection. With the ongoing practice and support of skilled facilitation, this approach becomes second nature and is the predominant technique used for exploring the experiences that arise in the narratives, perceived through the quality of mindfulness. Please refer to the *Scripts* section of the book for storytelling and listening guidelines employed by facilitators in leading participants through the Mindful Practice sessions (Krasner & Epstein, 2010).

Mindful Practice Outcomes

In 2009, the *Journal of the American Medical Association* published an article describing the outcomes of a year-long Mindful Practice program (at the time it was called *Mindful Communication*) for 70 primary care physicians (Krasner et al., 2009). This project was funded by the Physicians Foundation for Health Systems Excellence, a nonprofit 501(c)(3) organization that seeks to advance the work of practicing physicians and helps facilitate the delivery of healthcare. The second round of funding since the Foundation's creation focused, among other areas, on physician well-being. The project, undertaken under sponsorship of the New York Chapter of the American College of Physicians, recruited two cohorts of primary care physicians from the Rochester, New York, community, with Internal Medicine, Family Medicine and Pediatric specialists.

These two separate cohorts consisted of nearly 35 physicians each and included 52 hours of training, allocated as follows: Initial eight weekly sessions, each for 2.5 hours, with an all-day 7-hour silent retreat after the sixth weekly session. This program was followed by ten 2.5-hour monthly sessions. Each session included time allocated for the practice of formal mindfulness meditation, as well as time allocated for interpersonal dialogues based on sharing of narratives related to clinical experiences. The dialogues followed contemplative and reflective periods for participants to write about experiences relating the theme to their clinical lives and were presented as meditative practices themselves. Each session focused on a specific theme, integrated into the mindfulness meditation guidance as well as the reflective writing and dialogues. Home meditative practices, readings, and journaling were encouraged. Examples of themes and the kind of questions asked of participants are displayed in the table:

Topic	Write or tell a brief story about…
Awareness of pleasant or unpleasant sensations, feelings, or thoughts	A pleasant or an unpleasant experience during clinical work and its effect on the patient–physician relationship
Perceptual biases and filters	A surprising clinical experience (an experience that differed significantly from what you expected)
Burnout	An experience of noticing and responding to your own emotional exhaustion, depersonalization, and low sense of personal accomplishment
Meaning in medicine	A clinical encounter that was meaningful to you; what made it meaningful, what personal capacities did you have that contributed to the meaning
Boundaries or conflict management	A time when you effectively said, "No!" or set a clear boundary in clinical practice and still maintained a healing relationship
Attraction in the clinical encounter	A time when you were aware of attraction toward a patient and its influence on the dynamics of the physician–patient relationship
Self-care	A time when you faced choices about caring for yourself as opposed to caring for others
Being with suffering or end-of-life care	A clinical encounter involving being present to suffering: sadness, pain, uncertainty, end-of-life, and the awareness of your role as physician

Although many of the topics that were used as themes for the session involve stressful challenges in the practice of medicine, the instructions that guided the narratives and hence the dialogues allowed the participant to focus on successes and capacities. In this way, the concepts of Appreciative Inquiry were integrated into the sessions.

Outcomes were measured a few months before the intervention, at baseline, 2, 12, and 15 months after the beginning of the intervention and included the following:

1. The "2-Factor" Mindfulness Scale in which mindfulness is conceptualized as a multifaceted attribute relating to one's inner experience. We used the 2 factors instead of the subsequent 5 described by Baer, as they had been validated at the time of the study (observe and non-react) and appeared most relevant to clinical practice (Baer et al., 2008; Baer, Smith, Hopkins, Krietemeyer, & Toney, 2006).
2. The Maslach Burnout Inventory (Maslach, Jackson, & Leiter, 1998).
3. The Jefferson Scale of Physician Empathy, measuring three dimensions of empathy: compassionate care, perspective taking, and standing in the patient's shoes (Hojat et al., 2001).
4. The Physician Beliefs Scale which measures physicians' beliefs about psychosocial aspects of patient care (Ashworth, Williamson, & Montano, 1984).
5. The Mini-markers of the Big Five Factor Structure describes the five major personality structures (Saucier, 1994).
6. The Profile of Mood States (POMS) is a widely used instrument to assess six mood states (McNair, Lorr, & Droppleman, 1971).

The 1-year results are summarized below, reported in standardized mean differences:

Measure	Standardized mean difference	p-Value
Mindfulness—total score	1.12	<.001
– *Observe*	1.03	<.001
– *Nonreact*	0.88	<.001
Burnout—emotional exhaustion	0.62	<.001
– *Depersonalization*	0.45	<.001
– *Low personal accomplishment*	0.44	<.001
Empathy—total	0.45	<.001
– *Standing in patient's shoes*	0.36	.003
– *Perspective taking*	0.38	.001
Physician belief scale	0.37	.001
Mini-markers—conscientiousness	0.29	<.001
– *Emotional stability*	0.40	<.001
POMS—total mood disturbance	0.69	<.001
– *Depression*	0.55	<.001
– *Anger*	0.76	<.001
– *Fatigue*	0.81	<.001

It is worth noting several things. Pre-intervention and baseline measures confirmed stability of these tools before the program began. Nearly all of the changes measured were observed at 2 months, and persisted throughout, and 3 months after the conclusion of the intervention. In fact, the changes in mindfulness were largest at the 15-month assessment. Additionally, the mini-markers scale was used to assess whether certain personality types could predict changes in outcomes. There were indeed no correlations, yet unexpected was the finding of a statistically significant change in two of the personality markers, conscientiousness and emotional stability.

An analysis of these findings confirms what other mindfulness-based interventions have regularly demonstrated in terms of personal well-being (Brown, Ryan, & Creswell, 2007). Of particular interest are the effects on physician burnout and on factors that can collectively be considered markers of a patient-centered orientation to care. Notably, the improvements in empathy, the increased psychosocial orientation demonstrated by the Physician Belief Scale, and the personality factors of increased conscientiousness and emotional stability reflect practitioners who became more capable of being present and relationship-centered in their clinical encounters with patients.

The changes in burnout, personality, mood disturbance, and empathy were moderately correlated with the changes in mindfulness, with r-values ranging from 0.25 to 0.39. These findings suggest the possibility of a mediating effect by mindfulness, and warrants further investigation. In this investigation, there was no randomization, and it could be that those practitioners drawn to this program had some interest in meditation, which makes them different than other of their colleagues. However, pre-intervention and baseline burnout scores placed this group of physicians in the moderate to high level of burnout category. Additionally, the investigators were very interested in the feasibility of this kind of program, intent on exploring what the effects would be on a cohort of physicians who would actually volunteer for a course such as this.

The intervention has been repeated among primary care providers in Spain, with similar results shown in burnout, empathy, mood, and mindfulness (Asuero, 2012). Since the 2009 publication, a number of other individuals and institutions have been using the curriculum in some manner to support educational activities either with medical students, physicians in training, practicing physicians, or mixed health professionals. A partial list includes the following locations and institutions:

Baystate Medical Center, Boston University, Brown University, Dalhousie University, Dartmouth Medical School, Drexel University, Duke University, East Carolina University, Georgetown University, Göteborg, Sweden, Hamilton Ontario Health Systems, Harvard Medical School, Hong Kong University, Jefferson Medical College, Mayo Medical School, McGill University, Oakland University, Ohio State University, Oregon Health Sciences University, Universidad Autónoma de Barcelona, University of Iowa, Université de Montreal, University of California San Diego, University of Massachusetts, University of Toronto, University of Wisconsin (personal communication).

A follow-up investigation was carried out, designed to determine what aspects of this educational intervention contributed to physicians' well-being and the care they provided. Investigators used structured interviews of participants, analyzing the responses using standard qualitative analytic tools (Beckman et al., 2012). Participants reported three main themes: (1) sharing personal experiences from medical practice with colleagues reduced professional isolation; (2) mindfulness skills improved the participants' ability to be attentive and listen deeply to patients' concerns, respond to patients more effectively, and develop adaptive reserve; and (3) developing greater self-awareness was positive and transformative, yet participants struggled to give themselves permission to attend to their own personal growth.

A number of quotes from that article highlight the personal transformations that participants experienced along those domains. One in particular is worth displaying here because it reflects not only a growing self-awareness but also the capacity for making choices when faced with challenging patients and challenging thoughts, thoughts created by the physician, that most of the time are experienced and often acted upon without awareness:

> *In general, I think that I am a pretty good listener. I will spend extra time with my patients if they need it, but I felt in some ways that it was kind of sucking me dry. I would be so empathetic, and then I would feel frustrated, like what else can I do?... I would think about patients at home, in the shower, thinking she can't get to her appointment, maybe I should pick her up and drive her.... I would empathize to the point of where I would be so in their shoes. I would start to feel the way that they felt and I mean, you know, take four of those in a row in a day, and I would be just wiped out ... and, they don't really want to hear about me and my processes.... It's not that I don't empathize with them anymore, but [now] I feel OK just to listen and be present with them ... and I think that in some ways that helps them more ... and that is a wonderful thing that you can do for patients.... I just needed to learn that myself, I guess.*

Mindful Practice: Future Directions

Since the publication of the JAMA article in 2009, there has been significant interest in the curriculum from medical educators, clinicians, and other health professionals. The developers of the curriculum have been offering workshops in retreat-like settings for those interested in using this kind of intervention in their work settings. To date, over 400 participants from the United States, Canada, Asia, Europe, South America, Africa, and Oceania have attended. Their professions include practicing physicians, medical educators, nurses, psychologists and therapists, physical therapists, and malpractice insurance executives.

With a growing number of individuals and institutions using Mindful Practice, there is the possibility of developing a more robust data base to ascertain suitability, feasibility, acceptance, and efficacy. Additionally, there is also an anticipation that the curriculum can and will be adapted to meet the specific needs of users. This intervention might find utility and effectiveness in the broader workplace. This setting can be investigated in a medical workplace with findings that may be extrapolated to other work places. The intervention can be designed to engage all levels of an organization, professionals, and nonprofessionals alike. Working together in this way, outcomes that are worth investigating include work satisfaction, job performance, absenteeism, presenteeism (Goetzel et al., 2004), worker health care utilization, and the extent to which the organization fulfills its mission and lives up to its vision.

Mindful Practice is a mindfulness-based intervention built on the cultivation of awareness and attention through contemplative practices while incorporating the sharing of narratives influenced by an appreciative inquiry approach. It holds promise for building resilience among health professionals who face an increasingly stressful and complex professional experiences. Additionally, empiric evidence suggests it enhances the adaptive reserve of physicians and also improves the quality of caring rendered by its practitioners. This final effect may have profound implications for the health and well-being of all.

Bibliography

Ashworth, C. D., Williamson, P., & Montano, D. (1984). A scale to measure physician beliefs about psychosocial aspects of patient care. *Social Science Medicine, 19*(11), 1235–1238.

Asuero, A. (2012). *Effectiveness of an educational program on mindfulness to reduce burnout and improve empathy in primary care professionals.* Barcelona, Spain: Universidad Autónoma de Barcelona.

Baer, R. A., Smith, G. T., Hopkins, J., Krietemeyer, J., & Toney, L. (2006). Using self-report assessment methods to explore facets of mindfulness. *Assessment, 13*(1), 27–45.

Baer, R. A., Smith, G. T., Lykins, E., Button, D., Krietemeyer, J., Sauer, S., … Williams, J. M. (2008). Construct validity of the five facet mindfulness questionnaire in meditating and nonmeditating samples. *Assessment, 15*(3), 329–342.

Beckman, H. B., Wendland, M., Mooney, C., Krasner, M. S., Quill, T. E., Suchman, A. L., & Epstein, R. M. (2012). The impact of a program in mindful communication on primary care physicians. *Academic Medicine, 87*(6), 815–819.

Beddoe, A., & Murphy, S. (2004). Does mindfulness decrease stress and foster empathy among nursing students? *Journal of Nursing Education, 43*, 305–312.

Bodenheimer, T. (2006). Primary care—Will it survive? *New England Journal of Medicine, 355*(9), 861–864.

Bodenheimer, T., & Sinsky, C. (2015). From triple to quadruple aim: Care of the patient requires care of the provider. *Annals of Family Medicine, 12*, 573–576.

Borrell-Cario, F., & Epstein, R. (2004). Preventing errors in clinical practice: A call for self-awareness. *Annals of Family Medicine, 2*, 310–316.

Brown, K., & Ryan, R. (2003). The benefits of being present: Mindfulness and its role in psychological well-being. *Journal of Personality and Social Psychology, 84*, 822–848.

Brown, K. W., Ryan, R. M., & Creswell, J. D. (2007). Mindfulness: Theoretical foundations and evidence for its salutary effects. *Psychological Inquiry, 18*(4), 211–237.

Buchbinder, S., Wilson, M., Melick, C., & Powe, N. (1999). Estimates of costs of primary care physician turnover. *American Journal of Managed Care, 5*(11), 1431–1438.

Carmody, J., & Baer, R. (2008). Relationships between mindfulness practice and levels of mindfulness, medical and psychological symptoms and well-being in a mindfulness-based stress reduction program. *Journal of Behavioral Medicine, 31*, 23–33.

Charon, R. (2001a). Narrative medicine: Form, function and ethics. *Annals of Internal Medicine, 134*, 83–87.

Charon, R. (2001b). The patient-physician relationship. Narrative medicine: A model for empathy, reflection, profession, and trust. *Journal of the American Medical Association, 286*, 1897–1902.

Cole, T., & Carlin, N. (2009). The art of medicine: The suffering of physicians. *The Lancet, 374*, 1414–1415.

Cooperider, D., & Whitney, D. (2005). *Appreciative inquiry: A positive revolution in change*. San Francisco, CA: Berrett-Koehler.

Croskerry, P. (2003). The importance of cognitive errors in diagnosis and strategies to minimize them. *Academic Medicine, 78*, 775–780.

Doherty, W., & Burge, S. (1989). Divorce among physicians: Comparisons with other occupational groups. *Journal of the American Medical Association, 261*(16), 2374–2377.

Downie, R. (2012). Paying attention: Hippocratic and Asklepian approaches. *Advances in Psychiatric Treatment, 18*, 363–368.

Dunn, P., Arnetz, B., Christensen, J., & Homer, L. (2007). Meeting the imperative to improve physician wellbeing: Assessment of an innovative program. *Journal of General Internal Medicine, 22*(11), 1544–1552.

Dyrbye, L., Thomas, M., Massie, F., Power, D., Eacker, A., Harper, W., … Shanafelt, T. (2008). Burnout and suicidal ideation among US medical students. *Annals of Internal Medicine, 149*(5), 334–341.

Dyrbye, L., Thomas, M., Power, D., Durning, S., Moutier, C., Massie, S. J., … Shanafelt, T. (2010). Burnout and serious thoughts of dropping out of medical school: A multi-institutional study. *Academic Medicine, 85*(1), 94–102.

Epstein, R. (1999). Mindful practice. *Journal of the American Medical Association, 282*, 833–839.

Epstein, R. (2003). Mindful practice in action (II): Cultivating habits of mind. *Families, Systems & Health, 21*, 11–17.

Epstein, R., & Krasner, M. (2013). Physician resilience: What it means, why it matters, and how to promote it. *Academic Medicine, 88*, 301–303.

Epstein, R. M., & Krasner, M. (2014). *Mindful practice: Enhancing quality of care, quality of caring, and resilience*. Rochester, NY: University of Rochester.

Flexner, A. (1910). *Medical education in the United States and Canada: A report to the Carnegie Foundation for the Advancement of Teaching. Bulletin no. 4*. Boston, MA: Updyke.

Forster, H., Schwartz, J., & DeRenzo, E. (2002). Reducing legal risk by practicing patient-centered medicine. *Archives of Internal Medicine, 162*, 1217–1219.

Freudenberger, H. (1975). The staff burnout syndrome in alternative institutions. *Psychotherapy Theory Research & Practice, 12*, 72–83.

Goetzel, R. Z., Long, S. R., Ozminkowski, R. J., Hawkins, K., Wang, S., & Lynch, W. (2004). Health, absence, disability, and presenteeism cost estimates of certain physical and mental health conditions affecting U.S. employers. *Journal of Occupational and Environmental Medicine, 46*(4), 398–412.

Grumbach, K., Osmond, D., Vranizan, K., Jaffe, D., & Bindman, A. (2003). Primary care physicians' experience of financial incentives in managed-care systems. *New England Journal of Medicine, 339*, 1516–1521.

Hojat, M., Mangione, S., Nasca, T., Cohen, M., Gonnella, J., Erdmann, J., ... Magee, M. (2001). The Jefferson scale of physician empathy: Development and preliminary psychometric data. *Educational and Psychological Measurement, 61*(2), 341–365.

Howe, A., Smajdor, A., & Stockl, A. (2012). Toward an understanding of resilience and its relevance to medical training. *Medical Education, 46*, 349–356.

Kearney, M., Weininger, R., Vachon, M., Harrison, R., & Mount, B. (2009). Self-care of physicians caring for patients at the end of life: "Being connected...a key to my survival". *Journal of the American Medical Association, 301*, 1155–1164.

Krasner, M., & Epstein, R. (2010). *Mindful communication: Bringing intention, attention, and reflection to clinical practice. Curriculum guide*. Rochester, NY: University of Rochester School of Medicine and Dentistry.

Krasner, M. S., Epstein, R. M., Beckman, H., Suchman, A. L., Chapman, B., Mooney, C. J., & Quill, T. E. (2009). Association of an educational program in mindful communication with burnout, empathy and attitudes among primary care physicians. *Journal of the American Medical Association, 301*, 1284–1293.

Ludwig, D., & Kabat-Zinn, J. (2008). Mindfulness in medicine. *Journal of the American Medical Association, 300*, 1350–1352.

Maslach, C. (1976). Burned out. *Human Behavior, 5*, 16–22.

Maslach, C., Jackson, S. E., & Leiter, M. (1998). Maslach burnout inventory. In C. Zalaquett & R. Wood (Eds.), *Evaluating stress: A book of resources* (3rd ed.). Lanham, MD: Scarecrow Press.

McNair, D. M., Lorr, M., & Droppleman, L. F. (1971). *Manual: Profile of mood states*. San Diego, CA: Educational and Industrial Testing Service.

Mechanic, D., McAlpine, D., & Rosenthal, M. (2001). Are patients' office visits with physicians getting shorter? *New England Journal of Medicine, 344*, 198–204.

Meier, D., Back, A., & Morrison, R. (2001). The inner life of physicians and care of the seriously ill. *Journal of the American Medical Association, 286*, 3007–3014.

Novack, D., Epstein, R., & Paulesn, R. (1999). Toward creating physician-healers: Fostering medical students' self-awareness, personal growth, and well-being. *Academic Medicine, 74*, 516–520.

Novack, D., Suchman, A., Clark, W., Epstein, R., Najberg, E., & Kaplan, C. (1997). Calibrating the physician: Personal awareness and effective patient care. *Journal of the American Medical Association, 278*, 502–509.

O'Connor, P., & Spickard, A. J. (1997). Physician impairment by substance abuse. *Medical Clinics of North America, 81*(4), 1037–1052.

Prins, J., Gazendam-Donofrio, M., Turbin, B., Van Der Heijden, F., Van De Wiel, H., & Hoekstra-Weebers, J. (2007). Burnout in medical residents: A review. *Medical Education, 41*, 788–800.

Rabow, M., Remen, R., Parmalee, D., & Inui, T. (2010). Professional formation: Extending medicine's lineage of service into the next century. *Academic Medicine, 85*, 310–317.

Safran, J., & Segal, Z. (1990). *Interpersonal process in cognitive therapy*. New York, NY: Basic Books.

Santorelli, S. (1998). *Heal thy self*. New York, NY: Bell Town.

Saucler, G. (1994). Mini-markers: A brief version of Goldberg's unipolar big-five markers. *Journal of Personality Assessment, 63*(3), 506–516.

Shanafelt, T. S. (2003). The wellbeing of physicians. *American Journal of Medicine, 114*(6), 513–519.

Shanafelt, T., Boone, S., Tan, L., Dyrbye, L., Sotile, W., Satele, D., … Oreskovich, M. (2012). Burnout and satisfaction with work-life balance among US physicians relative to the general US population. *Archives of Internal Medicine, 172*(18), 1377–1385.

Shanafelt, T. D., Bradley, K. A., Wipf, J. E., & Back, A. L. (2002). Burnout and self-reported patient care in an internal medicine residency program. *Annals of Internal Medicine, 136*(5), 358–367.

Shanafelt, T. D., West, C., Zhao, X., Novotny, P., Kolars, J., Habermann, T., & Sloan, J. (2005). Relationship between increased personal well-being and enhanced empathy among internal medicine residents. *Journal of General Internal Medicine, 20*(7), 559–564.

Shapiro, S., Astin, J., Bishop, S., & Cordova, M. (2005). Mindfulness-based stress reduction for health care professionals: Results from a randomized trial. *International Journal of Stress Management, 12*, 164–176.

Shapiro, S., Schwartz, G., & Bonner, G. (1998). Effects of mindfulness-based stress reduction on medical and premedical students. *Journal of Behavioral Medicine, 21*, 581–599.

Sibinga, E. M., & Wu, A. (2010). Clinician mindfulness and patient safety. *Journal of the American Medical Association, 304*, 2532–2533.

Spickard, A. J., Gabbe, S., & Christensen, J. (2002). Midcareer burnout in generalist and specialist physicians. *Journal of the American Medical Association, 288*(12), 1447–1450.

Stange, K., Piegorsh, K., & Miller, W. (2003). Reflective practice. *Families, Systems & Health, 21*, 24–27.

Treadway, K. (2008). The future of primary care: Sustaining relationships. *New England Journal of Medicine, 359*(25), 2086.

Weiner, E., Swain, G., Wolf, B., & Gottlieb, M. (2001). A qualitative study of physicians' own wellness-promotion practices. *Western Journal of Medicine, 174*, 19–23.

Williams, E., Conrad, T., Scheckler, W. P., Linzer, M., McMurray, J., Gerrity, M., & Schwartz, M. (2001). Understanding physicians' intentions to withdraw from practice: The role of job satisfaction, job stress, mental and physical health. *Health Care Management Review, 26*(1), 7–19.

Yarnall, K., Pollak, K., Ostbye, T., Krasue, K., & Michener, J. (2003). Primary care: Is there enough time for prevention? *American Journal of Public Health, 93*, 635–641.

Zuger, A. (2004). Dissatisfaction with medical practice. *New England Journal of Medicine, 350*(1), 69–75.

Zwack, J., & Schweitzer, J. (2013). If every fifth physician is affected by burnout, what about the other four? Resilience strategies of experienced physicians. *Academic Medicine, 88*, 382–389.

Chapter 22
Teaching Clergy and Religious

Donald R. Marks and Christine D. Moriconi

Mindfulness-Based Interventions for Clergy and Members of Religious Orders

The community of clergy and religious orders totals more than 350,000 people in the USA alone (Wells, Probst, McKeown, Mitchem, & Whiejong, 2012), comprising a diverse range of individuals with widely varying professional responsibilities and roles. Churches and religious organizations have varied expectations and requirements for members of the clergy (e.g., celibacy) which can present challenges for the development and maintenance of social support networks. Moreover, the vocational roles adopted by members of the clergy can be extraordinarily heterogeneous, with a single individual serving as, for example, liturgists, musical directors, parish and school administrators, accountants, spiritual directors, educators, researchers, scholars, individual and family counselors, activists, peer supports, and trusted confidants.

Given the diversity of their work, clergy and religious are confronted with nearly constant and often conflicting demands on their time and are often "on call" among "frontline" responders when people in their faith communities experience trauma, loss, or illness (Wang, Berglund, & Kessler, 2003). They routinely devote time, energy, effort, and compassionate concern to vulnerable individuals, including many who are unable to express appreciation or acknowledgment for the care provided (Unruh & Sider, 2005). In addition, they must contend with frequent administrative pressures regarding the maintenance of financial and institutional support, including

D.R. Marks, Psy.D. (✉)
Department of Advanced Studies in Psychology, Kean University,
1000 Morris Avenue, Union, NJ 07083, USA
e-mail: domarks@kean.edu

C.D. Moriconi, Psy.D., L.M.F.T., P.M.H.C.N.S-B.C., R.N.
Center for Contemplative Studies, West Chester University of Pennsylvania,
930 E. Lincoln Highway, Suite 100, Exton, PA 19341, USA
e-mail: cmoriconi@wcupa.edu

© Springer International Publishing Switzerland 2016
D. McCown et al., *Resources for Teaching Mindfulness*,
DOI 10.1007/978-3-319-30100-6_22

administrative burdens associated with fundraising and with management of facilities and staff, both paid and volunteer (Francis, Hills, & Rutledge, 2008). At the same time, expectations associated with the roles of clergy and religious as spiritual leaders, practitioners, and advisors often exclude important dimensions of self-care. Rev. Fulton J. Sheen's influential book, *The Priest Is Not His Own* (1963), offers just one example of ways that faith traditions can depict members of religious orders as always available and ceaselessly giving. Congregations and pastoral communities can have similar expectations regarding the exceptional holiness, selflessness, and exemplary moral conduct of clergy and those in religious orders (Proeschold-Bell et al., 2013; Rayburn, Richmond, & Rogers, 1986).

While the model of the self-sacrificing pastoral servant is inspiring for people of many faiths, efforts to live in keeping with this ideal may entail significant costs in both psychological and physical well-being, particularly for those lacking adequate support and resources for responding to high-stress situations. Contemporary guides to an effective way of life as a pastor (Hamman, 2014) or member of a religious order (D'Avila-Latourrette, 2012) may have become less insistent upon the virtues of self-abnegation compared to those of previous eras, yet the strategies offered for self-care are rarely informed by contemporary research regarding burnout or mindfulness- and acceptance-based interventions. The consequences of the work demands for clergy and members of religious orders have been much debated, with numerous researchers—beginning with Francis Galton's (1872) observations regarding the longevity of the English clergy in the nineteenth century—noting the potentially beneficial aspects of the contemplative and spiritual practices integrated in religious life. Nevertheless, clergy and religious, particularly those engaged in pastoral ministry, are susceptible to the emotional exhaustion, depersonalization, and diminished sense of personal accomplishment that Maslach (1978) has characterized as "burnout." Also, while it is not often openly discussed, compassion fatigue (Figley, 1995) may be an important risk factor for mental and physical health problems within the clergy (Kaldor & Bullpitt, 2001). According to Coetzee and Klopper (2010), compassion fatigue is the progressive and cumulative result of providing care for others without time for restorative self-care, leading to difficulties in accessing the emotion and motivation that inform the process of providing care. Compassion fatigue is a pervasive issue with all caring professions but is seldom discussed as a potential problem requiring active prevention. Instead, most clergy and religious wait until symptoms appear. Consequences for this delay are tremendous as they not only negatively affect the clergy and religious but all whom they serve.

A Mindfulness-Based Intervention Curriculum for Clergy and Religious

Recent research has demonstrated efficacy for mindfulness-based interventions, including mindfulness-based stress reduction, in addressing burnout or other forms of occupation-related psychological stress (Cohen-Katz et al., 2005; Geary &

Rosenthal, 2011; Goodman & Schorling, 2012; Rosenzweig, Reibel, Greeson, Brainard, & Hojat, 2003; Shapiro, Austin, Bishop, & Cordova, 2005; Shapiro, Brown, & Biegel, 2007; Shapiro, Schwartz, & Bonner, 1998). At the time of this writing, however, no other published research has explored the use of mindfulness-based interventions with clergy or members of religious orders. This paucity of research is surprising given the recognition that stress, burnout, and psychological distress are significant concerns among this population (see Faucett, Corwyn, & Poling, 2013; Francis, Louden, & Rutledge, 2004; Proeschold-Bell et al., 2013; Raj & Dean, 2005; Turton & Francis, 2007).

That said, the number of empirical studies involving mindfulness-based intervention for helping professionals in general is not large, and additional time may be needed for mindfulness-based interventions to gain acceptance before researchers working with clergy and religious develop interest in these interventions. In addition, individuals and institutions providing mental health care for clergy and religious are understandably cautious about conducting research and publicizing new, "novel" treatments. Expectations that clergy and members of religious communities epitomize good mental health, as well as notions that spiritual practices (e.g., prayer) alone should be sufficient to assuage any form of stress or psychological distress, may act to reduce opportunities to collect data regarding psychological outcomes of mindfulness-based interventions.

Data gathered from mindfulness-based interventions for helping professionals from various fields and vocations, however, suggest ways that mindfulness curricula could be adapted for use with clergy and members of religious orders (Symington & Symington, 2012). The curriculum described here has been developed specifically for use with groups of clergy and members of religious orders. For the past two years, this curriculum has been used with groups of clergy and members of religious orders receiving comprehensive mental health services for a variety of concerns, including symptoms of burnout, anxiety, and depression. This program, like many mindfulness-based interventions, draws its inspiration from MBSR as developed by Jon Kabat-Zinn (1990), and it also uses elements of acceptance and commitment therapy (ACT; Hayes, Strosahl, & Wilson, 2012) and compassion-focused therapy (CFT; Gilbert, 2009). These elements have been integrated to address particular concerns of those in religious life, including potential attitudes toward bodily experience and navigating one's relationships with judgments, rules, and expectations.

As in MBSR, the structure of the group intervention is based on the 8-week format, though sessions are typically 1.5 hours per week rather than 2.5 hours (see Table 22.1). The program can also include a retreat day or half day if feasible. The first four sessions and the retreat day are focused on learning mindfulness and exploring ways of bringing oneself into greater contact with present-moment experience. The other four sessions focus on deepening practice and self-care strategies. Sessions five through eight draw upon aspects of other mindfulness-based interventions (e.g., ACT, CFT) to highlight psychological and behavioral processes relevant to those in religious life. Themes for these sessions include self-compassion, responding to the expectations of others, values, and committed action. While the

Table 22.1 Mindfulness for clergy and religious, schedule of class themes by week	1.	Introducing mindfulness
	2.	Mindful eating
	3.	Body awareness
	4.	Mindful movement
	5.	Values
	6.	Willingness and acceptance
	7.	Compassion and self-compassion
	8.	Committed action

curriculum does involve education regarding mindfulness, burnout, and self-care, it is not merely or even primarily a psycho-education program. The emphasis throughout is on the practice of mindfulness and the use of relevant skills. The work of the group program is predicated on the assumption that the experiential practice both in the group and between group meetings can be generalized to other settings and situations.

Initial Assessment

The curriculum presented here was developed for individuals experiencing significant vocational stress, in ways that often contribute to psychological distress. Diagnoses of major depressive disorder, persistent depressive disorder, and generalized anxiety disorder are common. In many cases, participants have experienced trauma-related stress warranting diagnosis of posttraumatic stress disorder. In other cases, traumatization has occurred at second hand, through repeated exposure to congregants experiencing intense distress. This mindfulness program has been provided within a larger program of mental health services, but it could also be offered for those with lower levels of distress who are not engaged in other treatment.

As with MBCT (Segal, Williams, & Teasdale, 2013) and other mindfulness-based group interventions, it is useful to conduct individual interviews with each prospective participant. Specifically, it is important to discuss the following when considering whether the individual faces impediments to engaging usefully in the mindfulness program:

1. *The history of the person's experience of distress, including experiences of trauma and situational factors contributing to distress.* This discussion can provide useful information regarding the individual's willingness to reflect upon his or her own reactions to life events and emotional experiences. It includes assessment of the severity of current distress. Applicants articulating suicidal or homicidal ideation, engaging in self-harm (e.g., cutting), or lacking appropriate mental health support are examples of those for whom the program may be inappropriate. Decisions are best made case by case.

2. *Description of mindfulness practice, including some of the exercises used in the program.* Prospective participants often have ideas about mindfulness practice that are inconsistent with the philosophy informing mindfulness-based programs. Clergy and members of religious orders may even consider mindfulness practice incompatible with their faith tradition. For example, those in Christian religious life may view mindfulness as an Eastern devotional practice and consider engagement in mindfulness practice akin to participating in Buddhist or Hindu rites. Others may equate mindfulness with New Age spirituality and have reservations about its acceptability in their own faith traditions. Still others may view mindfulness practice as a "secularized" form of contemplative prayer, seeing the purpose of the practice as developing a closer relationship with God. It can be useful to define "mindfulness" as it is used in the course, while marking some of the differences between devotional practices and the practice of mindful awareness of present-moment experience. These issues will be addressed in the course itself as a more detailed understanding of mindfulness, and its potential functions develop through participation in the 8-week program. Discussion of such concerns at this initial meeting is important, however, since preconceptions regarding mindfulness can influence whether an individual is willing to participate and how he or she might show up for the group.

3. *The time commitment involved in participation and importance of consistent attendance.* Many individuals in religious life have demanding schedules. Surveys of Roman Catholic priests, for example, reveal that the typical workweek is 63 hours (Rossetti & Rhoades, 2013). The 8-week program described here demands 1.5 hour per week and a half-day (4-hour) or full-day (6-hour) retreat, as well as an average of 30 minutes per day of home practice, 6 days per week—a total time commitment of 40–42 hours. Many may believe that managing to "fit in" a few sessions and attempts at practice over the course of the 8 weeks would be helpful to them or at least more helpful than no participation at all. Whether this assumption is likely to be the case is not known. It is known, however, that the absence of some group members changes the group experience for others. One potentially detrimental consequence of sporadic attendance is that it suggests to other busy people in the group that partial participation is a potentially effective way to experience the group when there is no data to establish such potential effectiveness.

4. *The nonhierarchical structure of the group.* Members of clergy and religious orders are, in many cases, accustomed to living within a clearly defined hierarchy. In ways that resemble the function of rank in the military, hierarchical distinctions among those in religious life can have profound influence on interpersonal relationships (e.g., degree of familiarity acceptable). The use of first names rather than religious titles (e.g., Monsignor, Sister) is recommended, and it is important to disclose this practice to participants in advance of the opening session. Similarly, lay or civilian attire is recommended if feasible. This recommendation is made for two reasons: (a) some religious attire is not conducive to movement practices, and (b) religious attire conveys information concerning roles and ranks. Finally, whenever possible, unless there is a strong spirit

of collegiality or long-standing tradition of participatory decision-making, clergy or religious participants and their superiors should not be included together in the same group. Hierarchy is likely to influence the conduct and contributions of group participants. Although exploring this influence could be a useful group endeavor, particularly in the context of interventions for hierarchical hostility or conflict transformation (Lederach, 2003), these relational concerns are not the primary focus of this mindfulness program.

5. *What mindfulness has to offer, including evidence regarding psychological and physiological benefits.* Many prospective participants referred by a physician or mental health provider have received some information about the benefits of mindfulness. Others, however, particularly those who encountered mindfulness through popular media, may not have received clear information about outcomes associated with sustained practice. In many cases, individuals have encountered images of tranquil practitioners dressed in yoga gear and view the practice as a potentially blissful escape from emotional experience. While many participants may experience reduced reactivity and improvements in mood or anxiety symptoms during or after this mindfulness program, direct discussion of the health outcomes associated with mindfulness training, as well as acknowledgment that such outcomes cannot be guaranteed, allows for more fully informed consent.

Session One: Introducing Mindfulness

The first session has several important aims, including introducing members of the group to one another and to fundamental aspects of mindfulness practice. Although introductions may seem like a relatively straightforward process, concerns arise according to how participants wish to identify themselves. In keeping with the non-hierarchical structure of the group, it is advised that participants each receive a press-on nametag and be asked to use their first names. The instructor or co-instructors can model this behavior by wearing nametags and using their first names. In addition, groups often include a mix of participants who are accustomed to public speaking, including addressing large congregations extemporaneously, as well as participants who speak relatively infrequently and seldom to more than a small group. The balance of "air time" between these participants is useful to consider throughout the course of the group. It is also recommended that any introduction exercise that requires participation, such as going around the room with self-introductions, be brief, so that those who might speak at length are less inclined to do so and those who prefer not to speak are not coerced into an uncomfortable public presentation.

The introduction of mindfulness practice is often usefully conducted through an exploration of the ways that participants are living now. Specifically, group members are asked what they would like to gain from the program, and this discussion often leads to a useful exploration of ways that they are living that do not feel consistent with how they would prefer to live. The technique of "pop-corning" (i.e., spontaneous contribution to the group discussion) can be introduced prior to asking this question so that participants do not find it necessary to obtain permission to speak. Statements that participants make in this discussion often contain useful information about values (i.e., what matters most in life) that reappear over the course of the group. Themes of "busyness" and "time demands" frequently arise, along with concerns regarding how one is pressed to "multitask" and how little time is available for reflection and contemplation. Surprisingly, these concerns arise even among participants who are members of contemplative orders. In addition, themes of emotional exhaustion and compassion fatigue may arise, including self-critical comments regarding one's inability to meet others' expectations. Themes of frustration with institutional organization or hierarchy, which may be perceived as obstacles to effective ministry, may emerge. Alternatively, participants may characterize their experience of stress as the product of unreasonable expectations from those to whom they minister. A common concern throughout all of these initial comments, however, is how one responds in inherently stressful, high-demand, low-control contexts (Karasek, 1998).

Discussion of these themes can lead to a useful exploration of the definition of mindfulness. Introduction of "the triangle of awareness," thoughts, feelings, and emotions, is followed by an initial brief mindfulness practice. For this practice, the 3-minutes breathing space (Segal et al., 2013) or a longer variation on that exercise is recommended. This exercise introduces an alternative way of relating to experience—actively and attentively observing it, without responding to emotion-driven urges to judge or alter it. Participants are first invited to bring awareness to specific body sensations, including those associated with sitting in a chair, then to widen awareness gradually to include the whole field of body sensations. Next, awareness is narrowed, like a spotlight, as attention focuses on the breath, observing specific physical sensations associated with the coming and going of the breath. Finally, the awareness is widened again to note emotions that might be present and to observe thoughts arising and passing in the mind. Instruction throughout this practice allows for shifting of attention, acknowledging the pull of the mind to attend to other dimensions of experience and noting that wandering is "what minds do." Emphasis centers on cultivating a curious, gentle stance toward experience, being kind to oneself when the mind is restless, and sustaining attention is difficult.

Inquiry regarding participants' experience follows each exercise. Themes that arise early in the course often include obedience and devotion. Many religious orders underscore the importance of obedience and adherence to instruction. Given the many involuntary aspects of cognition and emotion, participants may notice frequent attention shifts and conclude that they are "not doing it right" or "no good at this." These initial discussions of obedience often create an opportunity to reiterate the gentle, nonjudgmental perspective adopted in mindfulness practice and to lay important groundwork for later discussions of self-compassion.

Homework following the first meeting includes a daily 30-minute seated meditation practice, structured consistently with the practice introduced in session. Participants receive a CD recording of the exercise and a log sheet for tracking daily practice.

Sessions Two Through Four: Exploring Dimensions of Mindfulness

The next three sessions examine specific dimensions of mindfulness, beginning with an emphasis on bodily sensations, shifting to mindful awareness of emotional experience, and then finally mindful attention to thoughts. In session two, participants engage in the raisin exercise (Kabat-Zinn, 1990), mindfully exploring sensory experiences associated with eating a single raisin, as an introduction to the practice of mindful eating and mindfulness in general. Obesity is one of the principal health concerns facing clergy and members of religious orders (Koller, Blanchfield, Vavra, Andrusyk, & Altier, 2012; Proeschold-Bell & LeGrand, 2010), and so-called stress eating is a prominent concern in populations facing high rates of chronic stress. Mindfulness-based eating awareness training (MB-EAT; Kristeller, Wolever, & Sheets, 2014) has been demonstrated to reduce disordered eating behaviors, and a single mindful eating exercise has been shown to decrease food-related impulsivity in obese individuals (Hendrickson & Rasmussen, 2013). The raisin exercise alone has been demonstrated to increase enjoyment and liking of food (Hong, Lishner, & Han, 2014; Hong, Lishner, Han, & Huss, 2011).

Homework for session two is continued use of the 30-minute seated practice introduced in session one, as well as implementation of a daily mindful eating practice. Participants are invited to divide one meal each day into two halves, eating one half mindfully using techniques introduced in the raisin exercise and the other half in their usual manner. They are asked to note differences in their experiences of eating in these two ways, attending to changes in bodily sensations, thoughts, and emotions. Log sheets are provided so participants can record daily completion of the seated practice and mindful eating exercises.

In session three, participants are introduced to the body scan exercise, a practice routinely used in the first week of MBSR. One reason for the delay in introducing the body scan is that many clergy and members of religious orders have histories involving discounting or harsh judgment of bodily experiences. Beginning the program with a lengthy body-focused practice could be overwhelming, particularly for those who have long embraced attitudes that minimize the body's importance. Even when participants have embraced a more holistic perspective regarding embodiment, subtle criticisms of the body can remain and give rise to stoic expectations regarding body sensations. In many traditions, the Neoplatonic distinction between the low or base body and the less corrupted or incorruptible mind or spirit remains (Nelson, 1978). Participants practicing mindfulness may find themselves employing strategies intended to control or maintain attention at the expense of bodily comfort. Christ's observation to Peter in the garden at Gethsemane, "The spirit is willing but the flesh is weak," (Matthew, 26:41) may arise as participants describe their practice experiences, and some may link the use of attention in mindfulness practices to vigilance and control of the body. The introduction of the body scan practice is also a useful place for exploration of self-compassion, noting the mind's tendency to evaluate experience and employ frames of "better" and "worse." Cultivating a kind and compassionate attention to experience is emphasized as a key dimension of mindfulness practice.

Homework following the third meeting is daily use of a 30-minute guided body scan CD. Log sheets are again provided so participants can record completion of the practice.

In session four, additional practices involving awareness of the body are introduced, including mindful stretching and mindful walking. The mindful stretching exercises employ simple and slow movements, with emphasis on maintaining awareness of sensation in the body as the practice unfolds. Health problems, including chronic pain and obesity, can limit what participants are able to do without significant pain or discomfort. The importance of fostering a compassionate, welcoming, and nonpunitive stance toward the body during these practices is critical. It is also important to develop variations of the movement practices that accommodate those with limited range of motion. Standing poses are appropriate, along with side-to-side turning and vertical reaching, as well as neck and shoulder rolls. In addition, body movements with strong sensory components, such as rubbing palms together to generate warmth, then applying warm palms softly to the face, can provide opportunities to bring awareness to the body and notice moment-to-moment changes in sensation. As instruction is provided, participants should be invited to move slowly and observe feedback from the body, including sensations of pain and stiffness, allowing the responses of their bodies to guide far to turn or stretch.

Homework following session four includes engaging in mindful physical activity, such as simple stretching or walking, for 15 minutes once per day. Log sheets are provided.

Retreat Day: Exploring Silence Anew

The retreat day can be either 4 or 6 hours in duration. It is conceptualized as a day of silence, in which participants make a commitment to enter silence together at the start of the day and to emerge from silence together at the close. Emphasis is placed on the choice to set aside other interests and obligations for the day or half day, not answering cell phones or email and not watching television or engaging in work or errands. In many cases, participants must arrange for someone to cover for them during the time they will be away from their duties and untethered from the electronic world. The process of making coverage arrangements can be arduous for participants who are accustomed to supporting others nonstop and who have accustomed those around them to this pattern. Many participants will suggest reasons they cannot attend the retreat day (e.g., the congregation has no other resource). Holding their uncertainty about setting boundaries while continuing to highlight the importance of self-care, and the retreat day of silence, can assist participants in learning the skills and procedures needed to set limits and practice self-compassion. Participants, especially those who found scheduling the retreat most vexing, routinely express a sense of satisfaction and rejuvenation following the retreat day.

The use of silence to designate the sacred is already familiar to most clergy and members of religious orders (Flanagan, 1985; Szuchewycz, 1997). Many participants report that the silence has a profound familiarity to them, evoking memories of other retreat experiences. Many are aware of the ways that social speech and interpersonal communication can distract the attention from inner experience as it unfolds. Participants often describe qualities of "freedom" and "ease" they experience when spending time with one another in silence, responding with awareness and without perceived demands to inform or entertain or to salvage flagging conversations. The retreat day is devoted to a variety of embodied practices, including the body scan, mindful movement, and mindful eating. Finally, the practice of choiceless awareness (Kabat-Zinn, 2005), cultivating an expansive field of awareness, including all dimensions of experience without selecting a particular object of concentration, is introduced. The sense of the awareness as a vast space, limitless in dimensions, without a particular focus, almost paradoxically can lead to vivid experience of events, thoughts, body sensations, and other phenomena. A recent participant described it as "seeing with God's eye." After this practice, participants divide into pairs or groups of three to break the silence together and discuss their experiences throughout the day.

Sessions Five Through Eight: Exploring Values, Acceptance, and Self-Compassion

The second half of the curriculum provides additional opportunities for mindfulness practice while integrating themes of acceptance and self-compassion. Session five includes a consideration of values. As defined in ACT interventions (Dahl, Lundgren, Plumb, & Stewart, 2009; Hayes et al., 2012), values can be viewed as an answer to the question, "what do I want my life to be about?" Values are not goals or objectives but rather guides to the direction in which one wants to move in life. A value is a source of intrinsic reward, insofar as engaging in activity consistent with one's values is experienced as rewarding in and of itself. Values are freely chosen rather than imposed from without, and they are not derived from externally defined standards. Moreover, "failure" to complete a particular task or attain a given objective does not diminish a value. Rather, it is always possible to recommit to one's values and choose behavior that moves in a values-consistent direction. Making these behavioral choices can be challenging at times, giving rise to feelings of vulnerability and fear. At the same time, however, pursuing what matters in life can be deeply enlivening, promoting a deep sense of vitality and engagement. A distinction is drawn in this session between emotion-driven behaviors, which serve the primary purpose of changing emotional experience, and values-driven behaviors, which are chosen in the service of moving one's life in valued directions.

For clergy and members of religious orders, there are several challenges associated with identifying values and values-consistent behaviors. One problem concerns identification with external standards and expectations. While exploring values, many participants recognize ways that they have focused on obtaining the admiration or recognition of others, particularly superiors or parishioners. Conspicuous adherence to rules and moral codes of conduct may have been affirmed in religious formation and become a dependable source of validation. At the same time, however, the disconnection between these externally defined standards and the participant's personal values (including those that informed his or her choice of vocation) may contribute to a sense of aridity in ministry and spiritual practice. Identifying and choosing values from a broad range of domains (e.g., relationships, family, work, spiritual life, and health) can provide a rejuvenating connection with religious life and ministry. It can also, however, give rise to feelings of grief regarding lost opportunities and regret for time and effort devoted to goals that were not guided by freely chosen values. Some participants report that they do not feel that they have the freedom in their role or vocation to choose what matters most to them. In these cases, it is useful to acknowledge the perceived barriers and to suggest the possibility of continuing to identify and define values despite these obstacles. It may also be useful to ask, "If you had the freedom to choose what was most important, and what you were willing to take a stand for, what would that be?" The possibility of choosing one's behavioral responses to inner experience concludes this discussion and ties the practice of identifying values and values-driven behavior to the mindfulness practices learned in earlier sessions. Specifically, mindfulness allows for enhanced awareness of one's experience, including the choices one makes to change or alleviate unwanted aspects of that experience and the options one has for responding differently.

There are several exercises that facilitate identification and definition of values. The eulogy exercise (Hayes et al., 2012) can have profound resonance for clergy and members of religious orders. In this exercise, participants envision giving a eulogy for themselves at the close of life, highlighting the most moving events they experienced, as well as themes regarding the meaning and value of life they would want to emphasize. Next, participants are invited to discuss themes that arose during this exercise as the instructor lists them on a whiteboard. The group then identifies common themes that relate to values (e.g., caring for others, friendship, fostering loving relationships with God) and those that pertain primarily to emotional experience. In addition to the eulogy exercise, the Values Compass worksheet (Dahl, Wilson, Luciano, & Hayes, 2005), Values Bull's Eye (Lundgren, Luoma, Dahl, Strosahl, & Melin, 2012), and Valued Living Questionnaire (Wilson, Sandoz, Kitchens, & Roberts, 2010) are pencil-and-paper exercises that can assist participants in identifying values and making values-consistent choices. The values exercises can be completed as a group or in dyads with participants engaging in reflective listening as they share their results. It can be helpful to introduce the concept of mindful communication (Shafir, 2003) as part of this exploratory discussion, including the practice of observing changes in one's inner experience while listening to another, cultivating curiosity and openness toward the perspectives of others, and choosing words with consideration for how others respond.

Homework following the fifth session includes a daily worksheet identifying three or four values, rating the importance of these values, and assessing whether one's actions that day were accordance with that value. Note that many value worksheets highlight "marriage" or "intimate partner relationship" as value domains. Those working with celibate clergy and religious can retain these categories, allowing for discussion of emotions that arise in association with celibacy, or replace them with categories such as "celibate life" or "caring relationships in celibate life."

Session six focuses on willingness and the acceptance of inner experience. This session begins with a series of exercises exploring the consequences of efforts to control experience. This discussion is introduced with the "white bear" exercise (Wegner, 1989) in which participants are shown a slide of a polar bear, asked to attend to particular details in the picture for approximately 2 minutes, and then asked to devote as much effort as possible to not thinking about the white bear. An observation widely used in ACT interventions may be shared with the group: "If you don't want it, you've got it; if you don't want to think it, you've thought it" (Dahl & Lundgren, 2006, p. 68). As a follow-up to this discussion, a series of metaphorical exercises is provided to elucidate different stances toward inner experience, including thoughts and emotions. For example, the "quicksand metaphor" highlights potential differences between the struggle to extricate oneself inner experiences and the alternative of acceptance. In this exercise, participants discuss what happens as one struggles in quicksand, including the increased likelihood of being drawn into the mire. As the group explores the problem, the alternative of increasing surface contact with the quicksand (opening up to the experience so that one can be supported by the quicksand itself and float) typically arises. Other useful metaphors regarding the difficulty associated with controlling inner experience include the "man in the hole" metaphor (Hayes et al., 2012). In this imagined exercise, participants confront the dilemma of a man stuck in a hole whose only tool is a shovel. Still another variation on these themes can be found in the "polygraph metaphor" (Stoddard & Afari, 2014). In this exercise, participants are invited to imagine they are connected to ultrasensitive polygraphic machines that can measure the presence of any anxiety, including any changes in heart rate or perspiration. They are then asked to envision that they have been told that they must not be anxious and that if the machine senses the presence of any anxiety whatsoever, they will receive an intense electric shock—bringing the challenge of controlling one's inner experience into sharp focus.

The discussion that follows these exercises considers the feasibility of controlling one's thoughts or emotions, even in conditions when it would be highly desirable to do so (e.g., when it would avoid electric shock). The possibility is introduced that efforts to change inner experiences, such as anxiety, evoke ironic processes of mind (Wegner, 1989) or set up processes of psychological reactance that intensify the experience. Ways that the consequences of stress, including the experience of chronic autonomic arousal, could be exacerbated by efforts to control experience are explored. The illustration of these processes, for example, as presented in the discussion of "responding vs. reacting" in Kabat-Zinn's *Full Catastrophe Living* (1990, p. 337), can also assist in exploring ways that efforts to "dig out" often serve to exacerbate the stress reaction.

Homework following session six includes daily engagement in one of the mindfulness practices introduced earlier in the program, as well as daily observation of situations in which anxious arousal occurs. Participants are asked to consider the application of mindfulness, particularly mindful observation of body sensations, thoughts, and emotions, in these situations.

Session seven introduces the theme of self-compassion and adopting a perspective of kindness toward oneself and one's inner experience. The word "compassion" usually refers to other-directed feelings, responding to other peoples' suffering with kindness and assistance (Neff, 2003). These forms of compassion are well familiar to clergy and religious and often serve as motivating and sustaining influences for their work. This session, however, explores an expanded definition of compassion, applying to inner and outer experience, to self as well as others. This session begins with the Rumi poem, "The Guest House," which is used in MBCT (e.g., Segal et al., 2013) and other mindfulness-based interventions (e.g., Mirdal, 2012). Given the poem's themes of welcoming aversive emotional experiences (e.g., sorrow), participants often comment on the unusual nature of such an approach and the potential inconsistency with their previously held views of self-care. Welcoming emotions is then explored as an alternative to the struggles with inner experience highlighted in the previous session. Ways that one might "turn toward" such experiences, as opposed to reactively suppressing or avoiding them, are considered. The closing line of "The Guest House" suggests that difficult emotions could be "sent as a guide from beyond" (Segal et al., 2013, p. 273). In discussion of the poem, many participants wonder that Rumi is ascribing divine purpose to emotional travail. Others emphasize the guiding aspect of emotional experience (i.e., what we can learn from our feelings), a key component of what has recently been labeled "emotional intelligence" (Salovey, Detweiler-Bedell, Detweiler-Bedell, & Mayer, 2008). Still others consider the possibility of transformation that could result from adopting an accepting stance toward such experiences. On several occasions, participants have identified the kindness for aversive emotions that Rumi espouses with Christ's nonjudgmental stance toward those perceived as enemies or outcasts.

Following these discussions, loving-kindness practice is introduced (Shapiro & Carlson, 2009). The term "loving-kindness" used in CFT (Gilbert, 2009) and mindfulness-based interventions is a translation of a Pali word, *metta* (Germer, 2009). The practice of loving-kindness can take numerous forms, including forms that resemble petitionary prayer. Germer, for example, notes that the practice of *metta* could be considered a form of "secular prayer" designed to "cultivate unconditional love" (p. 154). In this practice, participants are invited to call to mind a person or being who evokes feelings of joy and caring. If a person is difficult to identify, a beloved pet may fill the bill. Although participants are not explicitly discouraged from using images of God or other figures of religious devotion in this exercise (e.g., saints), the instructions suggest a friend or loved one. The important aspect of the practice is that the mental image of the figure gives rise to spontaneous feelings of affection.

Next, participants are invited to hold this image in mind while saying silently, "May you be safe and protected. May you be healthy and strong. May you have joy.

May you live with ease." Instruction guides the participants to observe bodily sensations, thoughts, and emotions arising in response to the image and phrases. Following
this practice, participants are asked to bring an image of themselves, as they are at
the present moment, into the mind's eye and repeat the phrases once again, this time
using the first person: "May I be safe and protected. May I be healthy and strong.
May I have joy. May I live with ease." Again the practice is repeated slowly, with
emphasis on observing changes in inner experience. A third iteration invites participants to envision a person with whom they have experienced interpersonal difficulty. It can be useful for participants to identify a person for whom they nonetheless
have some caring feelings, perhaps a parishioner or someone to whom they minister, who has been a source of stress or challenge. The phrases of loving-kindness are
repeated again with the intention of cultivating compassion for this individual.
Participants are encouraged to notice subtle changes in their emotional experience,
including shifts in body sensations (e.g., changes in muscle tension), as well as
thoughts that arise in response to this practice. Finally, instructors may add a fourth
segment, in which participants envision a larger collective (e.g., the whole church;
all beings).

Homework following session seven includes daily loving-kindness practice. A
log sheet is provided to track completion and list those for whom they cultivated
loving-kindness (i.e., loved one, self, a difficult other, all beings, or a collective
group).

The eighth and final meeting focuses on taking committed action in accordance
with one's values (Hayes et al., 2012). The curriculum emphasizes that committed
action includes self-care practices (see Table 22.2) that support sustained engagement in values-consistent activities. Participants are invited to discuss ways they
plan to make aspects of the course part of their daily lives and to share their views
regarding whether the practices could prove useful in sustaining their commitments
to ministry or religious vocation. Obstacles participants have encountered in their
religious lives are discussed, along with the body sensations, thoughts, and emotions associated with those obstacles. Strategies for responding to these dimensions
of inner experience are explored, including observation, description, and nonjudgmental acceptance (allowing and turning toward). The acceptance-based metaphors (e.g., quicksand) are reviewed. More importantly, however, the experience of
obstacles is connected to values, as participants are encouraged to notice ways that

Table 22.2 Self-care strategies for clergy and religious	• Mindfulness- and compassion-focused meditations daily
	• Balancing time and commitments to self and others
	• Establishing boundaries in relationships
	• Retreats
	• Support within the clergy community
	• Psychotherapy to address ongoing or persistent distress

challenges arise as they commit themselves to engage fully in values-consistent activities. The relationship between committed participation in religious life and the experience of vulnerability (e.g., fear of rejection, feelings of inadequacy, social disapproval) is acknowledged. In discussion, participants consider whether they might be willing to accept and allow aversive inner experiences in the service of moving in valued directions. Awareness of willingness and the relationship between values and willingness are explored. In this session, the theme of "courage" is introduced, including Ambrose Redmoon's (1991) definition of this term: "Courage is not the absence of fear but the judgment that something else is more important than fear." Discussion highlights ways that participants are exercising courage each time they choose to pursue their values. One example of such courage would be taking the chance that demonstrating care (perhaps by listening to another's suffering or hardship) will make a difference, while simultaneously facing the risk that it may not.

Finally, as a concluding practice, participants engage in an exercise that explores the ACT process of self as context (Hayes et al., 2012), emphasizing flexible, adaptive perspective-taking. In this exercise, entitled "Hello, Old Friend" (see Part IV, Chapter 23, K for sample script), participants are invited to stand side-by-side in pairs. The instructor guides participants as they consider the many challenges and turning points that the person standing next to them has faced on his or her journey. Specific themes relating to vitality and engagement in religious life, as well as sources of vulnerability, may be incorporated. This practice serves as the conclusion of the program as a whole. Participants are invited to make their own choice whether they wish to stay a few moments and talk with one another or whether they wish to depart.

Themes and Challenges Specific to Clergy and Religious

One theme that frequently arises is the relation between mindfulness and devotional or contemplative prayer. Many participants describe an active prayer life and report that they often engage in silent, seated prayer. The similarity between the postures adopted in mindfulness practice and prayer may lead participants to shift quickly into other forms of practice. Often, when asked for comment on their experience during the mindfulness practice, the participants will volunteer information concerning images of God or other figures of devotion. In addition, they may describe use of a sacred word or phrase during contemplation, a practice associated with centering prayer (Keating, 2009), or describe a sense of God's presence.

Instructors are faced with a choice when responding to these comments. One option is to demarcate mindfulness as a secular practice, one that facilitates physical and psychological well-being, but distinct from spiritual contemplation. While this approach has the advantage of minimizing participants' tendency, particularly early in the program, to story their experiences in religious or dogmatic terms (e.g., "silence reminds me how thankful we should all be that God is with us today"), it can be difficult to sustain such a distinction. As the course progresses, participants almost invariably discover points of contact between mindfulness practices and their own spiritual traditions, including aspects of mindfulness, acceptance, and compassion informing their own faith traditions. Demarcating too starkly the distinction between a spiritual practice that a participant describes and a given mindfulness practice could be perceived as privileging one mode of practice over another and could suggest that the participant has "done it wrong" or has invalidated the participant's contribution. An alternative that offers potentially greater flexibility is to confine inquiry to the bodily sensations, thoughts, and emotions that arose in the practice without explicitly addressing the relationship between spiritual practice and mindfulness. A potential consequence of this choice, of course, is that members of the group could perceive the lack of inquiry regarding explicitly shared religious themes as a derogation of their own spiritual practices.

Another option is to create opportunities to consider similarities and differences between spiritual practices and mindfulness. Asking participants how they respond in prayer, if they notice the mind has wandered, can be a useful avenue for exploration. The nonjudgmental and non-goal-directed perspective of mindfulness can be emphasized, along with the possibility of praying mindfully. When working with Christian communities, a useful quotation when employing this approach can be Christ's comment in the Sermon on the Mount, "Learn from the way the wild flowers grow. They do not work or spin." (Matthew 6:28, *New American Bible, Revised Edition*), which highlights allowing and accepting experience, as well as non-driven ways of being. Indeed, a daily practice of "listening" in silence without goal or purpose is a mainstay in many religious traditions. Writing of the contemplative Thomas Merton, Matthews (2002) notes that "listening to silence" can help "rescue our everyday social relations from further suffering in a fractured culture" (p. 62). Listening in silence with attention, acceptance, and compassion may bring participants into contact with the pain and suffering they have witnessed, as well as with the deep joy they carry. That said, drawing strong parallels between spiritual practices and mindfulness practices used in the curriculum also has pitfalls. It could reinforce continued adherence to a devotional practice that differs significantly from mindfulness practice, particularly from the embodied practices. Facing these parallels at least to some degree, however, is helpful in making explicit the ways that participants are holding their feelings regarding mindfulness practice.

When exploring the values and compassion practices in this program, questions regarding one's relationship with God are likely to arise. It will be helpful for teachers to recall that for many clergy and religious, God *is* the significant other in their lives (Miner, Dowson, & Malone, 2013)—at once a source of love, meaning, and acceptance that is both personal and transcendent. Development of mindfulness and acceptance practices begins at the personal level, holding one's own experience without judgment. For those who focus their lives on devotion to God, such a self-focused practice may feel awkward or unfamiliar. It may be useful for participants to consider ways they have experienced God's presence through daily life and the world around them. Ignatian (from Saint Ignatius de Loyola, founder of the Jesuit order) spiritual exercises in the Roman Catholic tradition, for example, emphasize "finding God in all things" (Martin, 2010). Practitioners in the Ignatian tradition consider all of life worthy of attention, including both wanted and unwanted aspects of experience. Many religious traditions feature similar contemplative practices. Finding God in all things may offer a way of developing curiosity about experience, as well as profound appreciation for what it is, while also acknowledging the most deeply held value of devotional life.

Another theme that can arise in mindfulness groups with clergy and religious is one of "numbness," loss of feeling, or disconnection. It is useful to explore absence of sensation or emotion in the same open, accepting manner as the presence of feelings or body sensations. It is also important to consider the possibility that these experiences, while disconcerting, are common among those reporting burnout, trauma-related distress, and compassion fatigue. Clergy and religious may encounter numerous suffering individuals who relate their experiences of traumatic events in hopes of obtaining spiritual solace. Participants may have felt powerless to respond adequately to the severity of suffering they have heard or witnessed, leading to the sense that the distress they have encountered surpasses their resilience or capacity for restoration (Coetzee & Klopper, 2010).

Training in mindfulness- and acceptance-based strategies for responding to inner experience offers a potential means of promoting greater resilience in response to suffering. Evoking the pillars of mindfulness (Kabat-Zinn, 1990), emphasizing non-judgment, patience, acceptance, and non-striving, can be particularly useful when themes of emotional numbing and disconnection arise, allowing the development of practice to facilitate contact with inner experience rather than pressing for a specific insight or change. This theme of inner transformation through kindness toward suffering, even when the suffering is one's own, is consistent with both mindfulness practice and the practice of forgiveness common to many faiths. Mindfulness practice, with its emphasis upon patient, nonjudgmental acceptance of lived experience, can become a sustaining means of renewal and reconnection with feeling, helping maintain a life of caring engagement and spiritual fulfillment.

An Individual Case Study of Mindfulness-Based Therapy

The following narrative from an individual treatment case provides an example of the way a mindfulness- and compassion-focused approach to vocational stress could assist a member of a religious order.

"Sister Katherine" was the principal at a parochial grade school for a large urban Roman Catholic parish. The majority of the students in her school were not of her faith; most came from single-parent African-American families and reported no faith affiliation. Katherine was referred, by her superior, to psychotherapy for symptoms of depression related to impending closure of her school. Her presenting problems included difficulty sleeping, weight gain of 20 lb in the past year, and difficulty making decisions. Although not suicidal, she reported experiencing "a crisis of faith" and thoughts of leaving her vocation.

For the past 12 years, Katherine had provided a nurturing haven for many children and families in her community. In this work she seemed to thrive and shine. Now, facing an uncertain vocational future, she was feeling alone and abandoned. Exploration of compassion fatigue with Katherine seemed to elicit the central issues contributing to her distress. She was exhausted and overwhelmed. Coming to terms with her *present* sense of loss and the implication of the school's closing was the initial focus of therapy.

The use of mindfulness practices with a compassion focus assisted Sr. Katherine in remaining present with her experience of sadness and feelings of loneliness. Specific interventions included distress tolerance skills of dialectical behavioral therapy (DBT; Linehan, 1993), which are rooted in mindfulness meditation. These skills gave Sr. Katherine tangible tools to face her emotions without feeling "drowned" in them. Being with her distress, she was able to experience acceptance of her own emotional processes and also to experience the therapist's acceptance of her and her emotional experience. Exploring distress and vulnerability within the context of the therapeutic relationship conveyed respect for her experience of suffering and helped her experience emotions without judging herself harshly.

Once trust in the therapeutic relationship was established, Sr. Katherine's fears of abandonment could be addressed. For example, she reported a recurring fear that she could no longer find a sense of meaning in her life. Not knowing what would happen next, uncertainty fueled her anxiety. Fears associated with "not knowing" included her next assignment and worry that she would not feel connected to God in the way she "used to be." Rumination entangled her mind, body, and spirit. Mindfulness practice allowed for pausing, observing, and feeling where fear was manifesting in her bodily sensation. Inquiry in session allowed her recognition about the quality of fear, which shifted to anger, disappointment, or hopelessness and even curiosity.

As therapy progressed, inquiry continued to assist Sr. Katherine in identifying what might be within, facilitating self-exploration with therapist as a guide. Her moment-to-moment observation of experience allowed Katherine to encounter her feeling states with greater acceptance. As she practiced staying in the moment, the distress associated with not knowing whether she could regain her previous sense of faith, meaning, and self-worth gave way to a different perspective and an ability to view her distress as background as she looked to possible opportunities. This change in perspective represented a liberation from overwhelming fears of abandonment and opened the way for a new sense of connection with her life. Mindfulness practice provided the path to acceptance in an active sense.

The letting go process was the final phase of therapy, where the dialectical aspects of the therapeutic process proved most poignant. Holding on to a position as school principal had in many ways served as a shield for Sr. Katherine, protecting her from encountering her own detachment from herself. It had been easy for her to assume the principal role; it offered a structured identity, and the role became who she was. What she gained through mindfulness based and CFT was a sense of kindness toward many parts of her experience she had never acknowledged. New awareness of experience gave rise to acceptance, and viewing life nonjudgmentally and with curiosity proved liberating. At present, Sr. Katherine is studying to be a spiritual director. "You never know; you just never know" were her parting words to her therapist, spoken with a sense of openness to possibility.

The process of mindfulness-based and CFT begins with the self and ripples outward to assist in restoring resilience. This approach enables the therapist and the client to enter into a reflective dialogue using the attitudes of mindfulness to bring forth compassion in the therapeutic relationship, which at its conclusion enables compassion for self and others. The ongoing practice of compassion rooted in mindfulness practice may even foster a growth in spirituality (Greeson et al., 2011).

References

Coetzee, S., & Klopper, H. (2010). Compassion fatigue within nursing practice: A concept analysis. *Nursing and Health Sciences, 12*, 235–243.

Cohen-Katz, J., Wiley, S., Capuano, T., Baker, D. M., Deitrick, L., & Shapiro, S. (2005). The effects of mindfulness-based stress reduction on nurse stress and burnout: A qualitative and quantitative study, part III. *Holistic Nursing Practice, 19*, 78–86.

D'Avila-Latourrette, V.-A. (2012). *A rhythm of life: The monastic way.* Liguori, MO: Liguori.

Dahl, J., & Lundgren, T. (2006). *Living beyond your pain: Using acceptance and commitment therapy to ease chronic pain.* Oakland, CA: New Harbinger.

Dahl, J., Lundgren, T., Plumb, J., & Stewart, I. (2009). *The art and science of valuing in psychotherapy: Helping clients discover, explore, and commit to valued action using acceptance and commitment therapy.* Oakland, CA: New Harbinger.

Dahl, J., Wilson, K. G., Luciano, C., & Hayes, S. C. (2005). *Acceptance and commitment therapy for chronic pain.* Oakland, CA: New Harbinger.

Faucett, J. M., Corwyn, R. F., & Poling, T. H. (2013). Clergy role stress: Interactive effects of role ambiguity and role conflict on intrinsic job satisfaction. *Pastoral Psychology, 62*, 291–304.

Figley, C. R. (1995). *Compassion fatigue: Coping with secondary traumatic stress disorder in those who treat the traumatized.* New York, NY: Brunner/Routledge.

Flanagan, K. (1985). Liturgy, ambiguity and silence: The ritual management of real absence. *British Journal of Sociology, 35*, 193–223.

Francis, L. J., Hills, P., & Rutledge, C. F. (2008). Clergy work-related satisfactions in parochial ministry: The influence of personality and churchmanship. *Mental Health, Religion & Culture, 11*, 327–339.

Francis, L. J., Louden, S. H., & Rutledge, C. F. (2004). Burnout among Roman Catholic parochial clergy in England and Wales: Myth or reality? *Review of Religious Research, 46*, 5–19.

Galton, F. (1872). Statistical inquiries into the efficacy of prayer. *Fortnightly Review, 12*, 125–135.

Geary, C., & Rosenthal, S. L. (2011). Sustained impact of MBSR on stress, well-being, and daily spiritual experiences for 1 year in academic health care employees. *The Journal of Alternative and Complementary Medicine, 17*, 939–944.

Germer, C. K. (2009). *The mindful path to self-compassion: Freeing yourself from destructive thoughts and emotions.* New York, NY: Guilford.

Gilbert, P. (2009). *The compassionate mind: A new approach to life's challenges.* Oakland, CA: New Harbinger.

Goodman, M. J., & Schorling, J. B. (2012). A mindfulness course decreases burnout and improves well-being among health care providers. *International Journal of Psychiatry in Medicine, 43*, 119–128.

Greeson, J., Webber, D., Smoski, M., Brantley, J., Ekblad, A., Suarez, E., & Wolever, R. (2011). Changes in spirituality partly explain health-related quality of life outcomes after mindfulness–based stress reduction. *Journal of Behavioral Medicine, 34*, 508–518.

Hamman, J. J. (2014). *Becoming a pastor: Forming self and soul for ministry.* Cleveland, OH: Pilgrim Press.

Hayes, S. C., Strosahl, K. D., & Wilson, K. G. (2012). *Acceptance and commitment therapy: The process and practice of mindful change.* New York, NY: Guilford.

Hendrickson, K. L., & Rasmussen, E. B. (2013). Effects of mindful eating training on delay and probability discounting for food and money in obese and healthy-weight individuals. *Behaviour Research and Therapy, 51*, 399–409.

Hong, P. Y., Lishner, D. A., & Han, K. H. (2014). Mindfulness and eating: An experiment examining the effect of mindful raisin eating on the enjoyment of sampled food. *Mindfulness, 5*, 80–87.

Hong, P. Y., Lishner, D. A., Han, K. H., & Huss, E. A. (2011). The positive impact of mindful eating on expectations of food liking. *Mindfulness, 2*, 103–113.

Kabat-Zinn, J. (1990). *Full catastrophe living: Using the wisdom of your body and mind to face stress, pain, and illness.* New York, NY: Dell.

Kabat-Zinn, J. (2005). *Coming to our senses: Healing ourselves and the world through mindfulness.* New York, NY: Hyperion.

Kaldor, P., & Bullpitt, R. (2001). *Burnout in church leaders.* Adelaide, S.A.: Openbook.

Karasek, R. A. (1998). Demand/control model: A social, emotional, and physiological approach to stress risk and active behaviour development. In J. M. Stellman (Ed.), *Encyclopaedia of occupational health and safety* (pp. 34.6–34.14). Geneva, Switzerland: ILO.

Keating, T. (2009). *Intimacy with god: An introduction to centering prayer* (3rd ed.). New York, NY: Crossroad.

Koller, M., Blanchfield, K., Vavra, T., Andrusyk, J., & Altier, M. (2012). Assessing and meeting the health needs of Roman Catholic priests in the archdiocese of Chicago. *Journal of Prevention & Intervention in the Community, 40*, 219–232.

Kristeller, J., Wolever, R. Q., & Sheets, V. (2014). Mindfulness-based eating awareness training (MB-EAT) for binge eating: A randomized clinical trial. *Mindfulness, 5*, 282–297.

Lederach, J. P. (2003). *The little book of conflict transformation.* Intercourse, PA: Good Books.

Linehan, M. (1993). *Cognitive-behavioral treatment of borderline personality disorder.* New York, NY: Guilford.

Lundgren, T., Luoma, J. B., Dahl, J., Strosahl, K., & Melin, L. (2012). The Bull's-Eye Values Survey: A psychometric evaluation. *Cognitive and Behavioral Practice, 19*, 518–526.

Martin, J. (2010). *The Jesuit guide to (almost) everything: A spirituality for real life.* New York, NY: Harper Collins.

Maslach, C. (1978). Job burn-out: How people cope. *Public Welfare, 36*, 56–58.

Matthews, G. (2002). The healing silence: Thomas Merton's contemplative approach to communication. In *Merton Annual: Studies in Culture, Spirituality and Social Concerns* (pp. 1561–1576).

Miner, M., Dowson, M., & Malone, K. (2013). Spiritual satisfaction of basic psychological needs and psychological health. *Journal of Psychology and Theology, 41*, 298–314.

Mirdal, G. M. (2012). Mevlana Jalāl-ad-Dīn Rumi and mindfulness. *Journal of Religion and Health, 51*, 1202–1215.

Neff, K. (2003). Self-compassion: An alternative conceptualization of a healthy attitude towards oneself. *Self and Identity, 2*, 85–102.

Nelson, J. B. (1978). *Embodiment: An approach to sexuality and Christian theology.* Minneapolis, MN: Augsburg.

Proeschold-Bell, R., & LeGrand, S. H. (2010). High rates of obesity and chronic disease among United Methodist clergy. *Obesity, 18*, 1867–1870.

Proeschold-Bell, R., Miles, A., Toth, M., Adams, C., Smith, B. W., & Toole, D. (2013). Using effort-reward imbalance theory to understand high rates of depression and anxiety among clergy. *The Journal of Primary Prevention, 34*, 439–453.

Raj, A., & Dean, K. E. (2005). Burnout and depression among Catholic priests in India. *Pastoral Psychology, 54*, 157–171.

Rayburn, C. A., Richmond, L. J., & Rogers, L. (1986). Men, women, and religion: Stress within leadership roles. *Journal of Clinical Psychology, 42*, 540–546.

Redmoon, A. H. (1991). No peaceful warriors! *Gnosis, 21*, 40–46.

Rosenzweig, S., Reibel, D. K., Greeson, J. M., Brainard, G. C., & Hojat, M. (2003). Mindfulness-based stress reduction lowers psychological distress in medical students. *Teaching and Learning in Medicine, 15*, 88–92.

Rossetti, S. J., & Rhoades, C. J. (2013). Burnout in Catholic clergy: A predictive model using psychological and spiritual variables. *Psychology of Religion and Spirituality, 5*, 335–341.

Salovey, P., Detweiler-Bedell, B. T., Detweiler-Bedell, J. B., & Mayer, J. D. (2008). Emotional intelligence. In M. Lewis, J. M. Haviland-Jones, & L. Barrett (Eds.), *Handbook of emotions* (3rd ed., pp. 533–547). New York, NY: Guilford.

Segal, Z. V., Williams, J. M. G., & Teasdale, J. D. (2013). *Mindfulness-based cognitive therapy for depression*. New York, NY: Guilford.

Shafir, R. Z. (2003). *The Zen of listening: Mindful communication in the age of distraction* (2nd ed.). Wheaton, IL: Quest Books.

Shapiro, S., Austin, J., Bishop, S., & Cordova, M. (2005). Mindfulness-based stress reduction for health care professionals: Results from a randomized trial. *International Journal of Stress Management, 12*, 164–176.

Shapiro, S., Brown, K., & Biegel, G. (2007). Teaching self-care to caregivers: Effects of mindfulness-based stress reduction on the mental health of therapists in training. *Training and Education in Professional Psychology, 1*, 105–115.

Shapiro, S. L., & Carlson, L. E. (2009). Mindfulness and self-care for clinicians. In S. L. Shapiro & L. E. Carlson (Eds.), *The art and science of mindfulness: Integrating mindfulness into psychology and the helping professions* (pp. 107–117). Washington, DC: American Psychological Association.

Shapiro, S. L., Schwartz, G. E., & Bonner, G. (1998). Effects of mindfulness-based stress reduction on medical and premedical students. *Journal of Behavioral Medicine, 21*, 581–599.

Sheen, F. J. (1963). *The priest is not his own*. New York, NY: McGraw-Hill.

Stoddard, J. A., & Afari, N. (2014). *The big book of ACT metaphors: A practitioner's guide to experiential exercises and metaphors in acceptance and commitment therapy*. Oakland, CA: New Harbinger.

Symington, S. H., & Symington, M. F. (2012). A Christian model of mindfulness: Using mindfulness principles to support psychological well-being, value-based behavior, and the Christian spiritual journey. *Journal of Psychology & Christianity, 31*, 71–77.

Szuchewycz, B. (1997). Silence in ritual communication. In A. Jaworski (Ed.), *Silence: Interdisciplinary perspectives* (pp. 239–260). The Hague, Netherlands: Mouton de Gruyter.

Turton, D., & Francis, L. (2007). The relationship between attitude toward prayer and professional burnout among Anglican parochial clergy in England: Are praying clergy healthier clergy? *Mental Health, Religion & Culture, 10*, 61–74.

Unruh, H. R., & Sider, R. J. (2005). *Saving souls, serving society: Understanding the faith factor in church-based social ministry*. New York, NY: Oxford University Press.

Wang, P. S., Berglund, P. A., & Kessler, R. C. (2003). Patterns and correlates of contacting clergy for mental disorders in the United States. *Health Services Research, 38*, 647–673.

Wegner, D. M. (1989). *White bears and other unwanted thoughts*. New York, NY: Viking Penguin.

Wells, C. R., Probst, J., McKeown, R., Mitchem, S., & Whiejong, H. (2012). The relationship between work-related stress and boundary-related stress within the clerical profession. *Journal of Religion and Health, 51*, 215–230.

Wilson, K. G., Sandoz, E. K., Kitchens, J., & Roberts, M. (2010). The Valued Living Questionnaire: Defining and measuring valued action within a behavioral framework. *The Psychological Record, 60*, 249–272.

Part IV
Scripts and Practices

Chapter 23
Practices for the Classroom

A. Exploring Community

Donald McCown

This practice can be used to bring participants' attention to the sense of connection that is created within the group as the course progresses. Class 6 of MBSR is an appropriate moment for it, as the interrelationships of the class have been developing and the curriculum is focused for the session on interpersonal communication.

The practice begins as a sitting meditation, which the class has been working with for a number of weeks. The participants need to be sitting in a circle, or some approximation of one, which allows everyone to see the others in the class.

Guidance for the first 10–20 minutes is perhaps slightly more focused on noticing body sensations and possibilities of coming towards resting in posture and breathing. By reading the group, the teacher will recognize the optimal time for beginning the exploration. It might be spoken this way:

When you are ready, bringing your attention into your body, and your sense of the room. Is it possible… with your eyes closed or while still looking down… to sense the others who are near you? (Long pause.) Aware of the quality or qualities of the atmosphere… (Pause.) Maybe there is a word for what you find… maybe not… We're just exploring… there is no particular answer to find… Staying as much as possible in touch with the breath and the body… (Long pause.) Maybe you have a word or so… See if you can just put it away for now… If there's not a word, there's not a problem; sometimes we know things without words…

Now, tilting your head down, so that your eyes would be—or maybe are—looking down at the floor in the center of the circle… Our practice is not ending, we are simply moving into another phase… (Long pause.) When the time is right, if your

© Springer International Publishing Switzerland 2016
D. McCown et al. (eds.), *Resources for Teaching Mindfulness*,
DOI 10.1007/978-3-319-30100-6_23

eyes are closed, you could open them… and allow the visual dimension to be part of your experience… Perhaps that adds to your sense of the class gathered here… (Pause.) How is it for you now? (Long pause.)

And, if it seems like something you'd like to do, raising your head, using your eyes, and seeing the class… looking around… perhaps acknowledging the others with you in this practice. How is this for you? What are you noticing, in your body, in your thinking, and in your emotions? The practice is not ending… so staying with your experience… (Long pause.)

So, perhaps you have a word or two that you would like to share with the class gathered here… Just speak out when you would like to… And the rest of us can take some time to take it in… let's leave a little quiet after each person speaks, to really hear what has been said…

The teacher allows this process to take its natural course. Not pressing participants to speak, and joining with the participants in receiving in silence whatever is said. When the time is ripe, the teacher may point the way back to silence before ending the practice:

Now, coming to quiet… you may choose to close your eyes or to rest your sight on the floor… and bringing more focus to the body and the breath… knowing that you are sitting… knowing that you are breathing… (Long pause.) (Ring bells or gently suggest opening the eyes and stretching.)

The teacher may choose to engage dialogue and further explore the discoveries the class made in the practice, or choose to bring the practice to a close and move on.

B.   Life Space: Demonstrating Passive, Aggressive, Assertive Dispositions

Florence Meleo-Meyer

This practice explores permission to establish healthy boundaries and identify times of withdrawing from or taking more than one's own space. This practice emerged from my working with adolescent youth who were in residential treatment. Most came from abusive homes, and had lost trust in safe relationships as their boundaries had been trespassed multiple ways in their young lives. This practice supports the sense of respect for one's innate wholeness. As a therapist, I would demonstrate an individual's right to have respectful boundaries by using a pink hula-hoop. For an MBSR class, a rope shaped into a circle in the middle of the room suffices. Once the teacher has placed the circle on the floor she stands in the middle of the circle:

o Suggesting this as a metaphor for the right to respect one's personal life space. Different cultures measure this physical space uniquely.
o Expressing the value that every human being deserves to have natural, equal rights honored.

o Describing the power of claiming one's birthright by honoring oneself. Self-respect and compassion support the cultivation of respectful relationships.

In the passive scenario, the teacher moves from standing in the middle of the circle to shrinking to a small portion of the rim, demonstrating a withdrawal from one's full measure, by saying, "I do not matter. You are more important than me." She describes the sense of lack and unworthiness, which causes a sense of separation—a sense of not being "enough."

In the aggressive scenario, the teacher strides across the circle boundary into the others' space, claiming the rights of the other as well as her own. "What is mine is mine and what is yours is mine!" "I matter more than you."

In the assertive scenario, returning to the center once more, the teacher confirms the possibility of maintaining self-respect as well as respecting others. "We both matter, and we both deserve respect."

At this point, if possible, the teacher asks participants to come to standing and assume a posture of assertiveness. The teacher invites them to strongly sense the stable support of the floor beneath them, the uprightness of their own bodies and the possibility of a relaxed confidence in which one can move consciously rather than reactively, in any situation. Kabir, a fifteenth century poet and sage, expressed claiming one's birthright with these words: "Just throw away all thoughts of imaginary things and stand firm in that which you are."

C. Interpersonal Communication Practice

Antonella Commellato and Fabio Giommi

In the sixth and seventh session of our MBSR course, we explore interpersonal relationships and difficult communication issues.

We tend to split the theme into two parts: in class 6, we devote time to entering in relation through the eyesight and through words.

First, we guide a silent individual reflection on the difficult communications calendar, asking people to contemplate one of the events they noticed during the week and then asking them to share the experience in groups of three. Then, we ask them to find a companion and to sit together facing each other with eyes closed and in a meditative posture.

We then offer a short individual guidance on awareness of the face as a preparation for the exercise that will follow:

> Feeling the sensitivity of your face ...feeling the 'mask' that is usually superimposed. forehead ....eyes ...nose ... cheeks ... lips .... everything becomes alive.
> Feeling the movements of the face, not holding to anything.
> Has your the face become a fixed pattern, or is it dynamic, moving?
> What sensations are there in the face when you are not pretending nor defending anything?

Letting release come naturally, ... putting down the mask ... letting go of the effort that tenses and contracts our features.
The form of the face is changing, moment by moment. Just feeling the face ... nothing to 'do'. Letting things just be. Feeling the weight, the density of the eyes ... the delicate pulsating in the eyes.
Cheeks ... tongue ... palate .... simultaneously the whole mouth.
The space in the cavity of the mouth ... letting this internal space enlarge ... the tongue is alive the tip, the back, the sides, the top and the bottom of the tongue.
The whole face is alive and vibrating ... feeling what is tense and what is released ... welcoming everything.

We then invite people to gently open their eyes and keep their gaze on their companion's eyes until we ring the bell, after 4 or 5 minutes. The simple fact of being in interaction with somebody else, with another face, can destabilize, throw off one's vision of the space. We often start thinking that we are in a face-to-face relation which weighs as a judgment. The look of someone else almost always traps us in our heads, behind a face mask. But after the guided practice, people enter the exercise with a naked face, mindful of it almost from the inside.

After the bell rings and people close their eyes again, we invite a few minutes of silence. Then, asking them to keep the same companion, we give instructions for a short interpersonal mindfulness dialogue. The structure is as follows:

Each companion takes a separate turn speaking, and has 5 to 6 minutes to reflect on a given theme of contemplation while the listener keeps silent and receives with full awareness the companion's words without answering back or commenting.

After the first 5 to 6 minutes we ring the bell and invite silence and closing of the eyes for a couple of minutes.

Then, the roles are reversed—the first speaker becomes the new listener and the first listener becomes the new speaker.

After both companions have had the opportunity to give voice to their reflections, we ring the bell again and invite the participants to go back to silence and close their eyes for a few minutes. The exercise ends with 5 more minutes of open shared dialogue (without taking turns) in which they give voice to what remains to be said.

Possible themes of contemplation:

What makes you feel most vulnerable when in relation with others?
What blocks you from having the relationship you truly want to have?
What makes you feel connected to the others?

In seventh session, we explore the role of the nonverbal and the body in communication using the Aikido inspired set of exercises introduced by Jon Kabat-Zinn (see Chap. 5 for a description). In Italy, there is no cultural resistance to entering into physical contact even among people that do not know each other well, as there is in the case of MBSR participants in North America. Our participants tend to enter the "game" playfully and with an attitude both approachable and curious. They do not feel threatened if physical boundaries are crossed or released; they tend to view the exercises as funny, challenging, surprising and, most often, insightful.

D. Teaching Stories and Loving Kindness Practice

Diane (Dina) Wyshogrod

Rabbi Akiva Taught: This, Too, Is for the Best

Rabbi Akiva used to teach: "This too is for the best." Once he was traveling with a donkey, a rooster, and a candle. As night approached, he tried to find lodging in a nearby village, only to be turned away. Although he was forced to spend the night in the field, he did not complain, saying instead, "This too is for the best."

During the night, a wind came and blew out his candle, a cat ate his rooster, and a lion attacked and ate his donkey. Each time, Rabbi Akiva's reaction was "This too is for the best."

Very late that night, a regiment came and took the entire town captive. Rabbi Akiva, sleeping in the field, went unnoticed and thus was spared. When Rabbi Akiva realized what had happened he said, "Didn't I tell you that everything that is for the best?" After all, had his candle been burning, making him visible in the dark, had his cat or donkey been alive to make noise, or even for that matter, had he been lodging in the village, the regiment would have noticed him and he would have been captured along with the others.

From the Babylonian Talmud, Tractate Beraḥot 60b

Good Luck, Bad Luck, Who Knows?

Once there was a farmer who used an old horse to till his fields. One day, the horse escaped into the hills. The farmer's neighbors sympathized with the old man over his bad luck. The farmer replied, "Bad luck? Good luck? Who knows?"

A week later, the horse returned with a herd of horses from the hills. This time, the neighbors congratulated the farmer on his good luck. His reply was, "Good luck? Bad luck? Who knows?"

The farmer's only son started taming one of the wild horses. The horse threw him, and he broke his leg. This time everyone was sure this was really bad luck. The farmer said, "Bad luck? Good luck? Who knows?"

A few weeks later, the army marched into the village and drafted every able-bodied youth they found. When they saw the farmer's son with his broken leg, they left him alone.

Good luck? Bad luck? Who knows?

Loving-Kindness Meditation

Begin by sending these wishes/intentions to yourself:

May I be safe and protected.
May I be happy.
May I be healthy.
May I treat myself kindly and compassionately.
May I be free from suffering.
May I be peaceful.

Now send these wishes/intentions to others:

1. *Someone dear/important to you (traditionally called "the beloved")*
2. *Someone neutral*
3. *Someone with whom you have some issue/difficulty (traditionally called "the enemy")*

May you be safe and protected.
May you be happy.
May you be healthy.
May you treat yourself kindly and compassionately.
May you be free from suffering.
May you be peaceful.

Now expand these wishes outward and send them to family… friends… community…. co-workers … all beings … the entire world.

May we all/may all beings be safe and protected.
May we all/may all beings be happy.
May we all/may all beings be healthy.
May we all/may all beings treat our/themselves kindly and compassionately.
May we all/may all beings be free from suffering.
May we all/may all beings be peaceful.

מדיטציית חמלה

בשלב ראשון, מכוונים את הכוונות/משאלות האלי לעצמנו:

מי ייתן ואהיה מוגן/ת ובטוח/ה
מי ייתן ואהיה מאושר/ת
מי ייתן ואהיה בריא/ה
מי ייתן ואתייחס לעצמי בעדינות ובחמלה
מי ייתן ולא אדע סבל
מי ייתן וכן אדע שלווה

בשלבים הבאים, מכוונים את הכוונות/משאלות האלי לאחרים:
(1) מישהו משמעותי, יקר ("האהוב")
(2) מישהו ניטרלי
(3) מישהו שיש לנו קושי אתו (לפעמים משתמשים בכינוי "האויב")

מי ייתן ותהיה/י מוגן/ת ובטוח/ה
מי ייתן ותהיה/י מאושר/ת
מי ייתן ותהיה/י בריא/ה
מי ייתן ותתייחס/י אל עצמך בעדינות ובחמלה
מי ייתן ולא תדע/י סבל
מי ייתן וכן תדע/י שלווה ושלום

בשלב האחרון, מרחיבים את המעגל לכלול קרובים, חברים, מטופלים, עמיתים,
בני עירך/קהילתך/ארצך, כל הבריות, כל העולם כולו...

מי ייתן ונהיה כולנו מוגנים/ות ובטוחים/ות
מי ייתן ונהיה כולנו מאושרים/ות
מי ייתן ונהיה כולנו בריאים/ות
מי ייתן ונתייחס אל עצמנו בעדינות ובחמלה
מי ייתן ולא נדע סבל
מי ייתן וכן נדע שלווה ושלום

E. Life Practice

Timothea Goddard

This exploration is offered in Week 7 of the MBSR curriculum as a way of focussing people's intention to care for their lives in an immediate and pragmatic way. The Life Practice they choose is then undertaken between Class 7 and Class 8.

Introduction (Spoken)

So, this project of developing mindfulness skills is not just about paying attention, on purpose, non-judgementally. It is really about our lives and opening up more possibilities and choices of acting skillfully to look after ourselves and others. We hope that all this paying attention develops the wisdom to be able to make good choices.

Contemplation (Spoken)

Closing your eyes … bringing attention to an area in your life that is emerging as something you would like to attend to more, take better care of, maybe awareness of some different kinds of actions that might be needed in certain areas …. relationships, loved ones, work, ways of listening and speaking, how we spend our time, care of the body, eating, exercise, work, maybe reflecting on whether your work is reflecting what you really want to be doing, the community more broadly, your contribution there, is there something that you care about that you would like more involvement in.

Dyad sharing: Participants come together in pairs to explore their reactions and responses.

Plenary group sharing: Participants may choose to offer one word about the area of life they want to explore and/or change.

Second Contemplation (Spoken)

Let's now explore what might be one action, one behavioral shift, in this area of life that you could undertake this week. It could be the smallest thing … maybe making a phone call to connect, or changing the way you respond to emails, making your lunch each day, or turning off your computer before dinner … What might it be like to take one small action to attend differently to what matters to you in this one "wild and precious life"?

Dyad sharing: Participants come together in pairs to explore their reactions and responses.

Plenary group sharing: Participants may choose to offer a one-word (or so) description of the action to be undertaken this week.

Reinforcing intentions: Invite participants to all stand up and walk around the group, finding at least two others to declare their intentions for their life practice this week.

F. The Stressed Body Drawing: Group Activity and Discussion

Beth Robins Roth

This highly participatory activity engages SRP participants' lived experiences of body sensation to introduce concepts of stress physiology in the first or second SRP session. The instructor draws two large side-by-side outlines of the human body that represent the front and back view of the same person (see Fig. 23.1a). Participants are asked to recall a recent stressful event, and then name aloud the physical sensations that were present during the stressful experience. I begin with an example. "If I get stuck in traffic driving to work and realize I will be late, physical changes happen almost immediately. I start to get a headache and my jaw feels tight." I draw with colorful markers each of these sensations within the outline of the face and head. As participants offer examples of sensations that they notice in their bodies during stressful experiences, I add these sensations to the drawing. When both views of the body are largely filled in, the instructor names all the physical sensations that are now on the drawing (see Fig. 23.1b).

The completed drawing is used to facilitate an inquiry of pivotal concepts underlying the mindfulness program. The instructor points to the completed drawing:

Instructor: *What do you think of this person?*

Participant 1: *What a mess!*

Participant 2: *Looks too familiar!*

Instructor: *Yes, you've done a great job naming the body sensations that occur when stressed. Now my job is to connect this drawing to the fundamental principles of the SRP. I'm going to ask a series of questions. You all know the answers. First, how do so many physical changes happen so fast during a stressful experience?*

There is silence in the room.

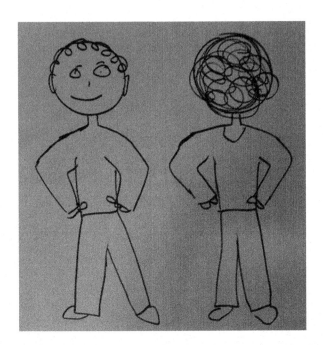

Fig. 23.1a

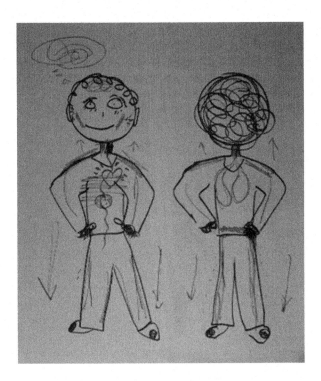

Fig. 23.1b

Instructor: This is not a trick question. Let's go back to my example. I'm driving to work on the highway, and traffic grinds to a halt. I'll be late to work. Suddenly, I'm getting a headache, my jaw is clenched, my shoulders are tight and elevated, my knuckles are purple from gripping the steering wheel, and I'm mildly nauseous. How did all this happen? Did an army of miniature people enter my car and start squeezing and pounding on my body?

Participant 1: Your mind. It's because of your mind.

Instructor: Thank-you! My mind perceived that I'd be late for work, and my brain immediately sent messages to my body that caused all these sensations to occur. Would you say then, that there is a strong relationship or a weak relationship between the mind and the body?

Participants: A very strong relationship!

Instructor: Absolutely, a very strong relationship. And would you say that the mind is powerful or weak?

Participants: Very powerful!

Instructor: The mind is very powerful. And is the mind promoting or harming our health by triggering this cascade of physical changes?

Participants: It's harming us.

Instructor: Exactly. This stress reaction is hard wired into us. It's part of our evolutionary heritage. It's what we call the Fight or Flight Response. It's designed to protect us in a dangerous situation. As someone mentioned when we were making the drawing, while the body is experiencing this flood of physical sensations, the mind can feel blank, or confused, or even far away. Animals living in the wild need to protect themselves from predators by mobilizing their entire system to fight back or run away. And that's why our minds can't think clearly when we are stressed. Our thinking mind would get in the way and slow down the instinctual reaction.

Participant 3: So that's why I can't think straight when I'm upset or stressed! I thought something was wrong with me.

Instructor: There's nothing wrong with you. It's your physiology, and your system is functioning perfectly…. So, to review, we see that our body experiences many changes in physical sensations during stressful moments. There is a strong relationship between the mind and the body. The mind is very powerful. And the mind is functioning in ways that are harmful to our overall health. Up to this point I've been talking about the mind–body relationship as if it is the mind that influences the body. But really it's a two-way street. The body also influences the mind. Let's go back to my example of being stuck in the traffic jam. I'm not aware of the physical changes while they are occurring. But soon I feel that I'm getting a headache, my jaw is tense, I'm holding my breath, my hands are gripping the steering wheel, and I have an upset stomach.

Instructor stands up and demonstrates gripping an imaginary steering wheel, shoulders elevated, jaw tight—as many points as possible.

Instructor: As soon as I become aware of all this, I know it doesn't feel good. So I say to my mind, "Oh come on, it's just a traffic jam. It's not the end of the world. Just relax." And does my mind obey?

Participants: No.

Instructor: No, it doesn't. Not because it doesn't want to, but because it doesn't know how. So I bypass the mind. I bring my attention to the body. In just a few seconds, I take a deep breath, resume regular breathing, open my mouth wide and close my mouth loosely. I take my right hand off the steering wheel and gently stretch the arm and hand, and place my softened fingers back on the steering wheel. What do you notice right now that's changed?

Participant 1: Your breathing is more normal.

Participant 2: Your face is relaxed.

Participant 3: Your shoulders have dropped and your arms are soft.

Instructor: And what has happened to my mind? I know you can't see my mind, but you all know what just happened.

Participant 4: Your mind has calmed down.

Participant 5: You're not as stressed.

Instructor: Exactly! My mind probably isn't 100% calm, but it's a lot calmer than it was. In just a few seconds, I softened or released a few tight places in my body. It's not possible to have a tight, tense body and a peaceful, calm mind. Or an upset mind and a comfortable relaxed body. And this is what I mean by "the mind–body relationship is a two-way street." The mind influences the body and the body influences the mind. In the SRP, we are retraining our minds and our bodies, using our intelligence to promote our health and well-being.

You can see that the role of physical sensation is really important. We will be training our attention to notice the body constantly, to learn what sensations are triggered by stress, and to feel the changes much sooner, when they are still small. Then we can intervene, breathe instead of holding the breath, open the jaw instead of clenching it, and soften muscles that have tightened. We learn what sensations accompany relaxation.

Instructor points to the squiggly line that represents confused thinking in the Stressed Body Drawing:

Instructor: We want to use conscious awareness and the rational mind to intervene right in the middle of stressful experiences. We want conscious choice about what to do or say next, before the stress reaction has really set in and we're on automatic pilot without access to our intelligence.

The completed drawing is used throughout the SRP to review, elaborate, and introduce new didactic information. I use it to explain stress physiology, the autonomic nervous system, the physiologic differences between stress and trauma, and the importance of the vagus nerve and the social engagement system. I also refer to it when we make lists of sensation vocabulary, and when each new mindfulness meditation practice is introduced. Some SRP groups give a name to the Stressed Body, and refer to it by name. Many SRP participants say that this powerful visual comes to mind during daily life, reminding them that automatic reactions can be replaced by consciously chosen responses.

G. Meditation on the Soles of the Feet

Nirbhay N. Singh and Monica Moore Jackman

Meditation on the Soles of the Feet (SoF) enables you to respond calmly during emotionally arousing situations, without resorting to verbal or physical aggression. It works well in situations that typically result in fight, flight, or freeze responses. This practice can be used as an antidote to internalized (e.g., worry, anxiety) and externalized (e.g., aggression) behaviors. The example below provides instructions for using the practice with an internalized behavior (i.e., anger) that often leads to an externalized behavior (i.e., aggression).

Rationale: When an incident occurs or a situation arises that typically makes you angry and you feel like either verbally threatening or hitting someone, it is important to let go of these feelings. *Meditation on the Soles of the Feet* is a simple way of moving your attention away from the emotionally arousing thoughts and feelings to a neutral place, the soles of your feet.

Initial Training in Soles of the Feet

1. Stand or sit in a comfortable position.
2. Rest the soles of your feet on the floor.
3. Close your eyes and focus your attention on your breath.
4. Breathe normally for a minute or two.
5. Now, think of a situation when you were angry, verbally aggressive, or physically aggressive.
6. Visualize the situation in your mind. Attend to the anger, verbal aggression, or physical aggression.
7. Now, refocus all your attention on the soles of your feet.
8. Move your toes, feel your shoes covering your feet, feel the texture of your socks or hose, the curve of your arch, and the heels of your feet against the back of your shoes. If you do not have shoes on, feel the floor or carpet with the soles of your feet.
9. When your attention is totally on the soles of your feet, gently open your eyes.
10. Practice this procedure until you are able to automatically focus your attention on the soles of your feet whenever you face an emotionally arousing situation, such as anger, aggression, anxiety, or worry.

Using the Skill

1. In daily life, situations will arise that may lead to anger, aggression, anxiety, or worry.
2. Try to recognize the first signs of arising anger, aggression, anxiety, or worry.
3. As soon as you are aware of arising anger, aggression, anxiety, or worry, focus your attention on the soles of your feet. Let your attention rest totally on the soles of your feet.
4. Move your toes, feel your shoes covering your feet, feel the texture of your socks or hose, the curve of your arch (in-step), and the heels of your feet against the back of your shoes. If you do not have shoes on, feel the floor or carpet with the soles of your feet.
5. If thoughts intrude, let them pass like clouds in the sky, without interaction.
6. Keep breathing naturally and focus all your attention on the soles of your feet.
7. When your attention is totally on the soles of your feet, you will realize that all feelings of anger, aggression, anxiety, or worry have disappeared.
8. When this realization arises, turn your attention to your daily activities.

Some Considerations When Using this Skill for Anger

1. Angry thoughts occur to all of us, but not all of us act on all of them. Also, anger can be justifiable and necessary depending on the context. So, we do not want to eliminate anger entirely.
2. Anger is strength because it provides us with information about the situation we are in, and alerts us to do something to change the situation.
3. Do not actively stop angry thoughts. They will stop naturally when the focus of your attention shifts fully to the soles of your feet.
4. Remember to breathe naturally. It is not necessary to take deep breaths.
5. This type of meditation can be done in any physical position.

H.   Self-Monitoring of Physical Pain

Lone Overby Fjorback and Else-Marie D. Elmholdt Jegindø

We introduce the practice of symptom monitoring in the MBSR program. If there are specific issues participants want to work with, for example, symptoms of pain, anxiety, or stress, they can note the symptoms down when they occur and rate their severity on the Symptom Monitoring Form (see below). While we do not review the form in class, for some patients it is a useful tool to become more familiar with their symptoms.

On the Symptom-Monitoring form, each day of the week is divided into four periods: morning, afternoon, evening, and night. Participants write down what they did and then rate the severity of symptoms on a scale of 0–10 (0 = no pain and 10 = worst pain).

For example: Monday morning: Work busy, already headache 5. Afternoon: Slept all afternoon, headache 3. Evening: Really quiet, relaxed at home, headache 1. Night: Sleep, woke up sometimes, but no headache.

Frequently, we think we know all about our symptoms or the things that irritate us. But often, we only know that the symptoms or problems are intolerable. The form gives an overview of the symptoms. To begin with, one must not try to alter the symptoms. The patients just need to register when they occur and their severity. Sometimes, registering the symptoms can be a frustrating experience. The symptom's very existence may make the patients unhappy or upset, so people try to avoid thinking about them. But if we want to eliminate symptoms, we have to know when and in what situations they arise. Patients should be encouraged to monitor symptoms also because the act of remembering to do so reveals those times when the symptoms are gone and when they are feeling better.

Symptom Monitoring Form for the Week

Note how irritating your symptoms are using the following scale:

No symptom=0 1 2 3 4 5 6 7 8 9 10=Worst imaginable symptom.
For each note write down a word describing the situation you were in.
For example, 8 bus, 7 cleaning, and 4 TV.

Date	Morning	Afternoon	Evening	Night

I. Listening and Looking Practice

Susan Bauer-Wu

During this practice, the person is directed to bring awareness to sounds and sights inside and outside. Try not to be overly directive and tell the person what he/she ought to be seeing or hearing. You may offer the person the opportunity to speak out loud and share what he/she is seeing and hearing. Simply listen, nod, and gently respond without judgment or getting into a dialogue.

Script/suggestions for prompts:

Listening

- *Settle into a comfortable position. If you'd like you may close your eyes as it may help you to better notice sounds.*
- *Scan your field of awareness for sounds close to you in the room. Notice what sounds immediately catch your attention.*
- *Try focusing now on just one sound.*

    - *Notice the qualities of the sound…the tone, pitch, loudness, and rhythm.*
    - *As you listen, tune into your body and notice if you can feel it resonating in your body, and if so, where do you feel it?*
    - *Notice thoughts or feelings that may arise as you attend to the sound.*

- *When you are ready, move your awareness to another sound close to you.* (Follow previous prompts).
- *Explore all sounds in your immediate vicinity in this way, and then expand your awareness to other sounds in the building.* (Follow earlier prompts)
- *After you have thoroughly explored the different sounds inside, now expand your awareness to the sounds outside.* (Follow earlier prompts)
- *Perhaps it's very quiet and you don't think you hear anything. Allow yourself to be still and to notice subtle sounds or lack of sound.*
- *Try not to get caught up in the stories surrounding the sounds or what the sounds mean, but listen to the essence of the sounds.*
- *Be aware of how the sounds affect sensations in your body, or not.*
- *Notice thoughts such as memories, plans, or conceptions that may arise in response to particular sounds.*
- *Notice emotions that surface in response to certain sounds.*
- *Try to keep your focus on the qualities of sound, and the changes in sound from one moment to the next, and to the silence between the sounds.*
- *After you have explored all of the different sounds outside, just allow yourself to rest for a few moments and notice how you feel right now.*

Looking

- *Settle into a comfortable position with your eyes closed.*
- *Once you are settled, gradually open your eyes. Without moving your head, begin by noticing the light, shadows, colors, shapes, and space.*
- *Gently and slowly expand your field of visual awareness and scan the room. Explore light, shadows, colors, shapes, and space. What do you notice?*

    - *Try not to get caught up in the stories of what the images mean or represent.*
    - *Try to stay with the qualities or essence of what you are seeing.*
    - *Are there memories or plans that come to mind?*
    - *What emotions are you feeling, if any?*
    - *If you find your mind running off into an elaborate story, acknowledge it with curiosity, then come back to the experience of seeing*

- *Once you've explored sights within the room, shift your position and look out-side.* (Follow similar prompts as previously. You may need to assist in bringing them near a window or door.)
- *After you have looked around outside very carefully and completely, close your eyes and allow yourself to just sit quietly for a few moments and notice how you feel right now.*

J. Making Mindful Choices: Cookies vs. Chips

Jean L. Kristeller and Andrea E. Lieberstein

The MB-EAT program, described in Chapter 19, contains many elements that focus on becoming more mindful about making food choices, whether for health value or simply to enjoy food more. The exercise below, from Session 5, is the first that introduces mindful choice; others include choosing among healthier foods (fruits and veggies); a wider range of snack-type foods; and facing the challenge of a buffet meal.

Introduction and Practice (15 minutes): Another aspect of **mindless** eating is grabbing the first food that's convenient—or which superficially "calls" us. Therefore, another aspect of mindful eating is stopping for a moment to tune into food choices, even when they are limited. Being aware of our preferences will likely increase our pleasure in eating one food versus another at a given moment. The foods chosen for this practice represent two very different tastes—sweet versus savory—butter cookies versus corn chips—but tastes that frequently present themselves as possible snacks either at home or at social gatherings. When such choices are made mindlessly, pleasure may be decreased, and you might continue to seek additional foods to eat or snack on, never feeling really satisfied. Another message being conveyed in this practice related to "outer wisdom" is that these foods, in small quantities, are not inherently "bad" foods, but ones they might be surprised at enjoying either more—or less—than they anticipate, once eaten slowly and mindfully. This practice (from Session 5) also integrates those from previous sessions: awareness of physical hunger, taste satiety, fullness, and considering nutritional value.

- Begin the practice by briefly explaining the purpose of the exercise, in regard to making mindful choices between types of food, summarizing from above, but avoiding reading verbatim. **Before starting to pass the food around, tell participants you will be passing plates around with two types of snack foods on each one, one sweet and one salty.** The first part of the practice will be to choose which type of snack they prefer to eat right now. **Do NOT tell them that they will also be offered some of the other snack in the second part.**
- Pass napkins or small paper plates around so that all participants have a place to put the snack they choose.
- As usual, ask everyone to prepare for the practice by clearing their laps, and then, to move into a mindful meditative state, slowing down their breath. Then, ask

them to rate how physically hungry they are on a scale of 1–10, with 10 being as hungry as possible; ask them to note to themselves "how they know." Eyes may be open or closed.

- Then, ask how full they are right now, again on a scale of 1–10, with 10 being as full as possible. What about body satiety on a scale of 1–10? Again, prompt them to be aware of "how they know."
- Before beginning to pass the plates, have them available and visible to all.
- The group should maintain a mindful state of silence as the plates are passed, keeping their attention focused internally except when making their own choice from the plate.

Guiding Awareness of Choice and Taste Satiety with Chips and Cookies

"Taking a few minutes to look at the food... (*Pause*)... Consider which flavor you would prefer at this particular moment... (*Pause*)... Reflect on how you made the choice... (*Pause*)... Then, please take MORE from the plate than you think you want to eat... (*Pause*)... **[Begin passing the plates now.]** While you are waiting for everyone to help themselves, observe what you have chosen ... (*Pause*)... Noticing its shape and color... (*Pause*)... Wondering where this food came from and how it came to you... noticing other thoughts and feelings (*Pause*)... **[wait another few moments after everyone has taken their snack food and then continue]** ... Now check in again and rate your hunger and your fullness from 1 to 10.... Now picking up a piece, and then closing your eyes... (*Pause*)... Smelling it... (*Pause*)... Feeling its texture against your lips... (*Pause*)... Biting into the food... (*Pause*)... Chewing it slowly... (*Pause*)... Being very aware of how and where in your mouth you experience the food... (*Pause*)... Being aware of how much you are enjoying the food... (*Pause*)... Notice, on your internal taste meter, your level of taste satisfaction, from 1 to 10... With each bite, noticing whether this goes up, down, or stays the same... is it going up as high as you might have expected? Or higher? Continuing to eat the rest of the cookie or chip in this way... (*Pause*)... Noticing the smell and texture... (*Pause*)... and how the flavor changes or stays the same... (*Pause*)... Enjoying the taste of the food as much as possible... (*Long Pause*)... Stopping when you have finished what is on your plate or when you no longer want any more... (*Pause*)... Now check in and rate your hunger and your fullness.... (*Pause*) .... Opening your eyes as you finish... **[Pass around the plate of food again]** .... Now you have a choice of taking more of what you've already had, or taking a little of the other food that you did not take originally... How are you making this choice? .... Lead yourself through eating this piece mindfully .... (Pause) ..... If you took the second food, how is it different from the first food?... (*Pause*)... If you took more of the first food, are there any surprises? ... (*Pause*)... With each bite, rating the pleasure of the taste on your taste meter, from 1 to 10... (*Pause*)...Noticing whether it goes up, down, or stays the same... is it going up as high as you might have expected? Or higher?.... Continuing to eat the food mindfully... (*Pause*)... And stop eating when you have eaten everything on your plate or you no longer enjoy the food... (*Pause*)... Whenever you finish eating, appreciating what you've taken into your body... (*Pause*)... Resting your hand on your stomach... (*Pause*)... Again being aware of any hunger or fullness you experience there... (*Pause*)...Noticing any judgments you may have.... (Pause)... now bringing yourself back into the space of the room....in the space of the circle...and when you are ready, gently opening your eyes."

Inquiry and Discussion of Mindful Choice Experience (10 minutes)

- Solicit comments about the experience. Begin with general comments, and proceed to asking specifically about each of the skills that are woven together in this exercise: awareness of hunger, awareness of fullness, awareness of satisfaction, awareness of taste satiety, and making choices. (**Write this list on the board if you wish.**) Ask which types of awareness (hunger, fullness, satisfaction, taste satiety, choice) were easier and which were harder.
- General: What was surprising? Interesting? Did anyone want to keep on eating? Did this feel difficult? What thoughts did they notice? What feelings?
- Ask about if they noticed changes in taste. Ask them how satisfied they felt with their snack on the taste satisfaction meter, from 1 to 10, with 10 being totally satisfied, and 1 being not satisfied at all. Draw the meter on the board. Ask them what might contribute to feelings of "satisfaction." Ask how this might be different for a particular food or for a meal.
- Most individuals will have been able to experience a sense of taste satiety (the process by which taste buds lose their ability to be sensitive to the flavor of foods, regardless of how pleasant the taste is.) **If someone expresses that they cannot notice a change in sensitivity to flavor, encourage them to keep trying at home.** You might also point out that taste satiety is different from "taste satisfaction" which involves their level of pleasure. Note that it may be so long that they have been unaware of tasting and savoring each bite of food that they may need more practice. Encourage everyone to try at home and experiment with different foods, with different amounts, and with different levels of hunger. Reference can be made here to learning to eat like a "gourmet" or drink like a wine connoisseur.
- **For "outer wisdom": What do they guess about the calorie levels of the two foods?** Have available the boxes/bags and/or labels from the foods with caloric content and serving size. Note that this is part of "outer wisdom." Note that people generally guess high and are surprised, particularly by the caloric value of the chips (5 calories each).
- **What might they guess about the nutritional value?** Note: people often presume that the chips are far less healthy than the cookies, and have more additives and preservatives. In fact, the chips have none, and are only corn, water, and oil. Other snack chips, however, may have a wider range of additives and preservatives. The cookies, however, have a long list of ingredients and additives. End the practice by encouraging everyone to explore how they might use both their "inner wisdom" and "outer wisdom" at home to inform their food choices.

K. "Hello, Old Friend"

Donald R. Marks and Christine D. Moriconi

This exercise explores the acceptance and commitment therapy (ACT) process of self as context (Hayes et al., 2012), emphasizing flexible, adaptive perspective-taking. Participants stand side-by-side in pairs as the instructor invites them to consider the challenges that the person standing next to them has faced throughout his or her life journey. Themes relating to vitality and engagement in life, as well as sources of vulnerability, may be incorporated.

Closing the eyes, if you are comfortable doing so, and if not, keeping them open and directing the gaze toward the floor. Now bringing into the mind's eye, an image of the person standing next to you today, envisioning the long journey that has led this person to here and now, standing beside you. Like you, this person came into the world as a profoundly vulnerable, nearly helpless little baby. He or she turned to the others nearby—mom, dad, sister, brother, or other caregivers—for love and nurturance, which was sometimes there or easily found and other times absent.

This person standing next to you grew through childhood and entered into the world around him or her, sometimes trusting and other times unsure. This person as a child encountered many people and had many experiences, including experiences in which others were kind and loving and experiences in which others seemed cruel or distant or cold. This person, like you, became an adolescent and navigated his or her way through relationships with others, sometimes feeling accepted, other times feeling rejected, or perhaps fearing that a rejection might happen at any moment. He or she also formed a relationship with God that is likely to have shifted and changed as time unfolded.

This person standing next to you then grew to be a young adult, faced with figuring out a way to make a life in the world—working, attending school, making friends, perhaps falling in love, and all the while putting the resources together to build a life. People that mattered to this person may have been supportive and encouraging or they may have been fearful or judgmental or unavailable. Losses and joys of nearly any imaginable kind may have occurred for this person. And in effort to make sense of it all, he or she may have judged or blamed himself or herself, or judged or blamed others, for things that happened. He or she may have felt like giving up at times. A whole world of experiences and events happened to this person as he or she grew to be the person standing next to you today.

Across the decades, billions of perceptions and hundreds of millions of decisions, with all of the changing thoughts and feelings that accompanied them, have led this person to be this very person, feeling what he or she feels at this very moment, standing next to you. Beside you, now, is someone with a deep richness of experience who, like you, has traveled an incredible journey. He or she, like you, may be as complex and varied as the universe itself.

At this point, each participant is asked to turn toward his or her partner and say, "*Hello, old friend. Thank you for what you bring to this vast world.*" After sharing this statement, participants are invited to return to silence and note the thoughts, feelings, and body sensations that are present.

The instructor then says to all the participants, "*Hello old friend. Thank you for what you bring to this vast world.*" Participants may then be invited to share their experiences in the practice with the group as a whole.

Chapter 24
Practices for Teacher Development

A. Self-Inquiry: Investigating Confirmation Bias

Willoughby B. Britton

Confirmation bias refers to the tendency to seek and find confirmatory evidence in support of already existing beliefs and ignore or reinterpret disconfirming evidence and is a major barrier to evidenced-based practice (Lilienfeld et al., 2013). Confirmation bias is a universal human tendency that applies to everyone, so what distinguishes the mindful person from an unmindful one is not the presence or absence of the bias, but rather the willingness to acknowledge and challenge the bias in the service of "seeing clearly." The following is an exercise for investigating the sources of our own confirmation biases.

1. Imagine that you have read about a new study that finds a positive benefit for mindfulness or meditation:

   (a) What happens in your body and mind?

   _____
   _____

   (b) What kinds of speech and action do you feel are most likely?

   ☐ Praise, promote, or share with others.
   ☐ Incorporate the study into MBI curriculum or clinical practice.
   ☐ Find and read the original article.
   ☐ Ignore, dismiss, or discount.
   ☐ Find fault with the authors or methodology.
   ☐ Other:_____

© Springer International Publishing Switzerland 2016
D. McCown et al. (eds.), *Resources for Teaching Mindfulness*,
DOI 10.1007/978-3-319-30100-6_24

2. Imagine that you have read about a new study that finds a negative effect for mindfulness or meditation:

   (a) What happens in your body and mind?

   _____

   _____

   (b) What kinds of speech and action do you feel are most likely?

   ☐   Praise, promote, or share with others.
   ☐   Incorporate the study into MBI curriculum or clinical practice.
   ☐   Find and read the original article.
   ☐   Ignore, dismiss, or discount.
   ☐   Find fault with the authors or methodology.
   ☐   Other:_____

Self-Inquiry:

   In an unbiased world, the boxes checked in response to both questions would be the same.
   What kinds of thoughts, body sensations, or emotions contribute to this bias?
   What would it mean to be unbiased?

B.   Teaching from 'Doing' and 'Being' Mode of Mind

Rebecca S. Crane and Barbara Reid

A key aim of the teacher-led dialogue in MBSR and MBCT is to explore and develop insight into habitual reactive patterns and to begin the process of opening up recognition of opportunities to respond and relate in new and conscious ways. The parallel process that is happening during the dialogue is that the teacher is aiming to bring mindfulness to their moment-by-moment processes so that responses to participants' contributions embody the very possibility that is under exploration.

Teachers are human and will naturally move in and out of reaction/response and connection/disconnection, but with an overarching intention to bring awareness to these moments and to consciously and repeatedly move towards the potential for skilful responding.

This work is mindfulness practice in action and is resourced and replenished by the teacher's daily formal meditation practice. Over time this learning-from-practice becomes an integral part of the 'being of the teacher'—i.e. embodiment of the attitudinal qualities identified by Kabat-Zinn (2013, pp. 21–30)—and the capacity to be in mindful relationship to experience becomes a natural part of the person of the teacher.

Through a development process that is founded on personal practice, the teacher thus learns to rest in 'being'. A key part of is his/her development as a teacher is also founded on how he/she integrates and interweaves being and doing modes of mind. Each of the domains within the *Mindfulness-Based Interventions*: *Teaching Assessment Criteria* (*MBI:TAC*) (Crane, Soulsby, Kuyken, Williams, & Eames, 2012) requires an integration of skills informed by both modes. For example, *Domain 1* (*Coverage, pacing and organisation of session curriculum*) relies strongly on the teacher's capacity to conceptually understand the curriculum components, to logically move through them, and to be organised and structured. However, these skills need to be balanced with a capacity to be highly sensitive, responsive and flexible (i.e., mindful) to the moment. *Domain 3* (*Embodiment of mindfulness*) could be considered as an overarching domain on which all other domains are founded and the development of embodiment is given particularly high priority in training programs. Embodiment is an expression of being mode of mind. The premise on which the teaching method is founded is that it is through embodiment that participants 'catch' and learn the potential of responding with kindly awareness to the moment. Whether the teacher's responses are predominantly fuelled by 'being' or 'doing' mode is thus thought to be critical to participant learning.

Here we consider two potential directions that class dialogue could take—first when the teacher's responses are orientated towards goal orientated 'doing' and second towards 'being' mode. (For further exploration on the theme of doing and being mode within skilful teaching see Chap. 17 of Mindfulness and the Transformation of Despair (Williams, Fennell, Barnhofer, Crane, & Silverton, 2014)).

In week 2 of both MBSR and MBCT, class participants have been practicing the body scan at home and start the session with this practice. This is followed by a period of class dialogue investigating the experience of this practice and of home practice during the week. When invited to share experiences of the home practice over the last week Bill was the first to speak. He was forthright and categorical in the way he expressed himself—seemingly not leaving much space for inquiry and exploration. His experiences of practice during the week had been demoralising and frustrating, and his annoyance was conveyed though the tone of his speech.

Bill: I basically couldn't do the practice this week. Every time I tried I just felt so annoyed and frustrated with myself and the CD. I can't see the point in doing it if it is making me feel worse.

Pause for a moment in your reading and imagine being the teacher in this scenario. Notice the sensations, emotions, and thoughts that are triggered. Are there any associations? Any sense of needing to find a solution or to change how Bill is feeling about his practice? Any worries about how the rest of the group are reacting to Bill? Take a moment to notice any reactions with friendly curiosity.

Dialogue 1: Responding from a driven-doing place

A teacher who has inner reactivity that propels a 'driven-doing' feel to choices might have an idea that it is important to get everyone in the class practicing and getting 'good' learning from the practice, or an idea that the participants should be enjoying the class and the practice, or that there should be a sense of positivity in the room etc. Her/his responses are likely therefore to be taking the dialogue in the direction of moving the participant to a different place—emotionally (feeling better about things) and behaviourally (finding practical solutions to the 'problem' of 'doing' the practice). Initial teacher responses might be:

Bill: I basically couldn't do the practice this week. Every time I tried I just felt so annoyed and frustrated with myself and the CD. I can't see the point in doing it if it is making me feel worse.

Teacher: It is really difficult to build practice into our everyday lives. Let's take a look together at what could help you here. (Generating ideas/problem solving solutions for enabling the participant to do the practice).

Teacher: What has helped others in the room to fit the practice into everyday life this last week? (Bringing the group on board with getting generating ideas).

Teacher: This sounds frustrating. How could you move towards feeling kinder towards yourself when things are feeling difficult? (Focusing on the 'problem' of self-criticism and generating ideas about how kindness could be brought towards experience).

There are many other possible ways to respond from a doing perspective. All however have some themes in common. This mode of mind likes to identify and address problems and to systematically work through the things that need addressing/ solving/doing. The teacher and the group will be adept at getting on board with addressing issues and problems in this way. It is tremendously familiar to all of us—and of course is effective in many spheres of our life. However, it is not a mode of mind which opens up possibility, wonder or inquiry. Each of the responses above are not be 'wrong' but could close down the potential for exploration.

Interestingly, driven-doing mode of mind can appear in a more subtle way when participants are reporting 'positive' experiences. Read the following class scenario and once again take time to pause and notice/imagine emotional, physical and cognitive responses to it that might be present if you were the teacher.

Following the sitting meditation in class 6 Sophie shared her experience of the practice. She reported that she had felt calm during the sitting. This was a strong contrast to her experiences of practice in the early part of the course which had a predominant theme of struggle. There had been moments during the practice when difficult thoughts arose with accompanying ripples of physical tension, hotness and an emotional response of anxiety. However, she had felt able to work calmly with these within the practice.

Within this practice, Sophie had been able to be present and responsive to her experience. How might a teacher in a driven-doing perspective relate to this? This mode of mind likes to reward success:

Teacher: Thank you for sharing this Sophie. It is wonderful to hear how well you are applying this new learning.

This has the potential to set up a dichotomy of good/bad and success/lack of success. Other students in the room may well be feeling that they are not the best students. It also sets Sophie up to hold up this experience as something to aspire towards in the future. It encourages a 'trying' approach. This mode of mind also likes to identify and share important 'teaching points'.

Teacher: Particularly good to hear that you were able to bring a sense of ease to moments that were not easy.

Of course, sharing teaching points is an important aspect of the teacher's task. This response could have easily been spoken from a being mode of mind place. However, there is a risk that the learning points come from a place of 'needing to accomplish the task of making teaching points'. From this place, there is a risk that the teacher might lose connection with the student as they store teaching points in memory in preparation for sharing them with the group. There is a risk that the group is not learning to inhabit a process of mindfully exploring experience but is using experience as a way of generating quick insights. These doing mode replies from the teacher risk closing the potential for inquiry down. They do not invite the teacher, the individual and the group to move together into collective exploration of the immediacy of experience. This capacity to explore experience in new ways is the skill which is likely to stay with participants beyond the end of the course.

Dialogue 2 — Responding from a being place

A teacher who is working 'in the moment' with mindful awareness of inner reactivity (i.e., is operating predominantly in 'being' mode) is likely to have a sense of being open to whatever participant reactions emerge, to be willing to openly investigate and to have a lack of investment in particular outcomes. Picking up once again on the examples above:

Bill: I basically couldn't do the practice this week. Every time I tried I just felt so annoyed and frustrated with myself and the CD. I can't see the point in doing it if it is making me feel worse.

From a place of 'being' the teacher will be moved to simply connect with where Bill is at and with what he is expressing.

Teacher: Thank you for sharing this — really important for us to hear the range of experiences with the practice that will be in the room. Could we explore this a bit together?
Bill: yes [nods]
Teacher: Before we move into that — how many of the rest of you found it difficult to do the practice during the week?
[looking around, some nods, laughter, teacher also puts her hand up]
It is very common for the practice to feel very challenging — so let's take some time to look at what challenges have been in the mix this week and how we have worked with them.
[turning back to Bill]
Would you mind sharing a bit more, Bill — what were your experiences during the week with practice…?

The door is thus opened to Bill, the teacher and the group to explore together the direct experiences that emerged in and around the practice. A sense of connection has begun to develop between group participants and with the teacher through the shared experience of difficulty, and a willingness to explore without a pre-set agenda has been established. The teacher is prioritising connection and exploration. Of course, the teacher will also have in her mind an aspiration that Bill connects to his original motivation for coming on the course and his intention to stay with the exploration through these 8 weeks. She will though hold the aspiration in ways that support her to navigate a direction of travel, and will keep placing priority on responding with mindful attention to what is arising in the moment.

What about Sophie in session 6 reporting her tremendously positive experiences of practice? It can be surprisingly challenging for mindfulness teachers who are trained to meet painful and difficult experience with open friendly interest, to also do this with positive and happy experiences! There is perhaps a caution about offering positive feedback because of the risk of introducing a dichotomy of 'doing it well' and 'doing it badly'. The teaching intention though remains the same—to honour experience as it is, and to offer space to exploration and connection. Rather than calling forth our natural compassion towards the pain of others, these moments call forth our natural pleasure for others when they experience ease and happiness.

Teacher: … So lots of different experiences through the practice, but it sounds like a sense of ease underneath it all.

Sophie: Yes—I somehow felt able to ride with what was happening.

Teacher: Could you say a bit more—you mentioned that you experienced some difficult thoughts and then some reactions to these in your body. Could you describe one of these moments?

Sophie: I had a thought at one point about a disagreement I had with a colleague this week. As soon as it came into my mind, I felt this stab of tightness in my belly. I nearly stood up and walked out. I could feel the impulse. But then I also noticed the feel of my breath in my abdomen and I immediately felt connected back here. It subsided really quickly.

Teacher: Ah—this is really interesting to notice—so it was like a moment of being catapulted out of connection with this moment, seeing the reaction to the thought and then reconnecting through the breath…and it sounds like you had several experiences of this during the practice.

Sophie: [laughing] Yes, lots!

Teacher: [shared laughter and then turning to the wider group] Is what Sophie is describing familiar to any of the rest of you?

Again, the gateway for collective inquiry is wide open. There are multiple choice points within the process. There were a number of directions that this dialogue could have fruitfully gone. The main intention throughout though was sustained—that of offering space for open exploration. Through this the aspiration is that participants will gradually internalise a new way of relating to themselves and their experience. A way that is not driven by pre-formulated ideas about how things should or could be, or driven by prematurely synthesising neat teaching points that are motivated more by ideas about the teaching than by the actual experience within the group.

C.   Considering Loss: Exercise for Mindfulness Teachers

Lucia McBee

Take a piece of paper and divide it into four quarters. Label the four sections: people, places, possessions, and activities. Then, in each section, write down three to five of the people, places, possessions, or activities that are most important to you right now.

When you have finished, take a moment and imagine that 10 years have passed. Look at your list and consider if any of the people would still be living. If not, cross them off the list. Then, consider the activities you enjoy. Cross off any activities that you would no longer be able to do in 10 years. Are there places you might not be able to visit in 10 years? If so, cross them off. Finally, look at the possessions you listed. In 10 years, will you still have access to them? If you are young, the only change you may note is the loss of a favorite grandmother. If you are older, you may realize that you are no longer able to enjoy certain activities—going to the movies, running. Maybe, you will no longer be able to travel to the mountains or exotic locations. Cross them off. Take a moment to sit with whatever sensations, feelings, or thoughts arise. You may want to jot them down.

Now consider that 10 more years have passed and follow the same steps as above. When you finish, pause to observe your feelings. Continue the exercise as long as appropriate for your age, moving ahead 10 years at a time.

Finally, consider the time at which you may have one or more physical or cognitive problems, and you can no longer live independently. Perhaps, you will need to move to a care facility. You probably will have a small room, maybe, shared with one or more people. Cross off any possessions that you would not be able to bring. Consider the activities and places that are important to you. Would any of them still be a possibility? Think about all of the limitations you might have. For example, if your favorite activity is reading, perhaps your vision problems may prohibit reading. If you wanted large print materials or books on tape, would they be available to you? Would you have to rely on someone to assist you with obtaining them? If you enjoy cooking and eating, consider that your diet may be restricted. If institutionalized, dependent on institutional food. Possibly even on pureed food or fed by a gastro tube. Even if you were able to continue living at home with assistance, your life would be changed in many ways, and you would most likely be dependent on others for basic needs. If you doubt this possibility, do some research or ask those who work in aging. If you prefer to deny it, or think you will plan a quick exit, join the majority of our population in their denial of aging. In any case, this scenario already impacts most elders over 75 to some degree.

The exercise provided considers the concrete, tangible losses that accompany aging. Yet, there is an additional dimension to explore: the intangible losses of independence, work, role, looks, and identity. For many elders, the loss of independence and the ability to contribute are the most devastating losses. What do you feel when considering these potential losses? How will your mindfulness practices allow you to be present to such losses in others, and in your own life?

Many hold the wish for the ideal: to live a long life, without pain and disability, and then go to sleep one night and not wake up. This ideal has become less and less likely; however, as modern medical technology has ensured that most of us will live longer, but often with more chronic conditions, pain, and disability, and often the need for family or professional caregivers. The practice of mindfulness, *learning to live with what is*, offers ways to travel this path with increased equanimity. For those interested in teaching mindfulness to frail elders and their caregivers, the practices may allow us to be present for our own the losses as well as those of frail elders and their caregivers.

D.   Trauma-Informed Mindful Dialogue

Trish Magyari

The Trauma-Informed Mindful Dialogue describes a method of aiding a participant who is experiencing distress and/or dissociation following a meditation or curricular exercise which may have been triggering for them. Their distress may be discovered through inquiry sharing, through observation, or by asking following inquiry: "Is there anyone who feels they went away during that exercise and hasn't come back? Or is still in distress?" While some of this dialogue might seem repetitive, it is precisely the accompaniment of the participant through the arc of their experience that makes this trauma sensitive.

The following exchange took place following the Unpleasant Event Inquiry in Class 4 in response to the teacher's question regarding "going away" or "in distress":

Sally raises hand, a bit sheepishly. She is a 45-year-old woman on full disability from multiple childhood traumas, including sexual trauma. She's an active participant in the class, often asking perceptive questions, not requiring any additional support up until this time.

Teacher: [Nods, makes eye contact, notices Sally's eyes appear a bit distant but otherwise OK]. "Those exercises are challenging to many people [normalizes]. Turns to Sally, says first name. "Are you OK working with this one-on-one for a few minutes?" [seeks permission while making it easy to say "yes"].

Sally: Nods.

Teacher: "Do you sense me here with you right now?"

Sally: Nods. [A "no" would require additional preliminary steps].

Teacher: "OK. Let's start by all taking some stress relieving deep belly breaths [Looks around at whole class briefly then returns her full attention to Sally]:

Deep breath in, and out, relaxing the jaw and the tongue on the l-o-n-g exhale."
[This can help activate the PFC].

Sally, I'll invite you to take a moment to check inside, notice what's happening now.
Feeling your body in the chair, your feet on the floor, noticing your body. . .feel-
ings. . .your mind. What is happening? [Teacher inquires about present moment
experience, instead of guiding back to what had been happening earlier].

Sally: [talking with eyes closed]. "I'm starting to settle down. My mind was racing
so fast, bouncing all over the place."

Teacher: "Your mind had been racing and now you are noticing some settling. Was
there a particular mind-habit that was active as it was bouncing around?"

Sally: Judging. Everything.

Teacher: "Your mind has been judging everything—about yourself?"

Sally: "Yeah. About myself."

Teacher: "The self-judging mind habit was really active."

Sally: "Yeah. Self-judging."

Teacher: "And now you're noticing some settling. When you say "settle down," is
that in your body, your emotions, or your mind?" [follows thread to presence, not
back to distress].

Sally: "Definitely my mind. It's slowing down. And my heart is slowing down,
too."

Teacher: "Your mind and heart are slowing down." [Reflects movement towards
presence].

Sally: "Nods."

Teacher: "Take a moment to check in with your body—what is happening right
now?"

Sally: "Uh, I'm not jumping out of my skin anymore."

Teacher: "Your mind isn't racing as much and you're more in your own skin."
[Reflect, pause] "Take a moment—what is that like, to have come back to your
body, your heart, and your mind after having been away from it just now?"
[Teacher states this as a fact, doesn't react to the reactivity of distress or
dissociation].

Sally: "It's a little scary."

Teacher: "Yeah. [Leans in, makes eye contact]. You feel a little bit scared. On a
scale of 1–10, where would you put that fear?" [Uses concrete scaling].

Sally: "About a 6."

Teacher: "A 6. And where or how do you sense that fear in your body?"

Sally: "It's in my chest and throat, it's really tight."

Teacher: "Thank you. Let's take another mindful sigh." [Teacher models self-
soothing, a break from the intensity; whole class participates without prompt-
ing]. "I'll invite you right now to put a hand over your heart as a gesture of your
friendly intent, a sign of your support for yourself [looks around again at whole
class], and this is for all of us, I invite everyone to practice offering kindness and
friendliness to whatever feelings are flowing through you right now—sadness,
anger, fear. Sally, I invite you to say to yourself "Fear, fear is present right now"
while also sensing yourself *with* yourself. And if there are words that sound kind
and friendly to yourself, you might offer them to yourself right now. [pause].

"Then when you are ready, move your attention to those tight places in the chest and throat. Nothing to change or fix, just moving in close, in a kind and friendly way, the way you'd stand near a friend who was having a hard day. Feel free to take deep breaths if you'd like [reminds of calming resource]. What's happening right now?"

Sally: "It's starting to loosen its grip."

Teacher: "Thank you—staying with those sensations of loosening, noticing what that feels like, that loosening."

Sally: "It feels good, better."

Teacher: "It feels better. What's happening with the fear now? What level would you put it at?"

Sally: "Uh, it's lower, maybe a 2."

Teacher: "Thank you. While you're still inside, check in with yourself and see if there is anything that those loosening muscles in your neck and throat would like you to know? Or ask for?"

Sally: [softly] "Patience."

Teacher: "Those muscles that felt tight with fear would like patience. Do you have a sense of how you could give that to yourself?"

Sally: "Uh, I really want to be here, some of the time it is starting to feel good. I never thought it would. But it's still scary. This is all so new. I guess I could give myself time and not get so mad at myself when my mind starts racing and I check out a little bit and instead put my hand on my heart to help myself come back. That really makes a difference."

Teacher: "Thank you. And are there also some words that sound good to yourself, perhaps one of the loving kindness messages or any other phrase?" [Teacher asks, but is OK with a possible "no" response—not everyone will have self-soothing words].

Sally: "I'm here with myself."

Teacher: "I'm here with myself." [Repeats out loud], "Feel free to say it to yourself a few more times, sensing the support you are offering to yourself while you do." [Pause]. Sensing your body in the chair, your feet on the floor, feel free to open your eyes when you're ready." [Teacher guides to presence reminding of the support of the chair and the floor].

Teacher: [Summarizing while maintaining eye contact]: "It's starting to feel good to be present, and it's also new and a bit scary, too. It helps you to name your fear, be patient with yourself and offer yourself kindness by putting a hand on your heart and saying "I'm here with myself."

Sally : "Yes."

Teacher: "How are you doing right now?" [checks in one more time].

Sally : "Better."

Teacher: "When you say, 'better' is that in your body, your mind, or your heart?"

Sally : "All of it."

Teacher: "All of it feels better when you are with yourself in a kind and friendly way, even when you are afraid. Just breathe with that sense of 'better' in your body, your heart, and your mind. [Pause] Does that feel like enough for right now or is there anything else that you'd like?"

Sally: "That's enough."

Teacher: "Thank you, I'm sure that was helpful to others in the class as well." [Notes others nodding. Teacher does *not* invite group sharing at this time as it often devolves into fixing or problem solving.]

Teacher: "Is there anyone else who feels they could use that kind of support right now, who isn't fully back yet or is in distress?" [Looks around circle, making eye contact with group. Notices some people with hands over their hearts or a bit misty-eyed, no one seems to be in distress.]

Teacher: [Seeing no one raise their hand or appear in distress, moves on to new class material.]

Sally went on to successfully complete the MBSR course with perfect attendance without requiring any additional one-on-one support. She is a regular attender at my MBSR grad classes and mindfulness practice groups.

E.   Mindful Practice Interview and Storytelling Guidelines and Suggestions

Michael S. Krasner

Narratives are chosen by the participants from their own personal experiences of caring for patients. Thus, the narratives are grounded in the real, lived experiences of the physicians, not in philosophical or rhetorical "what-if's" that impact on cognitive and emotional challenges.

Appreciative inquiry involves the art and practice of asking unconditionally positive questions that strengthen the capacities to apprehend, anticipate, and heighten positive potential. It is an inquiry tool that fosters imagination and innovation.

The quality of mindfulness, cultivated through the meditative practices, functions as an ever present lens through which personal stories are contemplated, written, shared, and discussed.

There are three major "technologies" employed in Mindful Practice for health care professionals—cultivating mindfulness through meditative practice, working with narratives related to clinically relevant themes, and engaging in interpersonal dialogues informed by appreciative inquiry. All focus on developing a range of communication skills to enhance the health care professional's capacity for storytelling and listening. Each has obvious consequences for the domain of patient care in terms of the clinician–patient relationship.

Health care professionals can train in the use of mindfulness, narrative, and appreciative inquiry by engaging in dialogues, as both an interviewer and a storyteller. These guidelines and suggestions are meant to support such exploration.

In these explorations, one person will act as storyteller/patient and one as a listener/interviewer. To help understand these roles, participants can refer to the written guidelines for each, which appear below.

Interviewer Guidelines

As interviewer, think of your role as exploring the mind and experience of your partner, helping to bring forward his or her thoughts, feelings, and wisdom.
Listen slowly and deeply: encourage your partner to tell his or her story.
Avoid interruptions. It is rare that one gets to tell a story without being cut off, and equally rare that one gets to listen without feeling compelled to analyze, reflect, and interpret. This is an opportunity to do both.
Invite elaboration and clarification.
Remember that you are an explorer whose objective is to learn all you can about your partner's stories and what made them possible.
Take the opportunity to ask questions that you are truly curious about, and in this way assist the storyteller in expanding the narrative.
Resist the temptation to interpret the story, or agree or disagree with the storyteller.
Avoid sharing similar experiences that you have had that the story reminded you of.
Use reflective questions and empathy when appropriate.

Storyteller Guidelines

As a storyteller, your role is to authentically share your narrative. Be sure to consider your awareness of thoughts, feelings, and sensations as you re-experience and reflect on the story, sharing not only the content and details of the story but also how you experienced it. You might want to address:
What happened?
What helpful qualities did you bring to that moment?
Who else was involved, and how did they contribute?
What aspects of the context made a difference?
What lessons from this story are useful to you?

Representative Appreciative Inquiry Questions

What do you think were the core factors that made this success possible?
What did you do or bring to that event that contributed to its success?
Who else was involved and what did they contribute?
What was it about the setting or situation that made a difference?
What lessons do you take from his experience?

Appreciative Inquiry Guidelines

Stated in the affirmative
Built on the assumption of an individual/organization as full of possibilities
Presented as an invitation

Phrased in rapport talk, not report talk
Evoking essential values, aspirations, and inspiration
Valuing what IS, to spark appreciative imagination
Conveying unconditional positive regard

Representative Self-awareness Questions

What were you feeling in your body? What did your breathing feel like? Was there tension in your body? If so, where?
What about the experience was pleasant?
What about the experience was unpleasant?
What emotions were you experiencing?
What kinds of thoughts were you having?
When have you felt this way/found yourself in this situation before?
What aspects of this situation make you feel resourceful/satisfied? In what way?
What aspects of this situation made feel you uncomfortable or afraid? In what way?
What aspects of this person do you feel drawn to? Why?
What aspects of this person make you feel repelled or irritated? Why?

Representative Coaching Questions

How would you describe this situation? What is the story you're telling yourself? What other descriptions/interpretations/stories might be possible?
What worked? What didn't work as well as you might have wished?
What do you think [the other person] was thinking/feeling?
What was her/his goal? What strategy was she/he using? How did you respond? What other options did you have? What guided your choice?
What is your greatest hope [in this situation]? What is your biggest fear?
What were you doing that might have been contributing to the situation?
What has helped you in similar situations in the past?
What other forces may be operating here? Who else has a stake in this?
Where are you feeling stuck? What will help you move forward?

Responses that Help Expand the Narrative

Silence
Tell me the story
Go on/tell me more
Reflect/Echo
Express empathy
Paraphrase and summarize. For example—Let me see if I have this correct. You said that…

After the Exercises: Themes for Reflective Questions

Attentive Observation. *Help learners note not only what they observe about the patient/presenter, but also their own thought processes and emotions, including the judgments that they make based on those observations. Focus on biases,* *judgments, and heuristics; recognize their consequences ([avoidance of] errors, [lack of] miscommunication, etc.). Using their awareness of their own thoughts and feelings to understand and resolve the clinical issues at hand. Suggested questions:*

What did you notice that was unusual?

If there were data that you ignored, what might they be?

What interfered with and what facilitated your ability to be attentive and observant?

Critical Curiosity. *Help learners approach two parallel tasks—clinical reasoning and understanding the patient's life situation. The basis for this exercise is that students who are curious and interested in their patients are more likely to express caring, make wise decisions concordant with patients' values, and notice clinical features that others ignore. Suggested questions:*

What about this situation was surprising or unexpected?

What are you assuming about this patient that might not be true?

How might your previous experience affect how you are approaching this patient?

How did you manage to avoid premature closure?

Beginner's Mind (Informed flexibility). *Learners will examine how taking a fresh look at a situation can alter a diagnostic impression and psychosocial formulation, and, by extension, permit the clinician to better appreciate and care for the patient.*

What would a trusted peer say about how you are managing this situation?

Is there another way in which you can put (did put) together this patient's story?

Presence. *Learners will discuss situations in which they were either—really present for the patient and family, or somehow distracted or distant. They will describe their emotional reactions (e.g., what moved them most about the story), and how those reactions affected their relationship with the patient and clinical outcomes.*

How did you prepare me before seeing a patient (student)?

What moved you most about this situation?

How did this encounter affect your relationship with this patient?

Were there any points at which you were particularly present? Or distracted or uninvolved?

References

Crane, R. S., Soulsby, J. G., Kuyken, W., Williams, J. M. G., & Eames, C. (2012). The Bangor, Exeter & Oxford mindfulness-based interventions teaching assessment criteria (MBI-TAC) for assessing the competence and adherence of mindfulness-based class-based teaching. Retrieved from http://www.bangor.ac.uk/mindfulness/documents/MBI-TACJune2012.pdf.

Kabat-Zinn, J. (2013). *Full catastrophe living: Using the wisdom of your body and mind to face stress, pain and illness.* New York, NY: Delacorte.

Lilienfeld, S. O., Ritschel, L. A., Lynn, S. J., Cautin, R. L., & Latzman, R. D. (2013). Why many clinical psychologists are resistant to evidence-based practice: root causes and constructive remedies. *Clinical Psychology Review, 33*, 883–900.

Williams, J. M. G., Fennell, M. J. V., Barnhofer, T., Crane, R. S., & Silverton, S. (2014). *Mindfulness and the transformation of despair: Working with people at risk of suicide*. New York, NY: Guilford. (See in particular chapter 17 on what creates skilful teaching).

Index

© Springer International Publishing Switzerland 2016
D. McCown et al., *Resources for Teaching Mindfulness*,
DOI 10.1007/978-3-319-30100-6

Printed by Printforce, the Netherlands